CLINICAL LABORATORY
INVESTIGATION AND PSYCHIATRY

Clinical Laboratory Investigation and Psychiatry

A Practical Handbook

Russell Foster PhD MRCPsych

Centre for Neuroimaging Sciences
Institute of Psychiatry
King's College
London, UK, and

The Institute of Liver Studies
King's College Hospital
London, UK

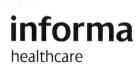

Informa Healthcare USA, Inc.
52 Vanderbilt Avenue
New York, NY 10017

Library of Congress Cataloging-in-Publication Data

Clinical laboratory investigation and psychiatry : a practical handbook / edited by
Russell Foster.
     p. ; cm.
   Includes bibliographical references and index.
   ISBN 978-0-415-47844-1 (pbk. : alk. paper)   1. Mental illness–Diagnosis. 2.
Diagnosis, Laboratory. I. Foster, Russell.
   [DNLM: 1. Mental Disorders–diagnosis. 2. Clinical Laboratory Techniques. 3. Mental
Disorders–drug therapy. 4. Psychotropic Drugs–analysis. WM 141 C6415 2008]
   RC473.L32C55 2008
   616.89'075–dc22

                                                  2008033946

ISBN-13: 978-0-415-47844-1 (Paperback)

For Corporate Sales and Reprint Permissions call 212-520-2700 or write to: Sales
Department, 52 Vanderbilt Avenue, 7th floor, New York, NY 10017.

Visit the Informa Web site at
www.informa.com

and the Informa Healthcare Web site at
www.informahealthcare.com

Composition by Exeter Premedia Services Private Ltd, Chennai, India
Printed and bound in the United States of America.

This book is dedicated to improving the lives of all those affected by mental disorders, especially patients and those caring for them — *Os rhôi barch ti gei barch.**

**Welsh proverb: If you give respect you will receive it.*

Contents

Preface

Despite the many myths, legends, anecdotes, and apocryphal stories that frequently surround psychiatry and its practitioners, it nonetheless remains a branch of medicine, albeit with influences from a wide range of other, diverse fields. It should therefore come as no surprise that the pathology laboratory plays an important role in the diagnosis and management of a number of psychiatric disorders. While there is at present no single, specific laboratory test for any psychiatric disorder, the laboratory nevertheless helps clinicians to exclude important, treatable causes of psychiatric morbidity and assists with appropriate treatment strategies. For example, whilst a psychotic patient may be initially thought to have schizophrenia, the laboratory can assist in the exclusion of diverse causes of psychosis such as infection, neoplasm, or sequelae of substance abuse. In addition, many of the medications used to treat this psychotic patient may have a range of adverse metabolic effects, which are amenable to, or indeed require, laboratory monitoring.

At present there does not appear to exist any specific single book in current use that addresses the often close association between laboratory medicine and mental health. There are, however, at least two previously published volumes dedicated to laboratory testing in psychiatry. The first of these[1] provides an excellent, if perhaps out of date, overview of the field, but is not intended as a handbook for front-line clinicians. The second one[2] is designed as a pocket handbook but is, again, out of date and does not, for example, consider the metabolic associations or therapeutic drug monitoring aspects of the newer psychotropics.

The current book therefore aims to fill this gap, and is intended as a basic guide to laboratory aspects of mental illness in the non-pregnant general adult population, generally taken to include the age range from 18 to 65. It focuses specifically on those aspects of psychiatry amenable to laboratory involvement and is not designed as a definitive textbook of general medicine, laboratory medicine, pathology, psychiatry, or psychopharmacology. Whilst it aims to span and complement these related disciplines, appropriate specialized texts or expert advisors should always be consulted for further information as required. The reader should also note that treatment will not be discussed in this book (except briefly in Chapters 3 and 5) as this should be undertaken after consultation with the appropriate experts and/or those with appropriate experience.

This book aims to cover the bulk of the important disorders that will be seen by the general-adult psychiatrist. Rarer conditions and most organic brain syndromes (neuropsychiatric syndromes) are excluded as these are covered in appropriate detail elsewhere. Additionally, other important investigations (imaging, electrophysiology) are not described here as they are felt to fall outside the remit of the pathology laboratory.

It is hoped that this book will initially be of utility for those two usually disparate groups of professionals, namely pathologists and psychiatrists. Additionally, the book should prove useful for general practitioners, pharmacists, nurses, medical students, doctors in training, laboratory staff, specialists in internal medicine, researchers, and others. To help non-mental-health workers understand psychiatric nosology, details of selected psychiatric conditions are included in order to assist, at least in part, in understanding the complexity of psychiatric disorders and presentations and why clinicians may request particular tests and investigations.

Where appropriate, definitions of specific psychiatric disorders will be based mainly on ICD-10 (International Statistical Classification of Diseases and Related Health Problems, 10th Revision) criteria with only occasional reference to DSM-IV (Diagnostic and Statistical Manual of Mental Disorders, Fourth Edition). Equally, details of selected medical presentations will be included to provide useful background as well as to assist with appropriate laboratory investigation and diagnosis.

Whilst every effort has been made to reflect current knowledge and minimize errors, it should be recognized that both psychiatry and laboratory medicine are ever-changing fields, and no liability can be accepted for inaccuracy, incompleteness, injury, damage, or loss. Where possible, the most recent guidance published by the UK National Institute for Health and Clinical Excellence (NICE) will be quoted.

Finally, this book is all my own work and is an entirely independent production. I have not received any commercial or institutional support, sponsorship, or other input and consequently have no declarations of, or conflicts of, interest.

Russell Foster
May 2008

References

1.   Gold MS, Pottash ALC. Diagnostic and Laboratory Testing in Psychiatry. New York: Plenum Publishing Corporation, 1986.
2.   Rosse RB, Giese AA, Deutsch SI, Morihisa JM. Concise Guide to Laboratory and Diagnostic Testing in Psychiatry. Washington, DC: American Psychiatric Press, 1989.

Acknowledgements

The team at Informa, especially Lindsay Campbell and Timothy DeWerff, for their unwavering support in making this project a reality.

The help and support provided by members of the Clinical Biochemistry laboratory at King's College Hospital, London, especially Drs Jamie Alaghband-Zadeh and Roy Sherwood, are gratefully appreciated.

The staff of the Medicine Information Service at the Pharmacy, Maudsley Hospital, London, are also thanked for assistance in obtaining hard-to-find information about psychotropics.

Drs Ruth and Chris Ohlsen at the Maudsley Hospital are thanked for their constant enthusiasm, encouragement, and support.

Kate Williams, head of nutrition and dietetics at the Maudsley Hospital, is thanked for enlightening chats and expert input.

Dr Peter Haddad is thanked for his enthusiam and helpful discussions.

Dr Simon Adelman is thanked for his helpful comments and support.

Dr David Ball is thanked for helpful discussions about laboratory and psychiatric aspects of alcohol abuse, and the many vagaries of purchasing property in London.

My colleagues at the Centre for Neuroimaging Sciences, Institute of Psychiatry, are thanked for the congenial atmosphere and numerous cups of tea.

My colleagues at King's College Hospital, especially in the Departments of Psychological Medicine (Drs C Maddoc, M Tarn, and D Tracy) and the Institute of Liver Studies, are thanked for ongoing support and interest.

The helpful and friendly staff at the Institute of Psychiatry library deserve a special mention for putting up with a certain gentleman who took up semi-permanent residence in the place and who persistently asked in an odd and obscure manner for odd and obscure tomes at odd and obscure times of the day and night....

How to use this book

Part One consists of eight chapters describing specific syndromes, medications, and special topics with guidelines for choosing appropriate laboratory tests. Each chapter is followed by a list of selected references to provide the reader with sources of additional information. Part Two is a glossary of the most common laboratory parameters with specific guidance on interpretation within a psychiatric context. No management advice is provided except in Chapter 3 ('Selected psychiatric medication-associated syndromes and emergencies'), as this is covered in greater detail elsewhere and should always include expert advice from those with appropriate knowledge and experience of managing the disorder in question.

List of abbreviations

ALP	alkaline phosphatase
ALT	alanine transferase
APTT	activated partial thromboplastin time
AST	aspartate transaminase
Ca	calcium
CFS	chronic fatigue syndrome
CNS	central nervous system
EDNOS	eating disorder not otherwise specified
eGFR	estimated glomerular filtration rate
ESR	erythrocyte sedimentation rate
FBC	full blood count
G6PD	glucose 6 phosphate dehydrogenase deficiency
GGT	gamma glutamyl transferase
Hb	haemoglobin
INR	international normalized ratio
K	potassium
LFT	liver function tests
MAOI	monoamine oxidase inhibitors
MCH	mean cell haemoglobin
MCHC	mean cell haemoglobin concentration
MCV	mean cell volume
Na	sodium
NICE	National Institute for Clinical Excellence
NMS	neuroleptic malignant syndrome
RBC	red cell count
SIADH	syndrome of inappropriate ADH secretion
SLE	systemic lupus erythematosus
SSRI	selective serotonin reuptake inhibitor
T3	triiodothyronine
T4	thyroxine
TCA	tricyclic antidepressant
TDM	therapeutic drug monitoring
TFT	thyroid function tests
TIBC	total iron-binding capacity
U&E	urea and electrolytes (including creatinine)
VL	viral load

Reference ranges (blood)

The following ranges are those currently used by the Maudsley Hospital, London, and King's College Hospital, London, and are intended as a guide only. For convenience, only the most commonly requested routine blood parameters are included and are listed in alphabetical order. For blood parameters not listed below appropriate expert advice should be sought. For selected cerebrospinal fluid (CSF) and urine parameters, see Chapter 8.

Parameter	Responsible department	Range	Units
Activated partial thromboplastin time	Haematology	23.8–32.2	s
Alanine transferase	Biochemistry	5–55	IU/l
Albumin	Biochemistry	35–50	g/l
Alkaline phosphatase	Biochemistry	30–130	IU/l
Ammonia	Biochemistry	10–47	μmol/l
Amylase	Biochemistry	15–80	IU/l
Aspartate transaminase	Biochemistry	10–50	IU/l
B12	Biochemistry	180–1100	ng/l
Basophils	Haematology	0.0–0.10	$\times 10^9$/l
Bicarbonate	Biochemistry	22–30	mmol/l
Bilirubin	Biochemistry	3–20	μmol/l
Calcium (total)	Biochemistry	2.2–2.6	mmol/l
Carbohydrate-deficient transferrin	Biochemistry	1.9–3.4	g/l
CD4	Immunology	500–1500	$\times 10^6$/l
Chloride	Biochemistry	90–110	mmol/l
Cholesterol	Biochemistry	<5.2	mmol/l
C-reactive protein	Biochemistry	<5.0	mg/l
Creatine kinase	Biochemistry	10–150	IU/l
Creatinine	Biochemistry	45–120	μmol/l
Eosinophils	Haematology	0.0–0.4	$\times 10^9$/l
Erythrocytes (females)	Haematology	3.8–5.8	$\times 10^{12}$/l
Erythrocytes (males)	Haematology	4.5–5.8	$\times 10^{12}$/l
Erythrocyte sedimentation rate	Haematology	<20	mm/h
Ferritin (females)	Biochemistry	0–200	μg/l
Ferritin (males)	Biochemistry	0–300	μg/l
Folate	Biochemistry	3–13	μg/l

(Cont.)

Parameter	Responsible department	Range	Units
Gamma glutamyl transferase	Biochemistry	1–55	IU/l
Globulins	Biochemistry	25–35	g/l
Glucose (fasting)	Biochemistry	3.0–7.0	mmol/l
Glycated haemoglobin (HbA1c)	Biochemistry	<6.0	%
Haemoglobin (females)	Haematology	11.5–15.5	g/dl
Haemoglobin (males)	Haematology	13.0–16.5	g/dl
International normalized ratio	Haematology	0.9–1.2	—
Iron	Biochemistry	14–30	µmol/l
Lactate	Biochemistry	0.7–2.0	mmol/l
Lactate dehydrogenase	Biochemistry	91–232	IU/l
Lipase	Biochemistry	5–60	IU/l
Lipoprotein (HDL)	Biochemistry	>1.2	mmol/l
Lipoprotein (LDL)	Biochemistry	<3.5	mmol/l
Lymphocytes	Haematology	1.3–4.0	$\times 10^9$/l
Magnesium	Biochemistry	0.7–1.0	mmol/l
Mean cell haemoglobin	Haematology	25–34	pg
Mean cell haemoglobin concentration	Haematology	32.0–37.0	g/dl
Mean cell volume	Haematology	77–95	fl
Monocytes	Haematology	0.2–1.0	$\times 10^9$/l
Neutrophils	Haematology	2.2–6.3	$\times 10^9$/l
Packed cell volume (females)	Haematology	35–47	%
Packed cell volume (males)	Haematology	42–52	%
$PaCO_2$	Biochemistry	4.5–6.0	kPa
PaO_2	Biochemistry	12–15	kPa
Parathyroid hormone (normocalcaemic)	Biochemistry	0–60	U/l
pH	Biochemistry	7.35–7.45	—
Phosphorus	Biochemistry	0.8–1.4	mmol/l
Platelets	Haematology	150–400	$\times 10^9$/l
Potassium	Biochemistry	3.5–5.0	mmol/l
Prolactin (females)	Biochemistry	0–510	mU/l
Prolactin (males)	Biochemistry	0–410	mU/l
Protein (total)	Biochemistry	60–80	g/l

(Cont.)

Parameter	Responsible department	Range	Units
Prothrombin time	Haematology	10.3–13.3	s
Red cell distribution width	Haematology	11.0–15.0	%
Reticulocyte count	Haematology	50.0–150.0	$\times 10^9/l$
Sodium	Biochemistry	135–145	mmol/l
Thyroid stimulating hormone	Biochemistry	0.3–5.5	mU/l
Thyroxine (free)	Biochemistry	9–25	pmol/l
Total iron-binding capacity	Biochemistry	50–72	µmol/l
Transferrin	Biochemistry	2.1–3.6	g/l
Triglycerides	Biochemistry	<2.0	mmol/l
Triiodothyronine (free)	Biochemistry	3.0–8.0	pmol/l
Triiodothyronine (total)	Biochemistry	1.2–2.9	nmol/l
Urea	Biochemistry	3.3–6.7	mmol/l
Uric acid (urate)	Biochemistry	0.1–0.4	mmol/l
Viral load (HIV)	Microbiology	0	copies/ml
White cell count	Haematology	4–11	$\times 10^9/l$

Guide to blood collection tubes

Note: these are used as per the current laboratory guidelines at the Maudsley Hospital, London, and King's College Hospital, London. Other laboratories may have different protocols, and it is advisable to check local laboratory guidelines before sending samples for analysis.

Plain tube (gold top, no anticoagulant, for serum analysis)

Biochemistry:	B12
	endocrinology
	ferritin
	fluoride
	folate
	haematinics
	liver function tests
	porphyrins
	'routine' profile
	therapeutic drug levels
	thyroid function tests
	urea and electrolytes
Immunology:	autoantibodies
	complement
	immunoglobulins
microbiology:	serology

EDTA tube (purple top)

Haematology:	ESR
	FBC
	HbA1c
	lead
	sickle cell

Fluoride Oxalate (grey top); as potassium oxalate is used as an anticoagulant in these tubes, potassium cannot be determined in these samples

Biochemistry:	ethanol
	glucose
	lactate

Heparin tube (green top)

Arterial blood gases (pH, bicarbonate)
Vitamin B1
Vitamin C

Sodium citrate (blue top)

Haematology:	coagulation
	lupus anticoagulant
	prothrombin (INR)

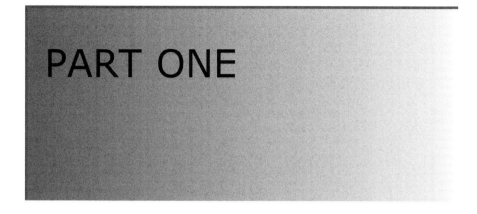

PART ONE

chapter 1

Introduction

Psychiatric disorders are common, and can be due to a wide range of aetiologies, some of which will remain unclear despite in-depth investigation.

In essence, all psychiatric diagnoses are diagnoses of exclusion, and the laboratory can assist the clinician in excluding treatable causes of psychiatric morbidity as well as helping to guide management.

In order to formulate a psychiatric diagnosis, the usual scheme of taking a history, examination (mental state examination *and* physical examination), and investigation are performed; a thorough psychiatric assessment will always include a physical examination and appropriate investigations where indicated and/or feasible (i.e. if the patient is able or willing to comply).

At present there is no single laboratory test for any specific psychiatric diagnosis. Rather, laboratory tests play a role in excluding organic pathologies (which may contribute to, or worsen the psychiatric presentation), or monitoring of treatment effects.

A number of tests have been mooted for certain psychiatric disorders; however, as yet none meets the requirement of a 'gold standard' test.

The requesting clinician should be aware of factitious illnesses and unusual reported symptoms/signs, and should, where possible, try to avoid 'over-investigation' in these patients. As these patients can often present management challenges, they may require specialist opinion(s).

The published literature is relatively sparse regarding laboratory testing for specific psychiatric presentations, with the majority of publications considering laboratory screening indirectly as part of general physical health monitoring in psychiatric patients. There is a review of the use of screening laboratory investigations by Anfinson and Kathol[1], who noted that extensive laboratory screening is not indicated for most psychiatric patients, but that screening may be of more relevance in older populations, those of lower socioeconomic status, patients with substance abuse problems, and those presenting with self-neglect, disorientation, or evidence of organic brain syndromes.

It should be noted that since the publication of the above paper, there has been an increased awareness of metabolic associations with psychiatric disorders; to reflect this, below is a brief review of the major studies considering laboratory testing/screening in general adult psychiatric populations.

Table Brief literature review of laboratory testing/screening in adult psychiatric patients

Reference	Study design	Number, type of patients	Laboratory investigations	Results
Barnes et al[2] (1983)	Prospective	$n = 147$, psychiatric outpatients	Biochemistry: 'SM-12 chemistries', T3, T4, urinalysis Haematology: FBC Immunology: VDRL (Venereal Disease Research Laboratory)	Abnormal laboratory findings in 50 patients: microhaematuria ($n = 5$), raised fasting blood sugar ($n = 4$), abnormal thyroid function ($n = 2$), glycosuria ($n = 1$), raised urea ($n = 1$)
Burke[3] (1978)	Prospective	$n = 133$, day hospital patients	'Routine urine, haematological, and biochemical investigations'	Physical disorder found in 50% of patients
Catalano et al[4] (2001)	Retrospective review of notes	$n = 349$, general hospital medical inpatients with psychiatric symptoms	Folate, thyroid stimulating hormone (TSH), syphilis serology, vitamin B12	Patients with a cognitive spectrum disorder: 5.9% had low B12, 26.9% had low folate, 5.6% had positive syphilis serology, 8.9% had abnormal TFT Patients with a mood spectrum disorder: 6.1% had low B12, 37.5% had low folate, 2.5% had positive syphilis serology, 5.0% had abnormal TFT
Dolan and Mushlin[5] (1985)	Retrospective review of notes	$n = 250$, psychiatric inpatients	FBC, SMA-7, SMA-20, TFT, urinalysis, VDRL	4% of patients had diagnoses based solely on laboratory testing

Table Brief literature review of laboratory testing/screening in adult psychiatric patients (Cont.)

Reference	Study design	Number, type of patients	Laboratory investigations	Results
Ferguson and Dudleston[6] (1986)	Prospective	n = 650, acute psychiatric admissions	Biochemistry: ALP, AST, bilirubin, calcium, creatinine, GGT, glucose, phosphate, potassium, protein, sodium, urea Haematology: Blood film, folate, FBC Immunology: VDRL Microbiology: ESR, urine culture/sensitivity	Laboratory abnormalities found in 17% of all laboratory tests performed; 39% of patients had abnormal results
Hall et al[7] (1978)	Prospective	n = 658, psychiatric outpatients	No details provided	Approximately 5.5% of patients had laboratory evidence of disease
Hall et al[8] (1980)	Prospective	n = 100, psychiatric inpatients	Biochemistry: '34-panel blood chemistry panel', urinalysis, heavy metal screen, urine drug screen, urine amino acids Haematology: FBC	46% of patients found to have previously undiagnosed medical morbidity
Honig et al[9] (1989)	Prospective	n = 218, psychiatric outpatients	Biochemistry: 'SMA-20' (20 item automated panel), TSH, T3, urinalysis Haematology: ESR, FBC Immunology: syphilis serology	69% of patients showed non-clinically significant laboratory abnormalities; 9.7% of patients showed laboratory abnormalities which resulted in a new diagnosis

Koran et al[10] (2002)	Prospective	n = 289, new psychiatric admissions	Biochemistry: albumin, ALP, bilirubin, calcium, cholesterol, creatine kinase, creatinine, free T4, glucose, glutamic oxaloacetic transaminase, glutamic pyruvic transaminase, iron, lactate dehydrogenase, magnesium, phosphate, potassium, protein, sodium, urate, urea, urinalysis Haematology: folate, FBC, vitamin B12 Immunology: syphilis serology	20% of patients found to have previously undiagnosed medical morbidity; 17% of patients had no laboratory abnormalities; one laboratory abnormality found in 27% of patients, 2 in 21%, 3 in 17% and 4–9 in 18%
Peet[11] (1981)	Survey of general adult psychiatrists	n = 100	Biochemistry: calcium, creatinine, electrolytes, glucose, liver function tests, thyroid function tests, urea, urinalysis Haematology: ESR, folate, FBC, vitamin B12 Immunology: syphilis serology	For inpatients: 14% of respondents did not carry out any routine laboratory investigations For outpatients: 96% of respondents did not carry out any routine laboratory investigations
Peet and Murphy[12] (1995)	Survey of general adult psychiatrists	n = 114	Biochemistry: calcium, creatinine, electrolytes, glucose, liver function tests, thyroid function tests, urea, urinalysis Haematology: ESR, folate, FBC, vitamin B12 Immunology: syphilis serology	For inpatients: 1.75% of respondents did not carry out any routine laboratory investigations For outpatients: 82% of respondents did not carry out any routine laboratory investigations
Roca et al[13] (1987)	Prospective	n = 42, psychiatric outpatients	Biochemistry: 'chemistries', urinalysis Haematology: FBC Immunology: syphilis serology	64% of patients found to have previously undiagnosed medical morbidity; 38.1% of patients had abnormal laboratory results

7

Table Brief literature review of laboratory testing/screening in adult psychiatric patients (Cont.)

Reference	Study design	Number, type of patients	Laboratory investigations	Results
Shatin et al[14] (1978)	Retrospective review of notes	$n = 4994$, psychiatric outpatients	Biochemistry: albumin, alkaline phosphatase, aspartate transaminase, bilirubin, calcium, chloride, CO_2 content, creatine kinase, creatinine, glucose, lactate dehydrogenase, phosphate, potassium, protein, sodium, urate, urea, urinalysis Cytology: vaginal (Pap) smear Haematology: FBC Immunology: syphilis serology	4.8% of all patients showed at least one laboratory abnormality at initial evaluation; 78% of patients with laboratory abnormalities had a diagnosis of schizophrenia; only 48% of abnormalities were followed up
Sheline and Kehr[15] (1990)	Retrospective	$n = 252$, new admissions	'Routine admission laboratory testing' (FBC, urinalysis, syphilis screening, SMA-20)	'New discoveries based on admission laboratory studies that led to changes in clinical management were found in 6% of admissions'
Sox et al[16] (1989)	Prospective	$n = 509$, patients in variety of inpatient and outpatient settings	Variable, depended on algorithm used Biochemistry: AST, albumin, calcium, cholesterol, free T4, potassium, sodium, T4, urine dipstick Haematology: FBC, vitamin B12	12% of patients found to have previously undiagnosed medical morbidity

Thomas[17] (1979)	Retrospective review of notes	*n* = 613, new psychiatric admissions	Biochemistry: ALP, AST, bilirubin, calcium, cholesterol, creatinine, glucose, phosphate, potassium, protein, sodium, TFT, urate, urea, vitamin B12 Haematology: blood film, folate, FBC, vitamin B12 Immunology: cardiolipin WR (Wasserman reaction), treponemal haemagglutination, VDRL Microbiology: ESR, urine culture/sensitivity	Laboratory abnormalities found in 13% of all laboratory tests performed; 27% of patients not actually screened
White and Barraclough[18] (1989)	Retrospective review of notes	*n* = 1007, psychiatric inpatients	Biochemistry: ALP, AST, bilirubin, calcium creatinine, GGT, glucose, phosphate, porphyrins, protein, sodium, potassium, urea Haematology: blood film, folate, FBC Immunology: autoimmune screen, syphilis serology	Laboratory abnormalities found in 10.2% of all laboratory tests performed; 40% of patients not actually screened
Willett and King[19] (1977)	Retrospective review of notes	*n* = 636, psychiatric inpatients	Biochemistry: ALP, AST, bilirubin, calcium, cholesterol, creatinine, glucose, LDH, phosphate, protein, urate urea, urine dipstick Haematology: FBC Immunology: VDRL	Laboratory abnormalities found in 5.9% of all laboratory tests performed; 26.9% of patients had abnormal results

9

In addition to the above, the literature contains a number of contributions which consider laboratory screening in individual psychiatric diagnoses; for details see individual syndromes in Chapter 2.

Investigations will be guided by the patient's history and physical examination but at a minimum all psychiatric patients should be investigated, at least initially, for the following.

Table	Basic laboratory screen for all psychiatric patients	
Domain	*Parameter*	*Notes*
Clinical biochemistry	Blood glucose	Hyperglycaemia and hypoglycaemia both affect mental state and are often easily correctable. Also, certain medications affect glucose metabolism and necessitate monitoring
	TFT	Both hyperthyroidism and hypothyroidism are associated with a wide range of medical and psychiatric presentations, especially in women over the age of 50
	LFT	Hepatic impairment is a caution for the majority of psychotropics, and LFT are especially important in patients with a history of drug and alcohol abuse
	U&E	Electrolyte imbalances may reflect underlying pathological processes. Renal impairment is a caution for the majority of psychotropics
	Creatinine	May indicate altered renal function. Renal impairment is a caution for a number of psychotropics
	Urinalysis	May reveal use of illicit drugs or pathological conditions, which can alter mental state
Haematology	Full blood count	May reveal anaemia, infection, or other pathology
Immunology	No specific tests	
Microbiology	No specific tests	

10

In individuals with a history of physical illness, chronic drug/alcohol use, or treatment with psychotropics, a wide range of other tests can be considered. These will be guided by history and physical examination and may include the following.

Table	Additional basic tests which may be of value in the baseline screening of psychiatric patients	
Domain	**Test**	**Notes**
Clinical biochemistry	Calcium	Both raised and lowered levels are associated with a range of psychiatric presentations
	Prolactin	Raised prolactin may commonly result from antipsychotic or antidepressant administration and during periods of stress, amongst others
	Vitamin B12 and folate	Deficiency is associated with a wide variety of presentations
	Urine dipstick	Cheap, easy test for a variety of medical conditions such as diabetes mellitus
	Urine drug screen	Aids in ruling out differential diagnoses
Haematology	No specific additional tests	
Immunology	Hepatitis serology Human immuno-deficiency virus (HIV) serology Syphilis serology	Aids in ruling out differential diagnoses
Microbiology	Midstream urine	May be especially useful to rule out urinary tract infection (UTI) as a cause of confusion in older patients

References

1. Anfinson TJ, Kathol RG. Screening laboratory evaluation in psychiatric patients: a review. Gen Hosp Psychiatry 1992; 14: 248–57.
2. Barnes RF, Mason JC, Greer C et al. Medical illness in chronic psychiatric outpatients. Gen Hosp Psychiatry 1983; 5: 191–5.
3. Burke AW. Physical disorder among day hospital patients. Br J Psychiatry 1978; 133: 22–7.
4. Catalano G, Catalano MC, O'Dell KJ, Humphrey DA, Fritz EB. The utility of laboratory screening in medically ill patients with psychiatric symptoms. Ann Clin Psychiatry 2001; 13: 135–40.
5. Dolan JG, Mushlin AI. Routine laboratory testing for medical disorders in psychiatric inpatients. Arch Intern Med 1985; 145: 2085–8.
6. Ferguson B, Dudleston K. Detection of physical disorder in newly admitted psychiatric patients. Acta Psychiatr Scand 1986; 74: 485–9.
7. Hall RCW, Popkin MK, Devaul RA, Faillace LA, Stickney SK. Physical illness presenting as psychiatric disease. Arch Gen Psychiatry 1978; 35: 1315–20.
8. Hall RCW, Gardner ER, Stickney SK, LeCann AF, Popkin MK. Physical illness presenting as psychiatric disease. II. Analysis of a state hospital inpatient population. Arch Gen Psychiatry 1980; 37: 989–95.
9. Honig A, Pop P, Tan ES, Philipsen H, Romme AJ. Physical illness in chronic psychiatric patients from a community psychiatric unit. The implications for daily practice. Br J Psychiatry 1989; 155: 58–64.
10. Koran LM, Sheline Y, Imai K et al. Medical disorders among patients admitted to a public-sector psychiatric inpatient unit. Psychiatr Serv 2002; 53: 1623–5.
11. Peet M. Laboratory screening for physical illness in psychiatric patients. Lancet 1981; 2: 529–30.
12. Peet M, Murphy B. Laboratory screening for physical illness in psychiatric patients. J Ment Health 1995; 4: 531–5.
13. Roca RP, Breakey WR, Fischer PJ. Medical care of chronic psychiatric patients. Hosp Community Psychiatry 1987; 38: 741–5.
14. Shatin L, Kymissis P, Brown W. Clinical laboratory abnormalities and their follow-up in a mental hygiene clinic. Br J Psychiatry 1978; 133: 150–5.
15. Sheline Y, Kehr C. Cost and utility of routine admission laboratory testing for psychiatric inpatients. Gen Hosp Psychiatry 1990; 12: 329–34.
16. Sox HC, Koran LM, Sox C et al. A medical algorithm for detecting physical disease in psychiatric patients. Hosp Community Psychiatry 1989; 40: 1270–6.
17. Thomas CJ. The use of screening investigations in psychiatry. Br J Psychiatry 1979; 135: 67–72.
18. White AJ, Barraclough B. Benefits and problems of routine laboratory investigations in adult psychiatric admissions. Br J Psychiatry 1989; 155: 65–72.
19. Willett AB, King T. Implementation of laboratory screening procedures on a short term psychiatric inpatient unit. Dis Nerv Syst 1977; 38: 867–70.

Further reading

Broderick KB, Lerner B, McCourt JD, Fraser E, Salerno K. Emergency physician practices and requirements regarding the medical screening examination of psychiatric patients. Acad Emerg Med 2002; 9: 88–92.

Gold MS, Pottash ALC. Diagnostic and Laboratory Testing in Psychiatry. New York: Plenum Publishing Corporation, 1986.

Livingstone C, Rampes H. The role of clinical biochemistry in psychiatry. CPD Bull Clin Biochem 2004; 6: 59–65.

Lukens TW, Wolf SJ, Edlow JA et al. Clinical policy: critical issues in the diagnosis and management of the adult psychiatric patient in the emergency department. Ann Emerg Med 2006; 47: 79–99.

Pomeroy C, Mitchell JE, Roerig J, Crow S. Medical Complications of Psychiatric Illness. Washington, DC: American Psychiatric Press, 2002.

Rosse RB, Giese AA, Deutsch SI, Morihisa JM. Concise Guide to Laboratory and Diagnostic Testing in Psychiatry. Washington, DC: American Psychiatric Press, 1989.

Schiffer RB, Side RC, Klein RS. Medical Evaluation of Psychiatric Patients. London: Springer, 1988.

Stoudemire A, Fogel BS, eds. Psychiatric Care of the Medical Patient. New York: Oxford University Press, 1993.

Zun LS. Evidence-based evaluation of psychiatric patients. J Emerg Med 2005; 28: 35–9.

chapter 2

Laboratory aspects of specific psychiatric disorders

At present there are no specific laboratory tests which are diagnostic for any individual psychiatric disorder, and there is equally no clear consensus as to how individual patients presenting with psychiatric symptoms should be investigated in the laboratory.

Laboratory tests should therefore be selected based on each patient's history, mental state examination, and physical examination.

Different tests may be selected depending on whether the patient is presenting *de novo* or with an established diagnosis or treatment regimen; laboratory screening aims to identify underlying medical causes as well as features resulting as a sequela of the disorder (e.g. effects of general neglect) or those specific to the disorder, including effects of treatment.

It should be further noted that presentations may be complicated by alcohol and substance abuse, which can also be monitored by appropriate laboratory investigations (see Chapter 7).

The following psychiatric disorders and their laboratory features are described in this chapter:

- anxiety disorders
- bipolar affective disorder
- chronic fatigue syndrome
- delirium
- dementias
- depression
- eating disorders
- obsessive–compulsive disorders
- personality disorders
- schizophrenia

- somatoform disorders
- stress reactions
- suicide/deliberate self-harm.

Note: the suggested laboratory investigations for each disorder are only recommendations, and tests should always be selected based on clinical presentation/index of suspicion of pathology together with local protocols and expert advice as appropriate.

For each condition described in this chapter the following information will be provided:

- definition
- diagnostic criteria
- differential diagnosis
- laboratory investigations (including NICE guidelines where appropriate).

Anxiety disorders

Definition

Anxiety is an emotional state which is unpleasant for the sufferer and is frequently accompanied by subjective experiences of fear, usually with physical symptoms and feelings of impending threat. It may occur when there is no clear external stimulus (such as in panic disorder), when there are discrete stimuli (such as in phobias), in a persistent state (such as in generalized anxiety disorder), or as part of a wide range of other disorders, both psychiatric and physical.

ICD-10 criteria (generalized anxiety disorder, F41.1)

Time frame At least 6 months in which there is prominent tension, feelings of stress, or apprehension.

Features At least one of points 1–4 and three of 5–24:

1. palpitations, tachycardia
2. sweating
3. shaking, trembling, tremulousness
4. dry mouth
5. breathing difficulty
6. choking sensation
7. chest pain
8. abnormal abdominal sensations
9. nausea
10. feeling dizzy or faint
11. feelings of derealization
12. feelings of depersonalization
13. fear of losing control
14. fear of dying

15. feeling hot or cold
16. numbness or tingling sensations
17. restlessness
18. feeling tense
19. difficulty swallowing
20. globus hystericus (feeling of lump in throat)
21. exaggerated startle response
22. difficulty concentrating
23. irritability
24. disturbed sleep pattern (difficulty in falling asleep due to excessive worrying).

Exclusion criteria Presentation not due to other psychiatric disorder (panic, obsessive–compulsive disorder, phobic disorder, hypochondriacal disorder) or physical disorder, organic mental disorder, or effects of substance intoxication or withdrawal.

Differential diagnosis

A wide variety of disorders can cause or exacerbate anxiety, and an exhaustive list could conceivably include almost every describable medical condition.

In addition, a very large number of drugs can cause anxiety, including those which are prescribed and those taken illicitly.

Psychiatric associations

Table Differential diagnosis of anxiety disorders: psychiatric causes	

Anxiety disorders	Adjustment disorder with anxiety
	Generalized anxiety
	Secondary anxiety as a result of:
	    death
	    dependence
	    intimacy
	    loss (self-control, self-esteem)
	    guilt
	    punishment
	    separation
	    situation
	    stranger

Other disorders	Acute stress reactions Adjustment disorders Agoraphobia Bipolar disorder Depressive disorders Mixed anxiety–depressive disorder Obsessive–compulsive disorder Panic disorder Psychotic disorders Specific phobia Post-traumatic disorders

Non-psychiatric associations

Table Differential diagnosis of anxiety disorders: non-psychiatric causes	
Medical conditions	Vascular: stroke, subarachnoid haemorrhage Infective: cerebral syphilis, chronic infections, encephalitis, human immunodeficiency virus (HIV), post-hepatitis Neoplastic: cerebral neoplasms, systemic malignancy, carcinoid syndrome Trauma: cerebral trauma, post-concussion syndromes Autoimmune: polyarteritis nodosa, rheumatoid arthritis, SLE, temporal arteritis Metabolic: B12 deficiency, hypoglycaemia, nicotinic acid deficiency, porphyria; Wilson's disease Endocrine: adrenal dysfunction, hyper-/hypothyroidism, parathyroid dysfunction, phaeochromocytoma; pituitary dysfunction Degenerative: multiple sclerosis, Huntington's disease Other: epilepsy, hyperventilation syndrome, hypoxia, mitral valve prolapse, postoperative, premenstrual syndrome
Substance intoxication	Amphetamine, amyl nitrate, caffeine, cannabis, cocaine, hallucinogens, theophylline
Substance withdrawal	Alcohol, antihypertensives, benzodiazepines, caffeine, opioids
Prescribed medications	Anticholinergics (e.g. benztropine), dopaminergics (e.g. levodopa, metoclopramide), stimulants (e.g. methylphenidate, aminophylline), sympathomimetics (e.g. epinephrine); miscellaneous (e.g. indometacin, metronidazole, oestrogens)

Laboratory investigations

When to perform laboratory investigations

- In order to make the diagnosis;
- In order to rule out possible organic differential diagnoses;
- In order to monitor physical health, especially with medical comorbidity or with medication treatment.

What laboratory investigations to perform

NICE guidelines As there is no specific laboratory investigation for any anxiety disorder, basic investigations should be guided by clinical presentation and are aimed at ruling out obvious differential diagnoses. The UK National Institute for Health and Clinical Excellence has published guidelines for anxiety disorders (http://guidance.nice.org.uk/CG22/guidance/pdf/English/ download.dspx) but makes no specific recommendations regarding laboratory investigation.

Most patients with anxiety will not manifest with an obvious physical cause, and most are not ultimately admitted to hospital.

Laboratory investigation is therefore based on history and physical examination, and routine blood testing is generally reserved for those individuals with medical morbidity, those presenting to hospital, and those with treatment resistance thought to be due to an underlying medical condition.

Table Recommended basic laboratory screen for anxious patients

Domain	Laboratory tests
Clinical biochemistry	Blood glucose C-reactive protein (CRP) U&E TFT Urinalysis (urine dipstick and possibly urine drug screening)
Haematology	FBC
Immunology	No specific investigations
Microbiology	

Additional tests may be considered, after obtaining expert advice, in selected patients to rule out other possible medical causes.

Table Additional laboratory investigations for anxious patients

Domain	Laboratory tests
Clinical biochemistry	Lipid screen Magnesium Porphyria screen Serum B12/folate Serum caeruloplasmin Urine 5-hydroxyindolacetic acid (5-HIAA) (for suspected carcinoid syndrome) Urine osmolality Urine toxicology (for heavy metals, substances of abuse, anabolic steroids; uroporphyrins, porphobilinogen) Urine vanillylmandelic acid (VMA) (in suspected phaeochromocytoma) Lumbar puncture/cerebrospinal fluid (CSF) analysis Faecal occult blood
Haematology	ESR Haematinics
Immunology	Autoantibodies (antinuclear antibody (ANA), Rh factor, Ro, La, U1 ribonuclear protein) HIV serology Syphilis serology
Microbiology	Blood/urine cultures

Additional non-routine (research) tests not normally performed:

Table Non-routine (research) tests and anxiety disorders

Carbon dioxide	Inhalation can precipitate attacks in predisposed individuals (secondary to respiratory alkalosis)
Lactate	Infusion of sodium lactate has been reported to induce panic attacks in over 70% of patients with panic disorder; it can also trigger flashbacks in post-traumatic stress disorder (PTSD)

Bipolar affective disorder

Definition

Bipolar affective disorders are a complex group of disorders characterized by recurrent episodes of altered mood, involving both elevation and depression. There may be individual episodes of hypomania/mania, or depression, and there is a related disorder, cyclothymia, which is less prolonged and severe than bipolar affective disorder.

Recurrent bipolar affective disorder can be further divided into bipolar I disorder (one or more manic/mixed episodes and usually one or more depressive episodes) and bipolar II disorder (recurrent major depressive and hypomanic episodes).

ICD-10 criteria (bipolar affective disorder, current episode hypomanic, F31.0)

Time frame   At least 4 days of elevated mood.

Features

1. The current episode meets the criteria for hypomania (F31.0), namely, mood is elevated/irritable above that which is normal for the individual and sustained for at least 4 days, with at least three of the following which lead to interference in normal daily personal functioning:

    i.   increased activity
    ii. physical restlessness
    iii. distractibility
    iv. poor concentration
    v.   decreased sleep
    vi. increased sexual energy
    vii. reckless/irresponsible behaviour
    viii. increased sociability/over-familiarity.

2. There has been at least one other previous affective episode (manic, hypomanic, depressed, or mixed affective).

Exclusion criteria   Single manic episode, other psychiatric disorders, organic brain syndromes, effects of psychoactive substances.

Differential diagnosis

A wide range of disorders have been reported to be associated with bipolar affective disorder.

Psychiatric associations

Table Differential diagnosis of bipolar disorder: psychiatric associations

Schizophrenia and psychotic disorders
Personality disorders
Schizoaffective disorders
Sleep disorders

Non-psychiatric associations

Table Differential diagnosis of bipolar disorder: non-psychiatric associations

Medical conditions	Autoimmune: rheumatoid arthritis, SLE Degenerative: dementias (Alzheimer's dementia, Parkinson's disease), Fahr's disease, Huntington's disease, multiple sclerosis Endocrine: adrenal insufficiency (Cushing's, Addison's), hyperaldosteronism, thyroid disorders (hyper- and hypo-), parathyroid disorders (hyper- and hypo-) Infection: HIV/acquired immunodeficiency syndrome (AIDS), post-viral fatigue/chronic fatigue syndrome, neurosyphilis, pneumonias, tuberculosis Metabolic: Wilson's disease, porphyria, uraemia, vitamin deficiencies (B12, folate, niacin, thiamine) Neoplastic: brain tumours, other cancers (pancreatic, gastrointestinal) Head trauma Vascular: stroke, migraine, Sjögren's arteritis, temporal arteritis Other: hydrocephalus, progressive supranuclear palsy, cardiopulmonary disease, narcolepsy, epilepsy
Substance intoxication/ withdrawal	Alcohol, amphetamines, corticosteroids, cocaine, hallucinogens, opioids, phencyclidine, procyclidine
Prescribed medications	Antidepressants, antivirals (didanosine, efavirenz, zidovudine), baclofen, bromocriptine, captopril, cimetidine, cyclosporine, isoniazid, levodopa, methylphenidate, yohimbine

Laboratory investigations

When to perform laboratory investigations

- In order to make the diagnosis;
- In order to rule out differential diagnoses;
- In order to monitor physical health, especially with medical comorbidity or with physical treatment methods particularly mood stabilizers (see Chapter 5 for details regarding therapeutic drug monitoring).

What laboratory investigations to perform

NICE guidelines As there is no specific laboratory investigation for bipolar affective disorder, basic investigations should be guided by clinical presentation and are aimed at ruling out obvious differential diagnoses. The UK National Institute for Health and Clinical Excellence has published guidelines for laboratory investigation of bipolar affective disorder (http://guidance. nice.org.uk/download.aspx?o=384826) and suggests the following tests.

The initial health check includes the following.

Table NICE-recommended basic laboratory screen for all bipolar patients

Domain	Laboratory tests
Clinical biochemistry	Blood glucose Creatinine LFT Lipid profile (over age 40 only) Prolactin (risperidone only) TDM (for carbamazepine and lithium) TFT U&E
Haematology	FBC
Immunology	No specific investigations
Microbiology	

Suggested further laboratory monitoring in medicated patients (see also Chapter 5) includes the following.

Table NICE-recommended reviews in medicated patients following initial screening

Time	Medication	Laboratory parameter	Notes
3-Monthly	Lithium	Lithium levels	Three times over 6 weeks following initiation of treatment and 3-monthly thereafter
	Olanzapine Quetiapine Risperidone	Glucose Lipid profile	Olanzapine is associated with increased risk of metabolic syndrome (see Chapter 5); NICE suggests that antipsychotic levels be done 1 week after initiation and 1 week after dose change until levels are stable and then 3-monthly
6-Monthly	Carbamazepine	Carbamazepine levels	NICE suggests that these be done 6-monthly
		FBC LFT U&E	Other laboratory tests may be required depending on clinical presentation
	Lithium	U&E	U&E may be needed more frequently if patient deteriorates or is on angiotensin converting enzyme (ACE) inhibitors, diuretics, or non-steroidal anti-inflammatory drugs (NSAIDs)
		TFT	Thyroid function, for individuals with rapid-cycling bipolar disorder; thyroid antibodies may be measured if TFT are abnormal
	Sodium valproate	FBC LFT	NICE suggests that these be done 'over the first 6 months'
Annually	All patients	Blood glucose TFT	Other laboratory tests may be required depending on clinical presentation
	Lithium	Glucose	
	Olanzapine	Glucose Lipid profile	
	Sodium valproate	Glucose	

Additional investigations will aim to rule out effects of comorbid medical conditions, substance use, or effects of prescribed medications; expert advice will be needed before investigation.

Table Additional possible laboratory investigations for bipolar patients

Domain	Laboratory tests
Clinical biochemistry	Calcium Magnesium Porphyria screen Serum B12/folate Serum caeruloplasmin Serum protein electrophoresis Urine osmolality Urine toxicology (for heavy metals, substances of abuse, anabolic steroids, urine steroid profile, uroporphyrins, porphobilinogen) Lumbar puncture/CSF analysis Faecal occult blood
Haematology	ESR Haematinics
Immunology	Autoantibodies (ANA and possibly also C3, C4, anti-dsDNA, Rh factor, Ro, La, U1 ribonuclear protein) HIV serology Syphilis serology Tuberculosis (TB) serology
Microbiology	Blood/urine cultures (including TB)

A number of other, non-routine investigations/findings have been reported in the literature which currently have no validated diagnostic validity and are thus not routinely performed apart from for research purposes.

Table Non-routine tests for bipolar affective disorder

Parameter	Notes
cAMP (cyclic 3'5'-adenosine monophosphate)	Increased urine levels have been reported in mania
Fractionated catecholamines	Increased urine levels of norepinephrine, epinephrine, and dopamine have been reported in bipolar affective disorders of long-standing
3-Methoxy-4-hydroxyphenylglycol	24-hour urine collections suggest levels lower in bipolar patients compared to those with unipolar depression. Low CSF levels have been mooted as a marker of decreased noradrenergic activity, possibly associated with increased suicidality
Taurine	Plasma levels have been reported to be increased in bipolar affective disorder
Thyroid stimulating hormone (TSH)	Elevated baseline TSH levels (<4 mU/l) have been found in some patients with rapid-cycling disorder; also, patients with bipolar disorder with elevated TSH levels may be at higher risk of antidepressant-induced rapid mood cycling
Rubidium	Rubidium has been investigated as a possible treatment in bipolar disorders and may enhance the antidepressant effect of lithium

Chronic fatigue syndrome

Definition

Chronic fatigue syndrome is a controversial entity in which the affected individual complains of persistent fatigue that is not readily attributable to any recognizable cause.

Clinical criteria (US Centers for Disease Control and Prevention, 1994)

Time frame   Fatigue must have lasted for at least 6 months.

Features

1. The fatigue is of clear or new onset;
2. The fatigue continues despite rest;
3. The fatigue has a major adverse impact upon activities (educational, occupational, personal, social);
4. At least four of the following symptoms have been present for at least 6 months:
    i. axillary/cervical lymphadenopathy (may be tender)
    ii. concentration/memory impairment
    iii. pain (headaches, joints, muscles)
    iv. poor-quality sleep ('unrefreshing' sleep)
    v. post-exertional malaise
    vi. sore throat.

Exclusion criteria   Alcoholism, fatigue secondary to continuing exertion, major psychiatric disorders (bipolar disorder, dementia, eating disorders, major depression, schizophrenia), obesity, organic medical conditions causing fatigue, substance abuse disorders.

Differential diagnosis

A great many disorders, both psychiatric and physical, have symptoms which overlap with chronic fatigue syndrome; selected examples are shown below.

Table Differential diagnosis of chronic fatigue syndrome (incomplete list)	
Psychiatric	Anxiety disorders (including agoraphobia, generalized anxiety disorder, and panic disorders) Depressive disorders (including dysthymia) Eating disorders Hypochondriasis Psychotic syndromes Sleep disorders (narcolepsy, sleep apnoea) Somatization disorders Substance abuse disorders
Non-psychiatric	Infections including Epstein–Barr virus, hepatitis, HIV, Lyme disease Neurological including myasthenia gravis, multiple sclerosis Multisystem disorders including autoimmune disease, coeliac disease, endocrine disease Respiratory disease such as asthma Toxicity due to heavy metals and solvents

Laboratory investigations

When to perform laboratory investigations

- In order to make the diagnosis;
- In order to rule out differential diagnoses;
- In order to monitor physical health, especially with medical comorbidity or with physical treatments.

What laboratory investigations to perform
As there is no specific laboratory investigation for chronic fatigue syndrome, basic investigations should be guided by clinical presentation and are aimed at ruling out obvious differential diagnoses. The UK National Institute for Health and Clinical Excellence has published guidelines for laboratory

investigation of chronic fatigue syndrome (http://guidance.nice.org.uk/CG53/niceguidance/word/English/download.dspx) and suggests the following.

Table	Suggested basic laboratory tests in chronic fatigue syndrome	
Domain	*Test*	*Notes*
Clinical biochemistry	Calcium Creatine kinase Creatinine CRP Glucose (random) LFT TFT U&E Urinalysis	Tests aim to exclude common, treatable differentials such as anaemia, diabetes mellitus, infection/inflammatory disease, liver/renal dysfunction, thyroid dysfunction, etc. Over-investigation is not recommended
Haematology	ESR Ferritin FBC	Serum ferritin only in children/young people. May be measured in adults if FBC suggests iron deficiency
Immunology	Gluten sensitivity	Antigliadin and antiendomysium antibody screening suggested
Microbiology	None	Serological tests for specific infections such as borreliosis, HIV, hepatitis B, or hepatitis C may be appropriate based on history

Additional tests may be useful in specific cases, and should always be guided by clinical suspicion. Over-investigation is to be avoided. Possible additional tests could include serological tests (e.g. for cytomegalovirus, Epstein–Barr virus, HIV, syphilis, toxoplasmosis), faecal occult blood, or autoantibodes.

Additional (non-routine) investigations A great number of parameters have been examined in chronic fatigue syndrome and related disorders, although many findings remain controversial. A summary of some of the less controversial changes is shown below.

Table Possible laboratory changes in chronic fatigue syndrome	
Parameter	*Notes*
Antithyroid antibodies	Reported in association with hypothyroidism in a small proportion (<10%) of patients
Complement	Depressed levels in chronic fatigue syndrome have been reported
Cortisol	Decreased response following corticotropin challenge test has been reported in some patients
CRP	May be elevated in about 25% of patients with chronic fatigue syndrome
Homocysteine	Increased levels reported
Lead	Increased levels reported
Red cell distribution width (RCDW)	Increased width reported in females but not males
TGF-β	Increased levels of tumour growth factor (TGF) reported
TNF	Increased levels of tumour necrosis factor (TNF) reported

Delirium

Definition

Delirium, also known as acute confusional state, is a relatively persistent and sustained condition of global decrease in cognitive functioning, usually fluctuating, and due to an underlying organic (i.e. non-psychiatric) defect. Delirium due to treatable causes is usually reversible. The term should not be confused with delirium tremens, an alcohol withdrawal state.

ICD-10 criteria (F05.0)

Time frame   Rapid onset (versus gradual onset in other conditions such as dementia).

Features

1. Clouding of consciousness (reduced awareness of external environment);
2. Disturbed cognition (disorientation in time/place/person; impairment of recent memory);
3. Psychomotor disturbance (may include any or all rapid changes in activity and speech; increased reaction time and exaggerated startle reaction);
4. Sleep disturbance (insomnia, worsening of symptoms at night (sun-downing), disturbing dreams/nightmares).

Exclusion criteria   Excludes emotional disturbances/other psychiatric disorders with similar features.

Differential diagnosis

A large number of disorders can precipitate/mimic delirium, including both medical and psychiatric disorders; note that almost any prescribed or illicit drug may be associated with delirium.

Table Disorders which may precipitate or mimic delirium	
Psychiatric	Dementias Pseudodementia Schizophrenia Schizophreniform disorder Brief reactive psychosis Mood disorders Dissociative disorders Factitious disorders
Organic brain syndromes	Amnestic syndrome Organic hallucinosis, delusional syndrome, mood syndrome, anxiety syndromes
Non-psychiatric	Intracranial: epilepsy, infection (Creutzfeldt–Jakob disease (CJD), HIV, neurosyphilis, TB), trauma, tumours, vascular (Binswanger's disease, stroke, transient ischaemic attack (TIA), subdural), normal pressure hydrocephalus, Fahr's disease (idiopathic cerebral ferrocalcinosis) Extracranial: endocrine (hypo-/hyperglycaemia; hypo-/hyperthyroidism), hypoxia, infection (urinary tract infection (UTI), reproductive tract infection (RTI), sepsis), metabolic (electrolyte disturbance, hepatic dysfunction, malnutrition, uraemia, vitamin deficiency, Wilson's disease), toxic (intoxication/withdrawal of alcohol, prescribed drugs, illicit drugs, environmental toxins such as lead, mercury, and thallium), genetic (Huntington's disease, metachromatic leukodystrophy, multiple sclerosis) Vascular: SLE Other: cardiovascular disorders (arrhythmias, heart failure, myocardial infarction), irradiation, post-anaesthesia, postoperative, sensory deprivation, sleep deprivation

Drugs which may precipitate or mimic delirium (intoxication and/or withdrawal) include the following.

Table Examples of drugs associated with delirium (incomplete list – see Bazire, *Psychotropic Drug Directory*, for more details)
Non-prescribed/illicit: alcohol, amphetamine, anabolic steroids, caffeine, cocaine, ergot alkaloids, heroin, ketamine, lysergic acid diethylamide (LSD), mescaline, opiates, phenylcyclohexylpiperidine (PCP), peyote, quaaludes, etc.
Psychotropics: barbiturates, benzodiazepines, carbamazepine, clozapine, disulfiram, tricyclic antidepressants, buproprion, fluoxetine, fluvoxamine, lithium carbonate, methylphenidate, maprotiline, MAOIs, neuroleptics (especially phenothiazines), paroxetine, procyclidine, promethazine, trazodone, valproic acid, etc.
Non-psychotropics: amantadine, aminophylline, antiarrhythmics, antibiotics, anticonvulsants, antifungals, antihistamines, anti-inflammatories, antimalarials, antiparkinson agents, antispasmodics, antituberculosis agents, antivirals, atropine, baclofen, benztropine, buprenorphine, calcium channel blockers, captopril, chlorambucil, chloroquine, cimetidine, clonidine, codeine, colchicine, cycloserine, cytotoxics, dapsone, digitalis, diltiazem, disopyramide, ephedrine, erythropoietin, fentanyl, hydroxymethylglutaryl coenzyme A (HMG-CoA) reductase inhibitors, interferon-α, interleukin-2, levodopa, lidocaine, mefloquine, methodone, metoclopramide, morphine, naltrexone, ondansetron, paraldehyde, pergolide, phenelzine, phenytoin, pilocarpine, procainamide, propranolol, quinine, ranitidine, scopolamine, simvastatin, theophylline, thiazide diuretics, vinblastine, vincristine, zolpidem, etc.

Laboratory investigations

When to perform laboratory investigations

- In order to make the diagnosis;
- In order to rule out possible organic differential diagnoses;
- In order to monitor physical health, especially with medical comorbidity or with medication treatment.

What laboratory investigations to perform

NICE guidelines As there is no specific laboratory investigation for delirium, basic investigations should be guided by clinical presentation and are aimed at ruling out obvious differential diagnoses. The UK National Institute for Health and Clinical Excellence has not yet published guidelines for delirium.

Investigation will therefore be guided by history, mental state examination, and physical examination, with suggested baseline investigations to include the following.

Table Recommended basic laboratory screen for all delirious patients	
Domain	*Laboratory tests*
Clinical biochemistry	Blood glucose Calcium CRP LFT TFT U&E Urinalysis (urine dipstick and urine drug screening)
Haematology	FBC
Immunology	No specific investigations
Microbiology	Mid-stream urine (MSU)

Additional tests can be performed after obtaining expert advice and could include the following.

Table Additional laboratory investigations for delirious patients	
Domain	*Laboratory tests*
Clinical biochemistry	Arterial blood gases Cortisol Magnesium Porphyria screen Serum B12/folate Serum caeruloplasmin Serum protein electrophoresis Screening for specific drugs/toxins Urinalysis (urine osmolality, urine toxicology for heavy metals, substances of abuse, urinary steroid profile; uroporphyrins, porphobilinogen) Lumbar puncture/CSF analysis
Haematology	ESR Haematinics
Immunology	HIV serology Autoantibodies (ANA and possibly also C3, C4, anti-dsDNA, Rh factor, Ro, La, U1 ribonuclear protein) HIV serology Syphilis serology TB serology
Microbiology	Blood/urine cultures TB cultures

Dementias

Definition

The dementias refer to a variety of disorders in which there is both a global and a progressive decline in higher cognitive functions (cognition, intellect, personality) which occurs in clear consciousness and which is not consistent with a diagnosis of delirium.

Note: demented patients are more susceptible to delirium and a delirium can be superimposed on dementia.

There are a number of clinical features which differentiate dementia and delirium.

Table Features differentiating between delirium and dementia		
Feature	*Delirium*	*Dementia*
Affect	Anxious, labile, irritable	Not usually anxious but may be labile
Awareness	Impaired	Less impaired
Consciousness level	Fluctuating	Normal
Course	Fluctuating	Progressive
Duration	Acute (days–weeks)	Chronic (months–years)
History	Acute illness	Chronic illness
Memory	Recent memory impaired	Recent and remote memory impaired
Onset	Rapid	Usually insidious
Orientation	Impaired (may be periodical)	Intact (at least initially)
Perceptions	Hallucinations common (especially visual)	Hallucinations less common (may be more common in the evening or at night – 'sun-downing')
Psychomotor function	Variable (retarded, agitated, or mixed)	Usually normal
Reversibility	Can be reversible	Most forms are irreversible
Sleep	Frequent disruption of sleep–wake cycle	Less disruption of sleep–wake cycle

ICD-10 criteria (DCR-10 general criteria for dementia)

Time frame   At least 6 months of cognitive decline (see below).

Features

1. Decline in memory (inability to learn new information, both non-verbal and verbal. The degree of memory loss may be further classified as:

   i. mild, in which the memory loss interferes with everyday activities, though not to an extent as to be incompatible with independent living;
   ii. moderate, in which individuals cannot recall basic information and the degree of memory impairment is a serious impediment to independent living;
   iii. severe, in which there is complete inability to retain new information;

2. Decline in other cognitive functions (judgement, planning, organization, general information processing) which can be further classified as:

   i. mild, in which the decline in cognitive functioning causes some impairment in daily living but is insufficient to cause dependence on others;
   ii. moderate, in which the individual is unable to function without the assistance of others;
   iii. severe, in which there is a complete or almost complete absence of intellectual functioning;

3. There is an absence of clouding of consciousness, i.e. awareness of the environment is preserved;
4. There is a change in behaviour which manifests as at least one of lability of mood, irritability, apathy, or inappropriate social behaviour.

Exclusion criteria   The diagnostic criteria for delirium are not met; a super-imposed delirium precludes a diagnosis of dementia.

Differential diagnosis

Dementias are a diverse group of disorders with a wide variety of aetiologies.

Table Differential diagnosis of dementia	
Psychiatric	Depression Delirium Pseudodementia
Organic brain syndromes	Amnestic syndrome Dysphasic syndromes Frontal lobe syndromes Parietal lobe syndromes Subcortical dementias
General medical conditions	Autoimmune: arteritis, SLE Degenerative: Alzheimer's, Binswanger's, Creutzfeldt–Jakob disease, Huntington's, Lewy-body, multiple sclerosis, Parkinson's, Pick's Endocrine: Addison's disease, hypothyroidism, hypo-/hyperparathyroidism Infective: abscess, encephalitis, encephalopathies, HIV, neurosyphilis, prion diseases, opportunistic, tuberculosis Metabolic: anaemia, cardiac failure, hepatic failure, hypercalcaemia, hypernatraemia, hypoglycaemia, renal failure, vitamin deficiency (B12, folate, niacin, thiamine), Wilson's disease Neoplastic: intracranial mass lesions, primary and secondary neoplasms, paraneoplastic syndromes (especially bronchial carcinoma) Toxins: carbon monoxide, lead, manganese, mercury Trauma: haematoma, head injury, punch-drunk syndrome Vascular: multi-infarct dementia, subarachnoid haemorrhage, subdural haematoma
Substance abuse	Alcohol, most substances of abuse
Prescribed medications	Antihypertensives, corticosteroids, digitalis, opiates, psychotropics (especially in the elderly and for those with anticholinergic properties)
Other	Amyotrophic lateral sclerosis as part of normal aging, cerebellar/spinocerebellar degeneration, dehydration, hydrocephalus (normal pressure/obstructive), hypertension, hypoxia, irradiation, progressive subcortical gliosis, progressive supranuclear palsy, stroke

Laboratory investigations

When to perform laboratory investigations

- In order to make the diagnosis;
- In order to rule out possible organic differential diagnoses;
- In order to monitor physical health, especially with medical comorbidity or with medication treatment.

What laboratory investigations to perform

NICE guidelines As there is no specific laboratory investigation for dementia, basic investigations should be guided by clinical presentation and are aimed at ruling out obvious differential diagnoses. The UK National Institute for Health and Clinical Excellence has published guidelines for dementia (http://guidance.nice.org.uk/cg42/guidance/pdf/English) but makes no specific recommendations regarding laboratory investigation.

A suggested, basic 'dementia screen' for newly presenting patients is given below.

Table Recommended basic laboratory dementia screen

Domain	Laboratory tests
Clinical biochemistry	Blood glucose Calcium CRP LFT TFT U&E Urinalysis (dipstick)
Haematology	ESR FBC
Immunology	Syphilis serology
Microbiology	MSU

Additional tests to consider (after obtaining expert advice) may include the following.

Table	Additional laboratory investigations for patients with dementia
Domain	**Laboratory tests**
Clinical biochemistry	Magnesium Porphyria screen Serum B12/folate Serum caeruloplasmin Serum protein electrophoresis Screening for specific drugs/toxins Urinalysis (urine osmolality, urine toxicology for heavy metals, substances of abuse, urinary steroid profile; uroporphyrins, porphobilinogen)
Haematology	ESR Haematinics
Immunology	HIV serology Autoantibodies (ANA and possibly also C3, C4, anti-dsDNA, Rh factor, Ro, La, U1 ribonuclear protein) HIV serology Syphilis serology TB serology
Microbiology	Blood/urine cultures TB cultures

Additional, non-routine (research) tests may include the following.

Table   Non-routine (research) tests and dementia

Parameter	Notes
Amyloid precursor protein	Alzheimer's disease (AD) patients have CSF levels lower than normals (AD range $0.8\pm0.4\,\mu g/ml$, normal range $2.7\pm0.7\,\mu g/ml$)
Apolipoprotein E (apoε4)	Increased plasma levels may be associated with Alzheimer's disease
β-Amyloid peptide 42	CSF levels of Aβ42 have been reported to be significantly lower in Alzheimer's patients compared to controls
Cadmium	Raised levels found in some patients with Alzheimer's dementia
Clusterin (apoJ)	A multifunctional lipoprotein associated with amyloid β-protein in senile plaques in Alzheimer's
Homocysteine	Raised levels (associated with low folate intake and low folate levels) have been suggested to be associated with Alzheimer's dementia
Tau protein	CSF levels in Alzheimer's patients are 2–10 times those of controls

Depression

Definition

Depression is a common disorder in which the primary feature is pervasive lowering of mood, often accompanied by low energy levels, loss of enjoyment of activities which are usually pleasurable, and reduced/altered patterns of sleep, appetite, and libido.

There is no single, clear consensus on how to classify depression, and ICD-10 includes a number of subtypes with varying features.

ICD-10 criteria (depressive episode F32)

Time frame   At least 2 weeks' duration.

Features

1. lowered mood
2. reduced energy levels
3. deceased activity levels

and at least four of the following ('somatic' or biological symptoms):

4. loss of interest in normally enjoyable activities ('anhedonia')
5. decrease of or lack of emotional reactions to events that would usually elicit a reaction
6. early morning waking from sleep (2 or more hours before usual time)
7. mood worse in the morning (diurnal mood variation)
8. objective evidence of psychomotor agitation or retardation
9. loss of appetite
10. weight loss (at least 5% of body weight over the previous month)
11. loss of libido.

Exclusion criteria   No current or previous manic or hypomanic symptoms; episode is not due to organic brain syndrome or use of drugs or alcohol.

Differential diagnosis

A wide variety of psychiatric disorders, medical conditions, and drugs are associated with depression.

Psychiatric disorders

Table	Differential diagnosis of depression: psychiatric conditions
Adjustment disorders Anxiety disorders Bipolar affective disorder and other mood disorders Dementia/pseudodementia Eating disorders Personality disorders Puerperal disorders Schizophrenia and psychotic disorders Somatoform disorders	

Non-psychiatric disorders

Table	Differential diagnosis of depression: non-psychiatric conditions
Medical conditions	Vascular: stroke, subarachnoid haemorrhage Infective: brucellosis, cerebral syphilis, chronic infections, encephalitis, HIV, post-hepatitis Neoplastic: cerebral neoplasms, systemic malignancy (especially pancreatic), carcinoid syndrome Trauma: cerebral trauma, post-concussion syndromes Autoimmune: polyarteritis nodosa rheumatoid arthritis, SLE, temporal arteritis Metabolic: B12 deficiency, end-stage renal failure, hypercalcaemia, hypoglycaemia, hypomagnesaemia, iron-deficiency anaemia, malnutrition, nicotinic acid deficiency, porphyria; Wilson's disease Endocrine: adrenal dysfunction, Cushing's disease, hyper-/hypothyroidism, hyperparathyroidism, phaeochromocytoma; pituitary dysfunction Degenerative: multiple sclerosis, Huntington's disease, Parkinson's disease Other: chronic pain, dioxane poisoning, epilepsy, hyperventilation syndrome, hypoxia, malnutrition, postoperative, premenstrual syndrome, sexual dysfunction, spinal cord injury
Substance intoxication/ withdrawal	Amphetamines, alcohol, anabolic steroids, cannabis, cocaine (especially crack), narcotics, PCP
Effects of prescribed medications (incomplete list)	Amantadine, amphotericin, antihistamines, antivirals (abacavir, acyclovir, efavirenz, indinavir, nevirapine), baclofen, benzodiazepines, cimetidine, codeine, corticosteroids, cycloserine, dapsone, diazepam, digitalis, disopyramide, interferon, interleukins (especially IL-2), isotretinoin, levodopa, mefloquine, methsuximide, methyldopa, metoclopramide, metronidazole, oestrogens, pergolide, procainamide, progestins, propranolol, reserpine, sulphonamides, thiazides, topiramate, vinblastine, vincristine

Laboratory investigations

When to perform laboratory investigations

• In order to rule out possible organic differential diagnoses;
• In order to monitor physical health, especially with medical comorbidity or with medication treatment.

What laboratory investigations to perform

NICE guidelines As there is no specific laboratory investigation for depression, basic investigations should be guided by clinical presentation and are aimed at ruling out obvious differential diagnoses. The UK National Institute for Health and Clinical Excellence has published guidelines for depression (http://guidance.nice.org.uk/CG23/guidance/pdf/English) but makes no specific recommendations regarding laboratory investigation.

Due to the complex potential aetiology of depression, first-line tests are aimed at excluding obvious, treatable causes of depression.

Table Recommended basic laboratory tests in depression

Domain	Laboratory tests
Clinical biochemistry	Blood glucose Calcium CRP LFT TFT U&E Urinalysis (dipstick)
Haematology	ESR FBC
Immunology	No specific investgations
Microbiology	

Additional tests will depend on clinical history and presentation and may require appropriate expert guidance, but could comprise the following.

Table Additional laboratory investigations in depression	
Domain	*Laboratory tests*
Clinical biochemistry	Arterial blood gases Cortisol Magnesium Porphyria screen Serum B12/folate Serum caeruloplasmin Serum protein electrophoresis Screening for specific drugs/toxins Urinalysis (urine osmolality, urine toxicology for heavy metals, substances of abuse, urinary steroid profile; uroporphyrins, porphobilinogen) Lumbar puncture/CSF analysis Faecal occult blood
Haematology	ESR Haematinics
Immunology	HIV serology Autoantibodies (ANA and possibly also C3, C4, anti-dsDNA, Rh factor, Ro, La, U1 ribonuclear protein) HIV serology Syphilis serology TB serology
Microbiology	Blood/urine cultures TB cultures

Additionally, a number of non-routine, yet to be validated investigations have been described in depression.

Table Non-routine (research) tests and depression

Parameter	Notes
β-Endorphin	Increased plasma levels may be found in depression
cAMP (cyclic 3'5'-adenosine monophosphate)	Decreased urinary levels reported in depression
Catecholamines	Increased levels in plasma have been reported especially in patients with at least a 6-month history of depression
Cortisol	Increased secretion reported in depression
Dexamethasone	Patients with depression (up to 50% reported) may have abnormal findings on overnight dexamethasone suppression test (normal: <3µg/dl (<0.08µmol/l), Cushing's >10µg/dl (>276nmol/l), depression >5µg/dl (>138nmol/l))
5-HIAA (5-hydroxyindoleacetic acid)	Decreased urinary levels may be found in depression
MHGP (3-methoxy-4-hydroxyphenylglycol)	Decreased plasma levels reported in depression
TRH (thyrotropin releasing hormone)	TSH blunting (= 7mU/l) may be seen in response to TRH in depressive disorders. TRH is not routinely measured.
5-OH-tryptamine (5-HT, serotonin)	Decreased blood levels in severe depression
Prostaglandins	Increased levels may be seen
Tryptophan	Low serum levels of total and free tryptophan associated with major depressive disorder. Diets low in tryptophan may be associated with precipitation of depression in patients predisposed to this condition
Urate	Increased levels may be seen in CSF, plasma, and urine

Eating disorders

There are two major eating disorders seen in psychiatry, anorexia nervosa and bulimia nervosa. In addition, the increasingly recognized category EDNOS (eating disorders not otherwise specified) and the relatively rare disorder of pica may also present to psychiatrists. The effects of obesity are considered in Chapter 8.

Both major eating disorders can cause a number of complex medical complications which may affect every organ system.

Definitions

Anorexia nervosa A disorder in which there is morbid fear of fatness, distorted body image, and deliberate weight loss.

Bulimia nervosa A disorder characterized by a preoccupation with body image, with binge eating followed by compensatory purging/vomiting.

Pica The persistent eating of non-nutritive substances not considered as foodstuffs.

ICD-10 criteria

Anorexia nervosa (F50.0)
Time frame None specific.

Features

1. weight loss of at least 15% below the expected weight for height and age
2. self-induced weight-loss
3. perception/dread of being too fat leading to a self-imposed desire for low weight
4. multiple endocrine effects on hypothalamic–pituitary–gonadal axis leading to alterations in sexual potency and amenorrhoea.

Exclusion criteria The disorder is not due to known physical disorders which cause weight loss, nor to bulimia nervosa.

Bulimia nervosa (F50.2)
Time frame Specific features (recurrent overeating) at least twice a week for at least 3 months.

Features

1. recurrent episodes of overeating (large amounts of food eaten in short periods of time)
2. preoccupation with eating with compulsion/craving to eat
3. manoeuvres undertaken by the patient to counteract the effects of eating by at least one of self-induced vomiting/purging, alternating episodes of fasting/starvation, use of drugs such as appetite suppressants, thyroid preparation, diuretics, and insulin
4. fear of and self-perception of being fat.

Exclusion criteria Excludes overeating due to other psychological disturbances, other psychiatric disorders, and physical conditions affecting appetite.

Pica (F50.8)
No features are described in ICD-10; DSM-IV criteria for pica as an eating disorder of infancy or early childhood include the following criteria:

• criterion A: at least a 1-month history of persistent eating of non-nutritive substances
• criterion B: behaviour is not developmentally inappropriate
• criterion C: the condition is not part of a culturally sanctioned practice
• criterion D: if pica occurs only during the course of another psychiatric disorder, a diagnosis of pica should only be made if it is of sufficient severity to warrant independent clinical attention.

Laboratory investigations

When to perform laboratory investigations

• In order to rule out possible organic differential diagnoses;
• In order to monitor physical health, especially with medical comorbidity or with medication treatment.

What laboratory investigations to perform

NICE guidelines As there are no specific laboratory investigations for the diagnosis of anorexia nervosa or bulimia nervosa, basic investigations should be guided by clinical presentation and are aimed at ruling out obvious differential diagnoses. The UK National Institute for Health and Clinical Excellence has published guidelines for eating disorders (http://www.bps.org.uk/downloadfile.cfm?file_uuid=C1173310-7E96-C67F-D396-ADF1B891F5A3&ext=pdf) and makes specific recommendations regarding laboratory investigation.

Table NICE guidelines: suggested laboratory tests in anorexia nervosa

	Domain	*Test*
Basic screening tests	Clinical biochemistry	Creatinine Glucose (random) LFT U&E Urinalysis
	Haematology	ESR FBC
Further tests (in severe/ complicated cases)	Clinical biochemistry	Calcium Creatinine kinase Magnesium Phosphate Serum protein electrophoresis
Tests to determine differential diagnosis of weight loss and amenorrhoea	Clinical biochemistry	Follicle stimulating hormone (FSH) Luteinizing hormone (LH) Prolactin TFT

NICE GUIDELINES: SUGGESTED LABORATORY TESTS IN BULIMIA NERVOSA In patients with frequent vomiting or taking large quantities of laxatives (especially when underweight), fluid status (creatinine, U&E) should be assessed.

Metabolic abnormalities are common in eating disorders, and it should be noted that severe electrolyte excretion, especially in bulimia nervosa, may resemble Bartter's syndrome (excess excretion of renal electrolytes); the resulting condition has been termed pseudo-Bartter's syndrome.

A large number of possible laboratory abnormalities may occur in eating disorders, including the following.

Table Possible abnormalities in eating disorders amenable to laboratory monitoring

Domain	Condition
Metabolic	Acid–base disturbance (metabolic acidosis/alkalosis) Azotaemia Hypercholesterolaemia Hypertriglyceridaemia Hyponatraemia Hypoalbuminaemia Hypoglycaemia Hypokalaemia Hypomagnesaemia Hypophosphataemia Osteoporosis
Endocrine	Diabetes insipidus Menstrual disturbance/amenorrhoea Thyroid abnormalities (e.g. sick euthyroid syndrome)
Haematological	Anaemia Coagulopathies Leukopaenia Liver abnormalities (hepatitis, steatohepatitis) Thrombocytopaenia
Gastrointestinal	Pancreatitis Cardiac dysrhythmias Cardiomyopathy
Other	Hirsutism Nutritional deficiencies

The following laboratory investigations may be required in patients presenting with severe eating disorders.

Table Recommended first-line laboratory tests in patients presenting with a severe eating disorder

Domain	Laboratory tests
Clinical biochemistry	Calcium Creatine kinase (and isoenzymes) CRP LFT Lipid screen Magnesium Phosphate Serum amylase Serum lipase Serum osmolality TFT U&E Urinalysis (including electrolytes, osmolality) Vitamin B12/folate
Haematology	ESR FBC Haematinics
Immunology	No specific investigations
Microbiology	

Other, more specialized laboratory investigations may include urinary screens or stool analysis for laxatives (such as bisacodyl or phenolphthalein), or chromatographic analysis of diuretics, although these are not commonly performed. For osteoporosis, assessment of bone markers (markers of bone formation, e.g. osteocalcin, or markers of bone resorption, e.g. desoxypyridinoline) may be useful.

EDNOS The category of EDNOS (eating disorder not otherwise specified) is used to describe individuals who meet some, but not all, of the criteria for anorexia nervosa or bulimia nervosa. As there is considerable overlap between these disorders, any laboratory investigation should be guided by the clinical presentation of the patient. Note that NICE does not include guidance on laboratory investigation of EDNOS.

PICA Pica is the compulsive ingestion of non-nutritive substances not normally considered as food and which are not accepted as part of a normal diet. It is common in children and individuals with learning difficulties and can occur in pregnancy.

There is an association with lead poisoning (especially in children), helminthic infections, and iron-deficiency anaemia.

In pica associated with iron-deficiency anaemia, a lack of iron results in the ingestion of various substances such as clay (geophagia), ice (pagophagia), starch (amylophagia), and others. The ingestion of clay in particular can cause chelation of iron in the gut, thereby potentially contributing to iron deficiency and possibly potentiating the pica.

Laboratory investigation of pica is based on history and physical examination, with investigations to rule out obvious manifestations of the disorder.

Complications of pica can include effects of ingested poisons (such as lead), exposure to infectious agents (such as those in faeces and soil), effects on the gastrointestinal tract (such as haemorrhage) and direct nutritional effects (vitamin deficiency, excess consumption of e.g. trace metals with resulting toxicity).

There are no specific laboratory investigations for pica. Selection of laboratory tests will be based on history and physical examination.

Tests to be considered can include the following.

Table Suggested first-line laboratory tests in patients with suspected pica

Domain	Laboratory tests
Clinical biochemistry	Blood glucose CRP LFT Serum amylase TFT U&E Urinalysis
Haematology	ESR FBC Haematinics
Immunology	No specific investigations
Microbiology	

Further laboratory tests should be considered after obtaining appropriate expert advice.

Non-routine tests and eating disorders
A number of tests (not routinely performed) have been reported to be useful in the assessment of eating disorders.

Table Non-routine tests and eating disorders

Parameter	Notes
Acetoacetate (ketone body)	Increased in anorexia nervosa (blood, urine)
Aldosterone	Increased plasma levels in laxative/diuretic abuse and starvation
Apolipoprotein B	Blood levels increased in anorexia nervosa
Bicarbonate	Levels may be increased in bulimia, in patients abusing laxatives and those with psychogenic vomiting
Chloride	Levels may be decreased in binge–purge bulimia and in patients with psychogenic vomiting
Cholecystokinin	Patients with bulimia may have blunted levels versus controls; antidepressant treatment may normalize levels as well as increase satiety in some patients
Clomiphene	Little or no response (measured in serum) in clomiphene stimulation test in anorexia nervosa (in normal individuals, clomiphene blocks oestrogen feedback mechanisms, leading to a rise in circulating LH and FSH)
Cortisol	Plasma levels often elevated, blunted dexamethasone suppression tests in some patients
FSH	Decreased urine and serum levels in anorexia nervosa
Growth hormone (GH)	Increased serum levels in anorexia nervosa; in 'GH suppression after glucose' test partial suppression is sometimes seen in anorexia nervosa
Gonadotropin releasing hormone (GnRH)	Peak LH and FSH responses in serum reduced in anorexia nervosa
Isoleucine, leucine	Increased plasma levels in starvation (decreased levels in acute hunger)
LDL-C (low-density lipoprotein cholesterol)	Increased blood levels seen in anorexia nervosa
LH	Decreased serum levels seen in anorexia nervosa
Oestrogens (total)	Decreased serum total oestrogens seen in anorexia nervosa
Prolactin	Increased serum levels seen in anorexia nervosa
pH	Decreased urine pH in anorexia nervosa
Retinol (vitamin A)	High levels associated with anorexia
SHBG (sex hormone binding globulin)	Increased serum levels seen in anorexia nervosa
Valine	Decreased levels in protein malnutrition secondary to anorexia nervosa
Zinc	Low levels associated with appetite loss

Obsessive–compulsive disorder

Definition

Obsessions are thoughts, impulses, ideas, images, or feelings which are both persistent and recurrent and which are intrusive and senseless. They are the product of the patient's own mind, and the patient's attempts to ignore them often cause subjective distress.

Compulsions are voluntary actions which are performed reluctantly in response to obsessions, with at least an initial desire to resist. With resistance the individual experiences increasing levels of discomfort until the compulsion is performed. The act is not inherently useful or enjoyable and involves stereotyped behaviours which are repeated, often many times.

ICD-10 criteria (obsessive–compulsive disorder, F42)

Time frame Obsessions or compulsions or both present on most days for at least 2 weeks.

Features

1. The obsessions or compulsions are formed within the individual's mind and are recognized as her or his own;
2. They are repetitive and cause subjective distress to the patient, and at least one of them is acknowledged as excessive or inappropriate;
3. The patient tries to resist them, and at least one must be unsuccessfully resisted;
4. The experience of the obsession or compulsion is not in itself pleasurable, despite any temporary relief of tension;
5. The obsessions or compulsions interfere with normal individual functioning.

Exclusion criteria The disorder is not due to any other psychiatric condition such as schizophrenia or affective disorders.

Differential diagnosis

Both psychiatric and non-psychiatric causes have been described.

Table Differential diagnosis of obsessive–compulsive disorder	
Psychiatric	Affective disorders (especially depressive illnesses) Anorexia nervosa Body dysmorphic disorder Generalized anxiety disorder Hypochondriasis Personality disorder (especially anankastic/obsessive–compulsive type) Phobic disorders Puerperal illnesses Schizophrenia Tourette's syndrome and other tic disorders
Non-psychiatric (rare)	Anoxia Brain tumours (especially those in the region of the cingulate gyrus and lesions of the caudate nucleus) Dementias Head trauma Neuroacanthocytosis PANDAS (paediatric autoimmune neuropsychiatric disorders associated with streptococcal infections) Parkinson's disease Poisoning (carbon monoxide, manganese) Progressive supranuclear palsy Sydenham's chorea Temporal lobe epilepsy Von Economo's disease (encephalitis lethargica) Drug-induced: cocaine, clothiapine, clozapine, ?fluoxetine, ?atypical antipsychotics (*note*: akathisia and dystonic reactions may resemble obsessive–compulsive disorder (OCD))

Laboratory investigations

When to perform laboratory investigations

- In order to rule out possible organic differential diagnoses;
- In order to monitor physical health, especially with medical comorbidity or with medication treatment.

What laboratory investigations to perform

NICE guidelines As there is no specific laboratory investigation for diagnosis of obsessive–compulsive disorder (OCD), basic investigations should be guided by clinical presentation and are aimed at ruling out obvious differential diagnoses. The UK National Institute for Health and Clinical Excellence has published guidelines for OCD (http://www.bps.org.uk/downloadfile.cfm?file_uuid=C1173310-7E96-C67F-D396-ADF1B891F5A3&ext=pdf) and does make specific recommendations regarding laboratory investigation.

Investigations are aimed at ruling out any occult cause, in addition to possible effects of concomitant drug and alcohol use or (rarely) effects of prescribed medications.

Table Recommended first-line laboratory tests in patients presenting with obsessive–compulsive disorder

Domain	Laboratory tests
Clinical biochemistry	Blood glucose CRP LFT TFT U&E
Haematology	FBC
Immunology	No specific investigations
Microbiology	

Any additional laboratory testing should be performed based on clinical suspicion after obtaining expert advice.

Personality disorders

Definition (ICD-10, F60–69)

Personality disorders are a complex group of disorders characterized by maladaptive patterns of inner experience and behaviour which are persistent, and life-long, and deviate from the individual's cultural and societal norms.

Individuals with personality disorders frequently present with marked personal distress and may also behave in ways which are adverse to society. They suffer from a number of difficulties, including affective problems, poor interpersonal relationships, poor impulse control, and cognitive difficulties in the way they perceive and interpret themselves, other people, and the world.

Personality disorders are challenging to clinicians, and individuals suffering from these common presentations are complex and often difficult to investigate and manage. Furthermore, individuals suffering from personality disorders often have concomitant drug and alcohol abuse and may engage in various forms of deliberate self-harm.

According to DSM-IV, there are three main groupings of personality disorders, although a number of other subtypes have been described in both ICD-10 and DSM-IV.

Table DSM-IV groupings of personality disorders (PDs)		
Cluster	*Name*	*Examples of characteristic traits*
A (eccentric/ odd)	Paranoid PD	Cold affect, suspicious of others, hypersensitive to rebuffs, bears grudges
	Schizoid PD	Social withdrawal, restricted emotional expression, aloof, insensitive to social norms
	Schizotypal PD	'Magical' thinking, eccentricity, tangential thinking, inappropriate affect
B (dramatic, flamboyant)	Borderline	Unstable interpersonal relationships, impulsive acts, recurrent suicidal or self-harming acts
	Histrionic	Attention seeking, labile affect, grandiosity, exploitative actions
	Dissocial	Gross irresponsibility, incapacity for maintaining relationships, deceitfulness, proneness to blame others
C (fearful, anxious)	Avoidant	Social inhibition, persistent feelings of tension and inadequacy, restriction on lifestyle to maintain perceived physical security
	Dependent	Submissive and clinging behaviour, difficulty in decision making, undue compliance with the wishes of others, lack of self-confidence

Differential diagnosis

A number of conditions can cause changes in personality, including general medical conditions, certain psychiatric conditions, and the effects of illicit substances and prescribed medications. However, an overriding feature of personality disorders is that they are life-long and are not directly due to any single, identifiable cause. Hence, the differential diagnoses for individuals with personality disorders are primarily psychiatric.

Table	Differential diagnosis of personality disorders
Psychiatric conditions	Other personality disorders, schizophrenia, delusional disorders, somatization disorder, conversion disorder, phobic disorders, dysthymic disorders
Medical conditions	Intracranial: brain damage secondary to trauma, encephalitis, meningitis; cerebrovascular disease, neoplasms (frontal lobe dysfunction associated with impulsivity, poor judgement and lack of will; temporal lobe dysfunction can be associated with hypersexuality, violence, religiosity, Klüver–Bucy syndrome; parietal dysfunction can be associated with euphoria and denial) Extracranial: almost any medical disorder can cause non-specific changes in personality in vulnerable individuals; for list see schizophrenia section below
Substance intoxication/ withdrawal	Use of alcohol, stimulants (may produce paranoid features and predispose to violence)
Effects of prescribed medications	No clear evidence

Laboratory investigations

When to perform laboratory investigations

- In order to rule out possible organic differential diagnoses;
- In order to monitor physical health, especially with medical comorbidity, drug/alcohol abuse, or medication treatment.

What laboratory investigations to perform
NICE guidelines As there is no specific laboratory investigation for diagnosis of personality disorders, basic investigations should be guided by clinical presentation and are aimed at ruling out obvious differential diagnoses. The UK National Institute for Health and Clinical Excellence has not yet published guidelines for personality disorders, although has published guidelines for self-harm (http://guidance.nice.org.uk/CG16/guidance/cfm/English).

Laboratory investigations in individuals with personality disorders are often within normal ranges; however, laboratory tests may be useful in assessing general health, effects of self-harm, and effects of self-medication with alcohol and psychoactive substances, and establishing a baseline for later comparison.

There are no specific tests for personality disorder, and investigation will be determined by history and physical examination. It is stressed that over-investigation is not recommended, and in most cases is inappropriate.

The following minimum first-line tests are suggested.

Table Recommended first-line laboratory tests in patients presenting with personality disorders

Domain	Laboratory tests
Clinical biochemistry	Blood glucose CRP LFT TFT U&E Urinalysis (urine dipstick and possibly urine drug screening)
Haematology	FBC
Immunology	No specific investigations

Other investigations may be considered based on the results of the above, and on the patient's overall presentation as based on expert advice.

Non-routine tests and personality disorders
A number of tests (not routinely performed) have been investigated in individuals with personality disorders.

Table Non-routine (research) tests and personality disorders

Parameter	Notes
Hydroxyindoleacetic acid (5-HIAA)	Low levels reported to be associated with suicide attempts, impulsiveness, and aggression
17β-Oestradiol	Increased levels found in people who exhibit impulsive traits
Oestrone	Increased levels found in people who exhibit impulsive traits
Platelet monoamine oxidase	Low levels have been noted in some patients with schizotypal disorders; low levels have also been associated with increased sociability in both humans and monkeys
Testosterone	Increased levels found in people who exhibit impulsive traits

Schizophrenia

Definition

There is no single entity known as schizophrenia; rather, the term refers to a number of related conditions in which the patient suffers from abnormalities in thought processes, often accompanied by unusual behaviour and diminished social functioning.

ICD-10 criteria (general criteria for schizophrenia, F20.0–F20.3)

Time frame At least some time during most days for at least 1 month.

Features At least one of the features described in A or at least two of B below:

A.
1. thought disorder (thought broadcast, echo, insertion, withdrawal)
2. delusions (control, influence, passivity) clearly referred to movements of the body or body parts or specific thoughts, actions, feeling or sensations; delusional perception
3. third person auditory hallucinations (running commentary, two or more voices discussing the patient)
4. culturally inappropriate and unusual delusions such as having impossible powers or being in communication with beings from another world.

B.
1. ongoing hallucinations in any modality occurring daily for at least 1 month when accompanied by delusions or persistent overvalued ideas
2. disorders of thought form resulting in incoherent speech
3. catatonia
4. negative symptoms (affect, apathy, ambivalence, loosening of associations).

Exclusion criteria No other concurrent psychiatric disorder, presentation not attributable to organic brain disease or substance intoxication or withdrawal.

Differential diagnosis

There are a wide number of differential diagnoses, including other psychiatric disorders (psychotic and non-psychotic), drug and alcohol-induced disorders, and non-psychiatric (medical) conditions.

Table Differential diagnosis of schizophrenia	
Psychotic disorders	Subtypes including acute, affective, brief reactive, cycloid, schizoaffective, transient Delusional disorders including induced, persistent
Non-psychotic disorders	Depersonalization disorder, mood disorder, obsessive–compulsive disorder, personality disorder, pervasive developmental disorder, factitious disorder
Drug and alcohol-/medication-induced disorders	Any recreational agent including alcohol, amphetamine, cannabis, cocaine, ecstasy, LSD, phencyclidine, etc. Prescribed medications including antivirals (abacavir, amantadine, efavirenz, nevirapine), isoniazid, levodopa, salicylates at high concentrations, steroids
Non-psychiatric disorders	Autoimmune disorders: SLE Degenerative: early Alzheimer's disease Endocrine: congenital adrenal hyperplasia, Cushing's, hyper-/hypothyroidism, diabetes mellitus Head trauma and stroke Infections such as Creutzfeldt–Jakob, encephalitis lethargica, HIV, herpes encephalitis, meningitis (tuberculous) neurocysticercosis, subacute sclerosing panencephalitis, syphilis Neurological: epilepsy, head trauma, narcolepsy, tumours, degenerative disorders such as Friedrich's ataxia, Huntington's, Sydenham's chorea; stroke, subarachnoid haemorrhage, subdural haematoma, and ischaemic illnesses Systemic disorders: adrenoleukodystrophy, metachromatic leukodystrophy, metabolic disorders such as Wilson's disease and porphyria (acute intermittent, variegate), fever, postoperative, post-partum Toxic: heavy metal poisoning such as lead, mercury Vitamin deficiency such as folate (pteroylmonoglutamic acid) deficiency, cobalamin (B12), niacin deficiency (pellagra)

Laboratory investigations

When to perform laboratory investigations

- In order to rule out possible organic differential diagnoses;
- In order to monitor physical health, especially with medical comorbidity, drug/alcohol abuse, or with medication treatment.

What laboratory investigations to perform

NICE guidelines As there is no specific laboratory investigation for diagnosis of schizophrenia, basic investigations should be guided by clinical presentation and are aimed at ruling out obvious differential diagnoses. The UK National Institute for Health and Clinical Excellence has published guidelines for schizophrenia (http://guidance.nice.org.uk/CG1/?c=91523) but does not make specific recommendations regarding laboratory investigation.

Suggested baseline/screening for underlying medical comorbidity

This should be guided by the patient's presentation and physical examination, and should consider obvious treatable causes as well as effects of medication and possible environmental and medical associations of schizophrenia itself.

Table Environmental/medical associations with schizophrenia		
Domain	**Feature**	**Notes**
General	Avolition General neglect Poor housing/ homelessness	May be associated with poor access to appropriate health care as well as generally increased risk of illness, including cardiovascular, dental, dermatological, endocrine, gastrointestinal, infectious, neoplastic, respiratory, and trauma; rates of mortality related to medical causes are reported to be higher in individuals suffering from schizophrenia
Medical	Diabetes mellitus	Individuals suffering from schizophrenia are at higher risk of developing type II diabetes than the general population; this may be related to lifestyle factors, smoking, and use of neuroleptic medications
	Hypercholesterolaemia/ hypertriglyceridaemia	Associated with poor diet, sedentary lifestyle, smoking, and use of neuroleptic medication
	Obesity	May be related to poor diet, sedentary lifestyle, and neuroleptic treatment; obesity is a risk factor for a number of diseases, including cardiovascular disorders, diabetes mellitus, fatigue, and metabolic syndrome
	Polydipsia	Often not recognized, may result in water intoxication
	Poor diet	May lead to malnutrition or obesity, as well as specific nutritional deficiencies (see Chapter 8)
	Substance abuse	Can exacerbate both medical and psychiatric morbidity
	Tobacco use	Prevalence of smoking in individuals with schizophrenia has been estimated to be almost double that of the general population

The following laboratory investigations should therefore be considered in newly diagnosed or untreated patients.

Table Recommended basic laboratory screen for all schizophrenic patients

Domain	Laboratory tests
Clinical biochemistry	Blood glucose Calcium CRP LFT TFT U&E Urinalysis (urine dipstick and possibly urine drug screening)
Haematology	FBC
Immunology	No specific investigations
Microbiology	

Additional tests

Additional tests may be considered in selected patients (either those with suspected organic disorders or those with a history of treatment and/or treatment-resistance) to rule out possible medical comorbidity.

Table Additional laboratory investigations for schizophrenic patients

Domain	Laboratory tests
Clinical biochemistry	HbA1c (glycated haemoglobin) Lipid screen Magnesium Porphyria screen Prolactin Serum B12/folate Serum caeruloplasmin Urinalysis (urine osmolality, urine toxicology for heavy metals, substances of abuse, anabolic steroids; uroporphyrins, porphobilinogen) Lumbar puncture/CSF analysis
Haematology	ESR Haematinics
Immunology	Autoantibodies (ANA, Rh factor, Ro, La, U1 ribonuclear protein) HIV serology Syphilis serology
Microbiology	Blood/urine cultures

It has recently been reported that the incidence of 'metabolic syndrome', also known as 'insulin resistance syndrome' or 'syndrome X', may be higher in individuals with a diagnosis of schizophrenia (see Chapter 3 for further details).

Other blood investigations with psychiatric associations (not fully validated and therefore not commonly performed outside of research settings) include the following.

Table Non-routine tests described in schizophrenia

Test	Notes
Aldolase	A glycolytic enzyme, often *increased* in psychosis and schizophrenia, as well as a wide range of other conditions including disorders of skeletal muscle, acute hepatitis, myocardial infarction, pancreatitis, and neoplasia. Measured in serum, reference range <8 units
Carbon disulphide	Exposure reported to lead to psychosis
Caeruloplasmin	*Increased* levels have been reported in some patients
Cholinesterase	*Increased* serum levels reported in psychosis
Copper	*Increased* levels have been reported in some patients
Dehydroepiandrosterone (DHEA)	*Decreased* levels have been reported
GH	*Increased* GH response reported in schizophrenic patients challenged with dopamine agonists
GnRH	GnRH can be *decreased* in psychosis and schizophrenia
Homovanillic acid	Major dopamine metabolite, may reflect dopamine turnover in the brain; high levels may be a predictor of treatment responsiveness
5-Hydroxyindoleacetic acid	Association between low CSF levels and a variety of psychiatric disorders mooted but no clear specificity; not diagnostic
mRNA of α7 nAchR	Reduced mRNA levels of the α7 nicotinic acetylcholine receptor have been reported
Niacin	Deficiency associated with fatigue, apathy, and psychosis
Plasma cysteine/serine ratio	Raised ratio reported to be a marker of both presence and severity of psychosis
Prostaglandins	*Increased* serum levels reported in psychosis
Serine hydroxymethyltransferase	Enzyme reported to be deficient in psychotic patients
Unconjugated dehydroepiandrosterone	*Decreased* serum levels in psychosis reported
Urate	*Increased* serum levels reported in psychosis

Somatoform disorders

Definition

These are a complex group of disorders characterized by abnormal illness behaviour in which patients present with chronic physical complaints despite investigation and the ruling out of an organic cause.

A variety of disorders has been described:

- Chronic fatigue syndrome (myalgic encephalomyelitis (ME), neurasthenia): a condition of ongoing physical and mental fatigue lasting at least 6 months and in the absence of identifiable organic disease;
- Conversion disorder: loss of physical functioning suggestive of a physical disorder, but of psychological origin;
- Dysmorphophobia (body dysmorphic disorder): excessive concern (not of delusional intensity) about trivial or non-existent physical imperfections which are believed by the patient to constitute deformities;
- Factitious disorder (Munchausen's syndrome): the patient fabricates symptoms (physical or psychiatric), resulting in multiple attendances at A&E (Accident and Emergency) departments with frequent admissions and inappropriate treatments;
- Hypochondriasis: the patient interprets physical sensations as abnormal and becomes preoccupied with the thought of having a serious physical illness;
- Malingering: feigned physical illness in order to accomplish a specific goal (secondary gain), such as for financial gain or to avoid punishment;
- Pseudologia fantastica: a form of lying in which a person makes up extravagant lies and fantasies which they often appear to believe and can act upon; can be associated with Munchausen's syndrome;
- Somatization disorder (Briquet's syndrome): the patient presents repeatedly with multiple physical symptoms requesting investigation, in spite of repeated negative findings;
- Somatoform pain disorder: severe, chronic, and distressing pain not thought to be due to a physical disorder.

Somatization disorder is considered below as an example.

ICD-10 criteria (somatization disorder, F45.0)

Time frame At least 2 years.

Features

1. Multiple and variable physical symptoms not due to a known physical disorder, or, if a physical disorder is present, it is insufficient to explain the presentation;

2. Preoccupation with the symptoms; this causes distress and leads to multiple consultations and investigations (at least three);
3. Persistent refusal to accept reassurance that there is no obvious physical basis for the presentation;
4. At least six symptoms from the following, occurring in at least two organ systems:

   i. abdominal pain
   ii. nausea
   iii. bloated feeling
   iv. bad taste in mouth or excessively coated tongue
   v. vomiting
   vi. regurgitation of food
   vii. complaints of abnormal bowel motions
   viii. breathlessness at rest
   ix. chest pain
   x. difficulty or increased frequency of micturition
   xi. abnormal and unpleasant genital sensations
   xii. abnormal vaginal discharge
   xiii. skin disorders (discoloration, blotches)
   xiv. pain (joints, limbs, extremities)
   xv. unusual and unpleasant sensations (numbness, tingling).

Exclusion criteria No detectable physical basis for presentation; no concurrent psychotic, affective, or panic disorders.

Differential diagnosis

Note: the diagnosis of somatoform disorder is one of exclusion, and routine screening will rule out many of the possible, obvious causes.

Table Differential diagnosis of somatoform disorders	
Psychiatric	Affective disorders, anxiety disorders, other somatoform disorders, personality disorders, psychotic disorders
Medical conditions	Rule out obvious physical causes, e.g. endocrine abnormalities, malignancies, metabolic abnormalities (e.g. pantothenic acid deficiency), infections, neurological disorders, etc. Specific associations may include: Epstein–Barr virus and chronic fatigue; multiple sclerosis and weakness; porphyria and abdominal pain; undiagnosed HIV and general malaise; post-viral syndromes and fatigue
Drugs and alcohol	Substance abuse of any sort can contribute to symptoms, especially opioids and alcohol
Prescribed medications	Patients may have increased sensitivity to side-effects of, for example, aminocaproic acid, digoxin, digitoxin, NSAIDs

Laboratory investigations

When to perform laboratory investigations

- In order to rule out possible organic differential diagnoses;
- In order to monitor physical health, especially with medical comorbidity or with medication treatment.

What laboratory investigations to perform

NICE guidelines As there is no specific laboratory investigation for diagnosis of chronic fatigue syndrome, basic investigations should be guided by clinical presentation and are aimed at ruling out obvious differential diagnoses. The UK National Institute for Health and Clinical Excellence has published guidelines for chronic fatigue syndrome (http://guidance.nice.org.uk/CG53/guidance/pdf/English) but makes no specific recommendations regarding laboratory investigation.

Often, patients have been investigated countless times in various hospitals ('peregrinating patients'), and although collateral information is not always available immediately, it is not usually advisable to repeat more than basic blood tests in these patients.

Choice of investigations will be guided by history, mental state, and physical examination.

Table Recommended first-line laboratory tests in patients presenting with suspected somatoform disorder

Domain	Laboratory tests
Clinical biochemistry	Blood glucose CRP LFT TFT U&E Urinalysis (urine dipstick and possibly urine drug screening)
Haematology	FBC
Immunology	No specific investigations
Microbiology	

Further investigation will require expert advice and will aim to exclude organic disorders with a high index of suspicion. In general, complex investigations are best avoided in these patients.

Additional (non-routine) tests

A number of environmental agents have been found to be associated with abdominal pain and fatigue.

Table	Additional non-routine tests and somatoform disorders
Parameter	**Notes**
Carbon disulphide	Toxicity associated with fatigue, weight loss, and neurological symptoms
Chromium	Toxicity (via occupational exposure) associated with abdominal pain (see also Chapter 8)
Dioxane	Toxicity associated with anorexia, nausea, abdominal pain, weakness, and depression
Ethylene glycol	Toxicity associated with abdominal pain, metabolic acidosis, and renal failure
Lead	Toxicity associated with anorexia, abdominal pain, apathy, and irritability (see also Chapter 8)
Mercury	Toxicity associated with fatigue, apathy, headache, and neurological problems (see also Chapter 8)
Niacin (vitamin B3)	Deficiency associated with fatigue, apathy, and psychosis (see also Chapter 8)
Retinol (vitamin A)	High levels associated with fatigue, anorexia, and hepatomegaly (see also Chapter 8)
Vanadium	Toxicity associated with fatigue and cardiac disturbances (see also Chapter 8)
Zinc	Deficiency associated with abdominal pain, loss of appetite, skin rash, and diarrhoea (see also Chapter 8)

Stress reactions

Definition

Stress in the psychological sense involves loss or threat, and can manifest as a wide range of reactions to stressors. These can include emotional, autonomic, and psychological responses, and abnormal stress responses are exaggerated, often manifesting as intense reactions out of keeping with what is considered within the normal range for the individual's specific culture.

Categories include:

- acute stress reaction (including crisis reaction, combat fatigue, crisis state, psychic shock)
- post-traumatic stress disorder
- adjustment disorders.

ICD-10 criteria (acute stress reaction, F43.0)

Time frame Immediate onset of symptoms within 1 hour of exposure to stressor; if stressor is transient, symptoms should diminish within 8 hours. If the stressor is continuous, symptoms must diminish within 48 hours.

Features

1. There must be exposure to a stressor (physical or mental) of marked intensity;
2. Possible symptoms include any of the following:

    i. social withdrawal
    ii. narrowing of attention
    iii. aggression (verbal, anger, behavioural)
    iv. feelings of despair or hopelessness
    v. overactivity (often purposeless or inappropriate)
    vi. excessive grief (often uncontrollable).

The reaction may be classed as mild, moderate, or severe depending on the number of symptoms and the nature of the presentation.

Exclusion criteria There are no concurrent mental disorders (except generalized anxiety disorder and personality disorders) and the disorder does not occur within 3 months following resolution of any other mental disorder.

Differential diagnosis

A wide range of conditions may present with complaints of stress, often with comorbid anxiety, depression, or other psychiatric symptoms. The most common are summarized below.

Table Selected differential diagnoses of stress disorders	
Psychiatric	Anxiety disorders, depression, personality disorders
Medical conditions	Acute intermittent porphyria, Addison's disease, Cushing's disease, HIV/AIDS, neoplasms (intracranial, islet cell adenoma, pancreatic), hyperparathyroidism, hyperthyroidism, hypoparathyroidism, hypothyroidism, pernicious anaemia Rarer conditions: carcinoid syndrome, phaeochromocytoma, Wilson's disease
Drugs	All substances of abuse, many prescribed medications

In addition, it is recognized that stress can worsen many physical conditions, including the following.

Table Physical conditions affected by stress
Any chronic medical disorder, asthma, connective tissue disorders (rheumatoid arthritis, systemic lupus erythematosus), diabetes mellitus, gastrointestinal disorders (Crohn's disease, irritable bowel syndrome, peptic ulcer disease, ulcerative colitis), headaches, heart problems (angina, arrhythmias), hypertension, migraines, neoplasms, obesity, Reynaud's disease, skin disorders such as eczema, thyroid disorders, urticaria

Laboratory investigations

When to perform laboratory investigations

- In order to rule out possible organic differential diagnoses;
- In order to monitor physical health, especially with medical comorbidity, drug/alcohol abuse, or with medication treatment.

What laboratory investigations to perform
NICE guidelines As there is no specific laboratory investigation for diagnosis of stress reactions, basic investigations should be guided by clinical presentation and are aimed at ruling out obvious differential diagnoses. The UK National Institute for Health and Clinical Excellence has published guidelines for post-traumatic stress disorder (http://guidance.nice.org.uk/CG26/?c=91523) but makes no specific recommendations regarding laboratory investigation.

Stress can induce a wide range of familiar physiological changes which can affect choice of, and interpretation of, clinical laboratory investigations. These may include the following.

Table Some physiological parameters in stress amenable to laboratory measurement

Increased levels	Adrenocorticotropic hormone (ACTH) β-Endorphins Catecholamines Cortisol and other glucocorticoids Cytokines Glucagon Prolactin Vasopressin
Decreased levels	Follicle stimulating hormone Gonadotropin releasing hormone Insulin Killer T cells (chronic stress) Luteinizing hormone Testosterone levels (with prolonged stress) Thyroid hormones Total oestrogens

Basic laboratory investigations in a patient presenting with a stress reaction could include the following.

Table Recommended first-line laboratory tests in patient presenting with a stress reaction

Domain	Laboratory tests	Notes
Clinical biochemistry	Blood glucose	Usually increased; impaired glucose tolerance may be seen
	CRP	May be raised
	LFT	May show increased protein
	TFT	May reveal hyperthyroidism
	U&E	Urea may be increased in presence of normal creatinine
	Urinalysis (urine dipstick and possibly urine drug screening)	May help to reveal an underlying cause
Haematology	FBC	Eosinophils may be decreased
Immunology	No specific investigations	
Microbiology		

68

Additional tests aim to rule out possible medical comorbidities or effects of treatment and/or substance abuse.

Table Additional laboratory investigations for patients with stress reactions

Domain	Laboratory tests
Clinical biochemistry	HbA1c Lipid screen Lumbar puncture/CSF analysis Magnesium Porphyria screen Prolactin Serum B12/folate Serum caeruloplasmin Urinalysis (urine osmolality, urine toxicology for heavy metals, substances of abuse, anabolic steroids; uroporphyrins, porphobilinogen)
Haematology	ESR Haematinics
Immunology	Autoantibodies (ANA, Rh factor, Ro, La, U1 ribonuclear protein) HIV serology Syphilis serology
Microbiology	Blood/urine cultures

Non-routine (research) tests
A number of parameters have been investigated as possible markers of stress, although none as yet is specific to abnormal stress reactions.

Table Non-routine laboratory tests in the investigation of stress reactions

Parameter	Notes
Acetoacetate (ketone bodies)	Levels may be increased in stress reactions
Aldosterone	Levels may be increased in stress
Antidiuretic hormone (urine)	Levels may be increased in stress
Apolipoprotein B	Levels increased in emotional stress
Basophils	Levels may be decreased in stress
Cortisol	Levels increased in emotional stress
Free glycerol	Levels may be increased in stress
Globulins (α1 and 2)	Levels may be increased in stress
Growth hormone	Levels increased in emotional stress
17-Hydroxycorticosteroids	Levels may be increased in stress
Iron	Levels may be decreased in stress
17-Ketosteroids	Levels may be increased in severe stress
Low-density lipoprotein cholesterol	Levels may be decreased in acute stress
Myoglobin	Levels increased in long-term, prolonged stress
Neutrophil alkaline phosphatase	Levels may be increased in stress
Oxytocin	Levels may be decreased in acute stress
Prolactin	Levels may be increased in stress
Tissue plasminogen activator	Levels may be increased in stress
Triglycerides	Levels may be increased in stress
Zinc	Levels may be decreased in acute stress

Suicide/deliberate self-harm

Suicide and deliberate self-harm are common presentations in psychiatry at all stages of the act.

While suicide refers to intentionally self-inflicted death, a more common presentation is parasuicide, in which patients repeatedly try to harm themselves.

Psychiatrists usually see suicidal patients and those who deliberately self-harm before admission to hospital, but on occasion will need to manage the acutely suicidal individual and therefore will need to understand and interpret appropriate laboratory tests.

Patients who attempt suicidal acts do so in many ways, and the most common that is amenable to laboratory investigation is through drug overdose.

The most common agents implicated in parasuicide are paracetamol and salicylate, although a wide range of other agents may also be implicated. Other sources should be consulted for further details of these.

NICE has published guidelines for the management of self-harm (http://www.bps.org.uk/downloadfile.cfm?file_uuid=C11587F1-7E96-C67F-DD13-357E1AA3B75D&ext=pdf) and makes general reference to paracetamol and salicylate poisoning. More extensive details of investigation of poisoning with these two agents are given below.

Paracetamol overdose

Paracetamol overdose is common, and may not present with clinical signs in the first 24 hours.

Commonly, initial signs include nausea, vomiting, and anorexia. After this, usually within 48 hours, of ingestion, signs progress to include abdominal pain and hepatic tenderness. After 48 hours, jaundice, hepatic failure, renal failure, and encephalopathy may occur, which can lead to death.

Biochemical changes associated with paracetamol overdose include:

- raised INR (>3 associated particularly with poor prognosis, normal INR is 1.0)
- prothrombin time >36 s (normal is 14 s)
- serum creatinine >200 μmol/l (normal range 60–110 μmol/l)
- blood pH < 7.3 (normal range 7.35–7.45)
- abnormal LFT (elevated transaminases (AST and ALT) and bilirubin (normal range for AST 10–50 IU/l, normal range for ALT 5–35 IU/l, normal range for bilirubin 3–20 μmol/l))

- abnormal blood glucose (liver damage can cause hypoglycaemia (normal range for fasting glucose 2.8–6.0 mmol/l)
- possible hypokalaemia (may result in changes to electrocardiogram (ECG).

All patients with suspected overdose should be screened for paracetamol overdose, and the following baseline blood tests are recommended, to be repeated based on laboratory and clinical findings.

Table Important laboratory tests in suspected paracetamol overdose

Domain	Laboratory tests
Clinical biochemistry	Blood gases Blood glucose LFT Plasma paracetamol levels U&E
Haematology	FBC INR Prothrombin time
Immunology	No specific tests
Microbiology	

The upper limit of the therapeutic range for paracetamol depends on both plasma paracetamol concentration and time after ingestion. Blood samples should ideally be taken at least 4 hours post-ingestion.

An accepted normogram for treatment is as follows.

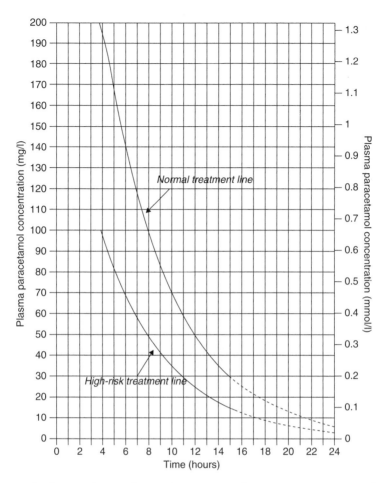

Figure Patients whose plasma paracetamol concentrations are above the **normal treatment line** should be treated with acetylcysteine by intravenous infusion (or, if acetylcysteine cannot be used, with methionine by mouth, provided the overdose has been taken **within 10–12 hours** and the patient is not vomiting). Patients on enzyme-inducing drugs (e.g. carbamazepine, phenobarbital, phenytoin, primidone, rifampicin, alcohol, and St John's wort) or who are malnourished (e.g., in anorexia, in alcoholism or those who are HIV-positive) should be treated if their plasma paracetamol concentrations are above the **high-risk treatment line.** The prognostic accuracy after 15 hours is uncertain but a plasma paracetamol concentration above the relevant treatment line should be regarded as carrying a serious risk of liver damage.

Graph reproduced courtesy of University of Wales College of Medicine Therapeutics and Toxicology Centre.

Salicylate overdose

Salicylate overdose is common, and can cause a variety of presentations, including deafness, tachycardia, tinnitus, tachypnoea, and vomiting, to coma.

Features of salicylism, especially at high plasma concentrations (>300 mg/l; >2.2 mmol/l) may include the following.

Table Clinical features of salicylism
Common (early): hearing impairment, hyperventilation, nausea, sweating, tinnitus, vomiting
Uncommon (later): arrhythmias, convulsions, coma, delirium, hyperthermia, impaired consciousness, psychosis, pulmonary oedema, renal failure, tetany

Biochemical changes associated with salicylate overdose include:

- initial respiratory alkalosis:
  common changes include **decreased** $[H^+]$, **increased** pH, **decreased** PCO_2, and **decreased** $[HCO^-_3]$
- this can be followed by a non-respiratory acidosis:
  common changes include **increased** $[H^+]$ with **decreased** pH, **decreased** PCO_2, and **decreased** $[HCO^-_3]$
- dehydration/electrolyte imbalance secondary to respiratory stimulation, increased sweating, and vomiting
- hypoglycaemia/hyperglycaemia due to increased glycolysis and/or gluconeogenesis
- rhabdomyolysis.

Table Important laboratory tests in suspected salicylate overdose	
Domain	*Laboratory tests*
Clinical biochemistry	Blood gases Blood glucose Plasma salicylate levels U&E
Haematology	FBC Prothrombin time
Immunology	No specific tests
Microbiology	

The upper limit of the therapeutic range for plasma salicylate is 2.5 mmol/l (35 mg/100 ml, 350 mg/l); levels above 3.6 mmol/l (50 mg/100 ml, 500 mg/l) suggest severe toxicity.

Further reading

General

Gold MS, Pottash ALC. Diagnostic and Laboratory Testing in Psychiatry. New York: Plenum Publishing Corporation, 1986.

Jacobs DS, DeMott WR, Grady HJ et al. Laboratory Test Handbook, 4th edn. Hudson, OH: Lexi-Comp, 1996.

Livingstone C, Rampes H. The role of clinical biochemistry in psychiatry. CPD Bull Clin Biochem 2004; 6: 59–65.

Rosse RB, Giese AA, Deutsch SI, Morihisa JM. Concise Guide to Laboratory and Diagnostic Testing in Psychiatry. Washington, DC: American Psychiatric Press, 1989.

Stoudemire A, Fogel BS, eds. Psychiatric Care of the Medical Patient. New York: Oxford University Press, 1993.

Anxiety disorders

Wise MG, Rieck SO. Diagnostic considerations and treatment approaches to underlying anxiety in the medically ill. J Clin Psychiatry 1993; 54 (Suppl): 22–6.

Bipolar affective disorder

Krishnan KR. Psychiatric and medical comorbidities of bipolar disorder. Psychosom Med 2005; 67: 1–8.

McElroy SL. Diagnosing and treating comorbid (complicated) bipolar disorder. J Clin Psychiatry 2004; 65 (Suppl) 15: 35–44.

Delirium

Bazire S. Psychotropic Drug Directory. Salisbury, UK: Fivepin, 2005.

Lipowski ZJ. Delirium: Acute Confusional States. New York: Oxford University Press, 1990.

Dementias

Massoud F, Devi G, Moroney JT et al. The role of routine laboratory studies and neuroimaging in the diagnosis of dementia: a clinicopathological study. J Am Geriatr Soc 2000; 48: 1204–10.

Mega MS. Differential diagnosis of dementia: clinical examination and laboratory assessment. Clin Cornerstone 2002; 4(6): 53–65.

Ross GW, Bowen JD. The diagnosis and differential diagnosis of dementia. Med Clin North Am 2002; 86: 455–76.

Depression

Perry MV, Anderson GL. Assessment and treatment strategies for depressive disorders commonly encountered in primary care settings. Nurse Pract 1992; 17(6): 25, 29–30, 33–6.

Phillips KA, Nierenberg AA. The assessment and treatment of refractory depression. J Clin Psychiatry 1994; 55 (Suppl) 20–6.

Rothschild AJ. Biology of depression. Med Clin North Am 1988; 72: 765–90.

Eating disorders

Herzog W, Deter HC, Fiehn W, Petzold E. Medical findings and predictors of long-term physical outcome in anorexia nervosa: a prospective, 12-year follow-up study. Psychol Med 1997; 27: 269–79.

Van Binsbergen CJ, Odink J, Van den Berg H, Koppeschaar H, Coelingh Bennink HJ. Nutritional status in anorexia nervosa: clinical chemistry, vitamins, iron and zinc. Eur J Clin Nutr 1988; 42: 929–37.

Wolfe BE, Metzger ED, Levine JM, Jimerson DC. Laboratory screening for electrolyte abnormalities and anemia in bulimia nervosa: a controlled study. Int J Eat Disord 2001; 30: 288–93.

Obsessive–compulsive disorder

Insel TR, Mueller EA 3rd, Gillin JC, Siever LJ, Murphy DL. Biological markers in obsessive-compulsive and affective disorders. J Psychiatr Res 1984; 18: 407–23.

Personality disorders

Oquendo MA, Mann JJ. The biology of impulsivity and suicidality. Psychiatr Clin North Am 2000; 23: 11–25.

Schizophrenia

Lewis ME. Biochemical aspects of schizophrenia. Essays Neurochem Neuropharmacol 1980; 4: 1–67.
Lieberman JA, Murray RM, eds. Comprehensive Care of Schizophrenia – A Textbook of Clinical Management. London: Martin Dunitz, 2001.
Voss SN, Sanger T, Beasley C. Hematologic reference ranges in a population of patients with schizophrenia. J Clin Psychopharmacol 2000; 20: 653–7.

Somatoform disorders

Dickinson CJ. Chronic fatigue syndrome – aetiological aspects. Eur J Clin Invest 1997; 27: 257–67.
Johnson SK, DeLuca J, Natelson BH. Assessing somatization disorder in the chronic fatigue syndrome. Psychosom Med 1996; 58: 50–7.

Stress reactions

Pollard TM. Physiological consequences of everyday psychosocial stress. Coll Antropol 1997; 21: 17–28.

Suicide

Sporer KA, Khayam-Bashi H. Acetaminophen and salicylate serum levels in patients with suicidal ingestion or altered mental status. Am J Emerg Med 1996; 14: 443–6.
Walker S, Johnston A. Laboratory screening of body fluids in self poisoning and drug abuse. Ann Acad Med Singapore 1991; 20: 91–4.

chapter 3

Selected psychiatric medication-associated syndromes and emergencies

There are a number of important psychiatric medication-associated syndromes that can induce changes in laboratory parameters; many of these, including overdoses and other forms of deliberate self-harm, are medical emergencies and are thus beyond the remit of this book. Other psychiatric emergencies, such as those related to violence and challenging behaviour, are similarly not included here, apart from a consideration of laboratory aspects of rapid tranquillization and physical restraint.

True life-threatening psychiatric emergencies related to direct metabolic derangements are comparatively rare, but include medication-associated syndromes and events related to physical restraints.

In the two most important syndromes, namely neuroleptic malignant syndrome and serotonin syndrome, the laboratory can play an important role in initial diagnosis and subsequent monitoring of management interventions.

There are a number of related syndromes, mostly related to prescribed medication, which can be distinguished mainly based on clinical features but also in some cases with the help of the pathology laboratory.

These syndromes include: neuroleptic malignant syndrome, serotonin syndrome, malignant hyperthermia, lethal catatonia, eosinophilia–myalgia syndrome, central anticholinergic syndrome, and other hyperthermic syndromes.

In addition there is a hypersensitivity syndrome related to anticonvulsants which has both clinical and laboratory features that clinicians need to be aware of.

In general, management will involve cessation of the offending substance with supportive measures and specific medications in some cases. It is advised that management of the following conditions be undertaken in a non-psychiatric setting by appropriately trained medical/anaesthetic staff.

For each of the conditions described in this chapter the following information will be provided:

- definition
- incidence
- psychiatric associations
- clinical symptoms
- clinical signs
- differential diagnosis
- laboratory investigations
- basic management.

Anticonvulsant hypersensitivity syndrome

Definition A multiorgan syndrome especially associated with anticonvulsant treatment and characterized by fever, rash, hepatitis, and haematological abnormalities.

If untreated, it can progress to multiorgan failure and death. It is also known as drug hypersensitivity syndrome with eosinophilia ('DRESS').

Whilst it is especially associated with anticonvulsant use, other medications have been implicated, including allopurinol, nevirapine, non-steroidal anti-inflammatories, and sulphonamides.

Incidence Approximately 1 in 5000–10000 patients taking an implicated agent.

Psychiatric associations Carbamazepine, lamotrigine, phenytoin, phenobarbital.

Clinical symptoms Fever, hepatitis.

Clinical signs Lymphadenopathy (tender), rash (usually macular and erythematous, although may generalize into erythroderma; generally involves face, trunk, and upper limbs). Facial and periorbital oedema may be present, splenomegaly may sometimes be apparent.

Differential diagnosis Cutaneous drug eruption, infectious mononucleosis, vasculitis.

Laboratory investigations

<table>
<tr><td colspan="3">Table Possible laboratory changes in anticonvulsant hypersensitivity syndrome</td></tr>
<tr><td>Event</td><td>Laboratory tests</td><td>Notes</td></tr>
<tr><td>Haematological abnormalities</td><td>FBC</td><td>Especially associated with eosinophilia and leukocytosis. Coagulopathy may also occur</td></tr>
<tr><td>Hepatitis</td><td>LFT</td><td>Hepatocellular pattern seen in about 50% of cases; LFT may take many months to resolve to baseline and presence of hepatitis suggests a worse prognosis</td></tr>
<tr><td>Renal dysfunction</td><td>U&E</td><td>Renal failure may rarely occur secondary to hepatorenal syndrome, especially with severe hepatitis</td></tr>
<tr><td colspan="3">Note: the measurement of blood levels of anticonvulsants is not considered helpful in the investigation of anticonvulsant hypersensitivity syndrome.</td></tr>
</table>

Management Treatment is largely symptomatic:

- stop the offending medication
- monitor routine biochemical and haematological parameters
- topical steroids/antihistamines may be helpful in some cases
- the condition may relapse.

Medication-associated syndromes

Central anticholinergic syndrome

Definition This is a rare syndrome due to medications which block central and peripheral muscarinic receptors. The syndrome shares certain similarities with neuroleptic malignant syndrome, delirium, and serotonin syndrome, and diagnosis is guided by history and physical examination.

Incidence Unclear.

Psychiatric associations Delirium; anticholinergics, antipsychotics (atypicals and phenothiazines), tricyclic antidepressants.

Clinical symptoms Cognitive changes (confusion, hallucinations, memory impairment), constipation, urinary retention.

Clinical signs Decreased sweating, dilated pupils, hyperthermia, tachycardia.

Differential diagnosis Delirium, drug intoxication, neuroleptic malignant syndrome.

Laboratory investigation There are no specific laboratory investigations for this syndrome, but laboratory investigations may play a role in ruling out comorbid medical conditions and likely differentials such as neuroleptic malignant syndrome (see below).

Management Treatment is largely supportive:

- stop the offending medication
- diazepam may be useful, as may physostigmine in cases of known anticholinergic poisoning
- no specific laboratory tests recommended: these should be determined as per clinical presentation
- in severe cases, monitor cardiac rhythm, blood pressure, and urine output.

Disulfiram–alcohol reaction

Definition   Disulfiram (Antabuse®) is a medication used in the treatment of chronic alcoholism in order to maintain abstinence. When consumed with alcohol it interferes with the metabolism of acetaldehyde, resulting in increased levels of the latter.

These increased levels of acetaldehyde result in subjectively unpleasant symptoms, which may appear within 30 minutes of ethanol ingestion and peak at 8–12 hours. Moreover, effects may last up to 2 weeks following discontinuation of the disulfiram.

Other agents also induce disulfram reactions with ethanol, including:

- industrial solvents
- certain mushrooms (*Coprinus atramentarius*, *Clitocybe claviceps*)
- antibiotics (metronidazole, sulphonamides, cephalosporins, nitrofurantoin)
- oral hypoglycaemics
- pesticides
- over-the-counter products and foods containing alcohol.

Incidence   Severe reactions considered rare, more likely with higher doses (actual frequency probably <0.1%).

Psychiatric associations   Alcohol detoxification.

Clinical signs and symptoms

Table   Clinical symptoms in mild disulfiram–alcohol reaction syndrome

Event	Notes
Flushing	Usually affects head, neck, and chest and is secondary to histamine-induced vasodilatation
Gastrointestinal symptoms: nausea, vomiting, diarrhoea, abdominal pain	Nausea and vomiting may be refractory
Throbbing headache Weakness, anxiety, confusion Vertigo, dizziness Orthostatic hypotension Diaphoresis Palpitations and dysrhythmias Pruritus	Effects usually self-limiting

Medication-associated syndromes

In overdose (>3 g) or with high blood ethanol levels (>120 mg/dl) the following symptoms and signs may occur.

Table Symptoms and signs in severe disulfiram–alcohol reaction syndrome

System	Event	Notes
Cardiovascular	Hypotension, tachycardia, arrhythmia, and dyspnoea	May be fatal
Gastrointestinal	Nausea, vomiting, abdominal pain, fetor	May be fetor (rotten-egg breath odour) secondary to sulphide metabolites
	Hepatitis (hypersensitive or toxic) or cholestatic jaundice	Peak at approximately 2 months of disulfiram treatment
Haematological	Agranulocytosis, eosinophilia, thrombocytopaenia, or methaemoglobinaemia	May not be initially evident
Ophthalmic	Optic neuritis	May lead to optic atrophy
Psychiatric	Hallucinations, agitated behaviour	Other, non-specific behavioural changes may be present
	Psychosis	Due to dopamine stimulation by limbic system
	Catatonia	More common in chronic toxicity
Neurological	Neuropathy	Central, peripheral sensory motor neuropathy and diffuse toxic axonopathy may occur
	Movement disorders	Choreoathetosis and parkinsonism may occur secondary to stimulation of basal ganglia by dopamine; excess dopamine enhanced excitotoxic effect of glutamate and calcium-mediated events also implicated
	Seizures	May herald coma
Skin	Exfoliative or allergic dermatitis	Peaks after 14 days of disulfiram treatment

Differential diagnosis Delirium, delirium tremens, head trauma, hepatic encephalopathy, hypernatraemia/hyponatraemia, hypoglycaemia, infection (encephalitis, meningitis, sepsis), intoxication (alcohol, other psychoactive substances, paracetamol/salicylate overdose).

Laboratory investigations

Table Possible basic laboratory investigations in suspected disulfiram–alcohol reaction syndrome

Investigation	Notes
Arterial blood gases Blood ethanol level Electrolytes and renal function tests Liver function tests Methaemoglobin level Paracetamol/salicylate levels Random blood glucose Serum osmolality	Investigations aimed at identifying treatable differentials

Additional, non-acute tests that may be considered include the following.

Table Additional laboratory investigations in suspected disulfiram–alcohol reaction syndrome

Test	Notes
Acetaldehyde levels	Toxic level >5.0 mg/l
CS_2 levels	Carbon disulphide is a disulfiram metabolite which is neurotoxic and may cause seizures; it is also hepatotoxic and cardiotoxic and inhibits cytochrome P450; normal range 0.02–0.60 µg/ml
DDC levels	Diethyldithiocarbamate is an active metabolite of disulfiram and depletes presynaptic norepinephrine, causes accumulations of dopamine and chelation of copper, and induces methaemoglobin production; normal range 0.3–1.4 µg/ml

Note: at present there is no accepted therapeutic range for disulfiram itself.

Management Treatment is largely supportive

- in severe reactions: treat symptoms of shock and fluid imbalance
- in some cases vitamin C (large doses), ephedrine sulphate, or antihistamines may be required
- routine monitoring of U&E suggested, especially in patients receiving digoxin due to risk of hyperkalaemia.

Eosinophilia–myalgia syndrome

Definition   This is a rare syndrome first described in 1989 in patients treated with L-tryptophan. It is thought that the triggering factor is the contaminant 1'1'-ethylidenebis[tryptophan].

Incidence   Extremely rare (<1%).

Psychiatric associations   Use of L-tryptophan as adjunct in treatment of depression.

Clinical signs

Table   Clinical signs in eosinophilia–myalgia syndrome

Feature	Notes
Dyspnoea	Non-specific finding, may appear early and become chronic
Hepatomegaly	Occasionally seen, may be late manifestation
Neurological	Sensory/sensorimotor deficiencies may be noted, usually in hands and feet
Oedema	May be facial or involve extremities, often appears early
Skin discolouration	May be late manifestation, 'peau d'orange' appearance common
Skin rash	Various forms seen, usually on face, neck, and extremities

Clinical symptoms

Table   Clinical symptoms in eosinophilia–myalgia syndrome

Feature	Notes
Arthralgia	Often appears early and involves large joints
Cough Breathlessness	May appear early on, cough is non-productive and usually self-limiting
Fatigue	Extremely common, especially in late stage
Muscle pain	Severe and generalized pain of back, legs, and shoulders which may include spasms and show a relapsing and remitting course
Neurological symptoms	A wide variety reported, usually altered sensations (burning feeling, paraesthesia)

Differential diagnosis Conditions associated with eosinophilia, including infectious diseases, allergic diseases, myeloproliferative/neoplastic disorders, cutaneous disorders, pulmonary diseases, connective tissue disorders, and immunodeficiency states.

Laboratory investigation

Table	Possible laboratory changes in eosinophilia–myalgia syndrome
Parameter	*Notes*
Aldolase	Usually elevated
Antinuclear antibodies	Low titres may be seen
Creatine kinase	Occasionally elevated
C-reactive protein (CRP)	Will usually be raised, especially in early disease
Eosinophilia	Usually markedly raised ($>10^9$ per litre)
ESR	Usually raised
Leukocytosis	Usually present
LFT	Non-specific abnormalities may occur, transaminases may especially be elevated

Management Treatment is largely supportive:

• stop offending agent
• prednisone may be helpful in some cases
• other treatment as per clinical presentation.

Lethal (pernicious) catatonia

Definition   Lethal catatonia (also called pernicious or Stauder's catatonia) is a rare syndrome with many similarities to neuroleptic malignant syndrome. Despite its name it is not invariably lethal, and may be due to neuroleptic treatment or to environmental toxins such as lead.

Incidence   Unclear, appears to be rare (<0.1%).

Psychiatric associations   Shares many features with neuroleptic malignant syndrome and may be related to antipsychotic treatment.

Clinical signs and symptoms

Table Clinical symptoms and signs in lethal catatonia	
Features	*Notes*
Early	
Motor excitement	May be first sign, involving marked agitation and behavioural alterations
Catatonia	A number of signs may be seen, including mutism, posturing, and possible catalepsy
Autonomic changes	May include diaphoresis, fever, hypertension, hyperthermia, or tachycardia
Late	
Fatigue	Fatigue is usually extreme
Hyperthermia Cardiac collapse/coma	If hyperthermia is untreated, it can result in cardiac embarrassment and death

Differential diagnosis   Delirium, infections (encephalitis, meningitis, sepsis), malignant hyperthermia, neuroleptic malignant syndrome, serotonin syndrome, thyrotoxicosis.

Laboratory investigation   Although there are no specific laboratory features of lethal catatonia, there may be changes in laboratory parameters secondary to autonomic instability, dehydration, or effects of medications. As it may closely mimic neuroleptic malignant syndrome or delirium, laboratory investigations should follow guidelines for these disorders.

Management   Treatment is largely symptomatic:

- rule out treatable medical disorders
- dantrolene and electroconvulsive therapy (ECT) may be useful
- monitor fluid balance and vital signs.

Malignant hyperthermia

Definition   Malignant hyperthermia is a rare disorder in which the following clinical features occur: hyperthermia, muscle rigidity, cyanosis, hypotension, and rhabdomyolysis. Drugs commonly associated with malignant hyperthermia include halothane, lidocaine, and succinylcholine.

It is thought to be an inherited disorder (autosomal dominant) and occurs during induction of anaesthesia. Untreated, it has a mortality of around 10%.

Incidence   Rare (<0.01%).

Psychiatric associations   May be seen in procedures requiring general anaesthetics such as ECT or psychosurgery.

Clinical signs and symptoms

Table Clinical signs and symptoms in malignant hyperthermia	
Feature	*Notes*
Cardiac dysrhythmia	Usually presents with tachycardia
Cyanosis	Due to pulmonary/cardiac embarrassment
Disseminated intravascular coagulation	May be seen in late stages
Hyperthermia	Usually a late sign
Hyper-/hypotension	Lability of blood pressure may be seen
Muscle rigidity	Affects skeletal muscle
Rhabdomyolysis	May be a late feature
Stupor/coma	May be seen in late stages
Tachypnoea	Exacerbated by metabolic acidosis

Differential diagnosis   Central core disease (a myopathy characterized by proximal muscle weakness thought to have a strong correlation with malignant hyperthermia), heat stroke, neuroleptic malignant syndrome; rarer differentials include glycogen storage diseases, lymphomas, myopathies, and osteogenesis imperfecta.

Test	Notes
Table Possible laboratory changes and malignant hyperthermia	
Arterial blood gases	To check for hypercarbia and metabolic acidosis
Clotting screen	To check for possible associated disseminated intravascular coagulation
Creatine phosphokinase	May be raised in susceptible patients, and may suggest underlying myopathy
Full blood count	Leukocytosis may be present
Halothane–caffeine contracture test	'Gold standard' test to diagnose malignant hyperthermia. A muscle biopsy is taken and the tissue bathed in a halothane–caffeine solution. The test is reported to be 100% sensitive and 85% specific
Plasma magnesium	Hypermagnesaemia may predispose to cardiac arrhythmia
Urea and electrolytes	To check for hyperkalaemia
Urinalysis	To check for myoglobinuria and other signs of rhabdomyolysis

Other conditions associated with hyperthermia

Hyperthermia may be secondary to medications such as atropine, lidocaine, meperidine, non-steroidal anti-inflammatory drugs (NSAIDs), or medical conditions such as phaeochromocytoma or thyrotoxicosis. Clinical features include hyperthermia, sweating, and general malaise.

Autonomic hyperreflexia may be accompanied by hyperthermia and may be induced by central nervous stimulants such as amphetamine or methylphenidate. Clinical features include excitement, hyperthermia, and hyperreflexia. Laboratory investigation aims to rule out suspected medical comorbidity or effects of drugs.

Management
- withdraw causal agent
- dantrolene may be helpful
- monitor potassium and creatine phosphokinase
- monitor urine output
- regular assessment of vital signs required
- treat medical complications (e.g. arrhythmias, metabolic disturbances).

Metabolic syndrome

Definition Metabolic syndrome, also called syndrome of insulin resistance, syndrome X, and Reaven's syndrome, consists of the association of central obesity with two or more of the four key features of the disorder (hypertension, hypertriglyceridaemia, raised fasting plasma glucose, reduced high-density lipoprotein (HDL)). The World Health Organization guidelines also include the feature of microalbuminuria.

Incidence Controversial; in schizophrenic patients treated with antipsychotics the published ranges vary between 22 and 54.2% (see De Hert et al in 'Further reading' at end of chapter).

Psychiatric associations Psychotic illnesses (especially schizophrenia); treatment with antipsychotic medication (especially atypicals); note that other medications have been associated with the development of metabolic syndrome including some antiretrovirals (stavudine, zidovudine) and steroids.

Clinical symptoms Frequently asymptomatic in early stages; in later stages signs and symptoms of underlying disorder may be seen.

Clinical signs Obesity, hypertension, signs associated with other associated medical disorders (acanthosis nigricans, haemochromatosis, polycystic ovary syndrome).

Differential diagnosis None specific; includes disorders with similar signs and symptoms such as diabetes mellitus.

Laboratory investigation

Table	Laboratory features of the metabolic syndrome	
Feature	*Laboratory investigation*	*Notes*
Disturbed glucose metabolism Disturbed insulin metabolism	Random blood glucose, HbA1c, glucose tolerance test, plasma insulin	May manifest as any of hyperinsulinaemia, impaired glucose tolerance, insulin resistance, or diabetes mellitus
Obesity	None specific	Particularly abdominal distribution
Dyslipidaemia	Plasma cholesterol/ triglycerides	Decreased HDL cholesterol and/or hypertriglyceridaemia
Hypertension	None specific	May not have any obvious clinical manifestations in early stages
Microalbuminuria	Urinalysis	May not be present; absence does not preclude the diagnosis

Management Depends on clinical presentation and severity; interventions may include lifestyle/dietary changes as well as specific interventions such as aspirin prophylaxis for prothrombotic states, specific measures aimed at lowering blood cholesterol, etc.

Neuroleptic malignant syndrome

Definition Neuroleptic malignant syndrome (NMS) is a rare, idiosyncratic, and life-threatening condition which is thought to be related to use of medications which block dopamine receptors and thereby induce sympathetic hyperactivity. Note that a considerable number of authors have published diagnostic/clinical criteria for neuroleptic malignant syndrome (e.g. Addonizio et al (1986), Adityanjee et al (1988), Caroff et al (1991), Friedman et al (1988), Keck et al (1989), Lazarus et al (1989), Levinson (1985), Pope et al (1986)); see review by Adityanjee et al (1999)* for further details. It should be noted that no single set of criteria has yet to be fully validated and adopted into clinical practice.

Incidence Approximately 0.2%.

Psychiatric associations Antipsychotic agents (all); occasionally with other agents.

Table Drugs implicated in the development of neuroleptic malignant syndrome

Class	Examples
Antidepressants	Monoamine oxidase inhibitors, tricyclic antidepressants, possible increased risk with amoxapine and nortriptyline; possible increased risk with paroxetine, especially when prescribed with olanzapine
Antipsychotics	All, possible increased risk with clozapine and risperidone
Miscellaneous agents	Metoclopramide, reserpine, tetrabenazine
Mood stabilizers	Lithium, especially in combination with antipsychotics
Psychoactive substances	Amphetamine, cocaine, phencyclidine
Discontinuation of agents which may lead to neuroleptic malignant syndrome	Amantadine, bromocriptine, levodopa

*Adityanjee et al (1999) Proposed research diagnostic criteria for neuroleptic malignant syndrome. Int J Neuropsychopharm 2: 129–144.

Clinical signs and symptoms

Table	Clinical features of neuroleptic malignant syndrome
Core features	Behavioural changes (patient may be mute or comatose, agitated or delirious) Diaphoresis Hyperthermia Impaired consciousness Lability of blood pressure 'Lead-pipe' rigidity Tachycardia
Associated features	Akinesia Dystonia Sialorrhoea Tachypnoea Tremor

Differential diagnosis Acute intoxication (amphetamine, cocaine), delirium, heat exhaustion, lethal catatonia, malignant hyperthermia, re-feeding syndrome, sepsis, serotonin syndrome, thyrotoxicosis.

Laboratory investigation

Table	Possible laboratory abnormalities in neuroleptic malignant syndrome	
Domain	*Parameter*	*Notes*
Clinical biochemistry	Blood gases	May reveal anoxia and/or metabolic acidosis
	Creatine phosphokinase	Elevated levels may be seen, reflecting myonecrosis from sustained muscle contractions (rhabdomyolysis)
	LFT	Raised liver enzymes (lactate dehydrogenase (LDH), ALP, AST) may be seen
	U&E	May reflect altered renal function
	Urinalysis	May reveal myoglobinuria (rhabdomyolysis)
Haematology	FBC	May reveal leukocytosis

Medication-associated syndromes

Management

- stop offending agent
- monitor and correct metabolic imbalances
- monitor temperature and cool the patient as required
- medications such as benzodiazepines, thiamine, dextrose, and/or naloxone
  may be needed
- monitor kidney function and urine output
- ECT may be helpful in some patients.

Serotonin syndrome

Definition   Serotonin syndrome is a disorder caused by the overstimulation
of serotonergic receptors following administration of a number of medications, especially antidepressants, including SSRIs, MAOIs, and TCAs. It is a
rare and idiosyncratic disorder which is nearly always observed following
administration of a serotonergic agent. Clinical features are based on the
triad of autonomic, cognitive/behavioural, and neurological symptoms. Note
that although several authors have published diagnostic/clinical criteria for
serotonin syndrome, no single set of criteria has yet to be fully validated and
adopted into clinical practice. Published criteria include the Hunter Serotonin
Toxicity Criteria (Dunkley et al (2004) The Hunter Serotonin Toxicity Criteria:
simple and accurate diagnostic decision rules for serotonin toxicity. Q J Med
2003; 96: 635–42) and the Sternbach Criteria (Sternbach H (1991) The
serotonin syndrome. Am J Psychiatry 148(6): 705–13).

Incidence   Unclear.

Psychiatric associations   Associated with a wide range of medications.

Table Agents associated with serotonin syndrome

Antidepressants	
Monoamine oxidase inhibitors	All (including moclobemide)
Norepinephrine and serotonin reuptake inhibitors	Duloxetine
Selective serotonin reuptake inhibitors	All (no data for escitalopram)
Serotonin and norepinephrine reuptake inhibitors	Venlafaxine
Serotonin agonists	Buspirone
Serotonin precursors	L-tryptophan
Tricyclic antidepressants	Clomipramine, imipramine
Others	
Miscellaneous	Bromocriptine, ginseng, iproniazid
Opioids	Pethidine, tramadol
Psychoactive substances	Amphetamine, dihydroergotamine, lysergic acid diethylamide (LSD)

Medication-associated syndromes

Clinical signs and symptoms

Table	Clinical features of the serotonin syndrome
Autonomic	Blood pressure lability Diaphoresis Dyspnoea Fever Tachycardia
Cognitive/behavioural	Changes in mental state (confusion, possible hypomania) and behaviour (agitation, insomnia) may be seen
Neurological	Akathisia Hyperreflexia Impaired coordination Myoclonus Tremor

Differential diagnosis

- psychiatric: catatonia
- medication-related syndromes: malignant hyperthermia, neuroleptic malignant syndrome
- drugs/medications: anticholinergics, amphetamine, cocaine, lithium, MAOIs, salicylates
- other: encephalitis, hyperthyroidism, meningitis, septicaemia, tetanus.

Laboratory investigation Although there are no specific laboratory findings in the disorder, a number of laboratory alterations may occur.

Table	Possible laboratory changes in serotonin syndrome	
Domain	*Parameter*	*Notes*
Clinical biochemistry	Bicarbonate	Decreased levels seen
	Creatine kinase (total)	Elevated levels seen
	Transaminases	Elevated levels seen
	Metabolic acidosis	May be seen
Haematology	Leukocytosis Disseminated intravascular coagulation	May be seen

Management Treatment is largely supportive:

- stop offending agent
- exclude treatable conditions
- benzodiazepines (diazepam or lorazepam) or dantrolene may be helpful
- in severe cases, cyproheptadine, methysergide, or propranolol may be helpful.

Syndrome of inappropriate antidiuretic hormone secretion

Definition A clinical syndrome characterized by water retention secondary to inappropriate secretion of ADH (antidiuretic hormone, arginine vasopressin). Note that although several authors have published diagnostic/clinical criteria for the syndrome of inappropriate anti-diuretic hormone secretion, on single set of criteria has yet to be fully validated and adopted into clinical practice. Published criteria include the Bartter and Schwartz Criteria (Bartter FC and Schwartz WB. The syndrome of inappropriate secretion of antidiuretic hormone. Am. J. Med. 1967; 42 (5): 790–806) and the Harragan Criteria (Harrigan MR. Cenebral salt wasting syndrome: a review. Neurosurgery 1996; 38: 152–60).

Incidence Unclear, but has been reported in up to 11% of acutely unwell psychiatric patients (see Siegler et al in 'Further reading' at end of chapter).

Psychiatric associations Has been associated with a variety of psychotropics including anticholinergics, all antidepressants/antipsychotics, benzdiazepines, and carbamazepine. Manifestations tend to present several weeks after starting implicated agents, although effects may be delayed following antipsychotic treatment.

It may also be a feature of medical illnesses including malignancy, metabolic disorders, miscellaneous CNS disorders such as head trauma and stroke, pulmonary disease, and some drugs including cytotoxics and opiates.

Clinical signs and symptoms

Table	Clinical signs and symptoms of syndrome of inappropriate antidiuretic hormone secretion
Signs	Cognitive changes (late) Coma (in later stages); may lead to death Seizures (late) Weight gain (early/chronic)
Symptoms	Anorexia (early/chronic) Headache (early/chronic) Lethargy (early/chronic) Muscle cramps (early/chronic) Weakness (early/chronic)

Differential diagnosis ADH-producing tumours, cerebral vascular accidents, delirium tremens, head trauma, infections (including encephalitis, Guillain–Barré syndrome, meningitis, pneumonia, tuberculosis), lung disease (asthma, pneumothorax); medications (e.g. amiloride, clofibrate, thiazide diuretics); post-surgery.

Laboratory investigation

Medication-associated syndromes

Table Laboratory investigation of syndrome of inappropriate antidiuretic hormone secretion		
Domain	*Laboratory tests*	*Notes*
Clinical biochemistry (blood investigations)	Cortisol	To rule out glucocorticoid insufficiency (normal adrenal function found in this syndrome)
	Glucose	To rule out osmolar diuresis
	U&E	To check for hyper-/hyponatraemia; normal renal function usually found in this syndrome
	LFT	To rule out liver failure
	Plasma osmolality	Decreased in this syndrome
	TFT	To rule out hypothyroidism
Clinical biochemistry (urine investigations)	Glucose	Raised glucose may suggest osmolar diuresis
	Osmolality Sodium	Concentrated urine with Na >20 mmol/l and raised plasma osmolality in the absence of hypovolaemia
Haematology	ESR FBC	To rule out possible treatable differentials

Management Fluid restriction may be needed as may other means of correction of hyponatraemia (*note*: over-rapid correction of hyponatraemia may result in central pontine myelinolysis; hence expert advice is required prior to any intervention).

Physical restraint and rapid tranquillization

Various types of physical restraint techniques are used in psychiatric/behavioural emergencies, and a number of adverse physical outcomes may result from these. While restraint is meant to be used only as a last resort by fully trained and experienced staff, the nature of the intervention means that on rare occasions adverse consequences may result.

A number of changes in laboratory variables may occur, either as a direct consequence of the physical restraint, or due to the use of administered medications. The most common adverse events are hypoxia and cardiac arrhythmias/arrest, which can, in rare situations, ultimately lead to death. *Note*: routine laboratory measurement is not usually indicated in uncomplicated restraints.

Table Possible laboratory changes directly related to physical restraint

Event	Pathology	Laboratory changes
Asphyxia	Hypoxia	Respiratory alkalosis, decreased carbon dioxide partial pressure, decreased oxygen saturation, increased 2,3-diphosphoglycerate, increased erythropoietin, increased lactate dehydrogenase, increased L-lactate
	Occlusion of carotid artery (bradycardia, hypoxia)	See above
Aspiration	Asphyxia	See above
	Acute pulmonary oedema	Respiratory acidosis, increased creatine kinase
	Pneumonitis	Moderate leukocytosis with left shift, hypoxaemia
Chest trauma	Arrhythmias	ECG; no specific laboratory tests
Catecholamine release	Arrhythmias	Metabolic acidosis

Medication-associated syndromes

Table Possible laboratory changes directly related to physical restraint (Cont.)

Event	Pathology	Laboratory changes
Exertion, prolonged stasis	Rhabdomyolysis	Feature of neuroleptic malignant syndrome; increased aldolase, decreased anion gap, increased creatine kinase, increased urine myoglobin; possible electrolyte imbalance (hypocalcaemia, hypokalaemia, hypomagnesaemia) Rarely: increased cardiac-specific troponin-T (peaks at 12–24 hours, normal range <0.2µg/l – can remain raised for up to 7 days)
Thrombosis	Pulmonary embolism	Decreased cholinesterase, increased creatine kinase, increased D-dimer test, positive ethanol gelation test, increased fibrin degradation products, positive fibrinopeptide A test, increased inorganic phosphate, increased lactate dehydrogenase isoenzymes
	Thrombophlebitis	Increased D-dimers; ESR or CRP may be helpful
	Deep vein thrombosis	Increased D-dimers; ESR or CRP may be helpful; positive fibrinopeptide A test, increased fibrinogen activator inhibitor, possible positive test for protamine paracoagulation, increased β-thromboglobulin
Other	Dehydration	Increased anion gap (metabolic acidosis), increased chloride, decreased potassium, increased sodium, increased total calcium, increased haemoglobin, increased urea nitrogen/creatinine ratio
	Fractures	Increased alkaline phosphatase isoenzymes, increased inorganic phosphate (healing fractures), possible increased total hydroxyproline
	Haemorrhage	Rarely severe; FBC and haematinics to monitor cases of severe bleeding

Further reading

General

Haddad P, Durson S, Deakin B, eds. Adverse Syndromes and Psychiatric Drugs – A Clinical Guide. Oxford: Oxford University Press, 2004.

Hallworth M, Capps N. Therapeutic Drug Monitoring and Clinical Biochemistry. London: ACB Press, 1993.

Jacobs DS, DeMott WR, Grady HJ et al. Laboratory Test Handbook, 4th edn. Hudson, OH: Lexi-Comp, 1996.

Taylor, D, Paton C, Kerwin R. The Maudsley Prescribing Guidelines, 9th edn. London: Informa, 2007.

Anticonvulsant hypersensitivity syndrome

Knowles SR, Shapiro LE, Shear NH. Anticonvulsant hypersensitivity syndrome: incidence, prevention and management. Drug Saf 1999; 21: 489–501.

Vittorio CC, Muglia JJ. Anticonvulsant hypersensitivity syndrome. Arch Intern Med 1995; 155: 2285–93.

Central anticholinergic syndrome

Hadad E, Weinbroum AA, Ben-Abraham R. Drug-induced hyperthermia and muscle rigidity: a practical approach. Eur J Emerg Med 2003; 10: 149–54.

Schneck HJ, Rupreht J. Central anticholinergic syndrome (CAS) in anesthesia and intensive care. Acta Anaesthesiol Belg 1989; 40: 219–28.

Eosinophilia–myalgia syndrome

Kazura JW. Eosinophilia-myalgia syndrome. Cleve Clin J Med 1991; 58: 267–70.

Lethal catatonia

Fleischhacker WW, Unterweger B, Kane JM, Hinterhuber H. The neuroleptic malignant syndrome and its differentiation from lethal catatonia. Acta Psychiatr Scand 1990; 81: 3–5.

Malignant hyperthermia

McCarthy EJ. Malignant hyperthermia: pathophysiology, clinical presentation, and treatment. AACN Clin Issues 2004; 15: 231–7.

Metabolic syndrome

De Hert MA, van Winkel R, Van Eyck D et al. Prevalence of the metabolic syndrome in patients with schizophrenia treated with antisychotic medication. Schizophr Res 2006; 83: 87–93.

Grungy SM, Cleeman JI, Daniels SR et al. Diagnosis and management of the metabolic syndrome. Circulation 2005; 112: 2735–52.

Neuroleptic malignant syndrome

Bhanushali MJ, Tuite PJ. The evaluation and management of patients with neuroleptic malignant syndrome. Neurol Clin 2004; 22: 389–411.

Physical restraint and rapid tranquillization

Mohr WK, Petti TA, Mohr BD. Adverse effects associated with physical restraint. Can J Psychiatry 2003; 48: 330–7.

Schillerstrom TL, Schillerstrom JE, Taylor SE. Laboratory findings in emergently medicated psychiatry patients. Gen Hosp Psychiatry 2004; 26: 411–14.

Serotonin syndrome

Birmes P, Coppin D, Schmitt L, Lauque D. Serotonin syndrome: a brief review. CMAJ 2003; 168: 1439–42.

Ener RA, Meglathery SB, Van Decker WA, Gallagher RM. Serotonin syndrome and other serotonergic disorders. Pain Med 2003; 4: 63–74.

Siegler EL, Tamres D, Berlin JA, Allen-Taylor L, Strom BL. Rick factors for the development of hyponatraemia in psychiatric inpatients. Arch Intern Med 1995; 155: 953–7.

Medication-associated syndromes

chapter 4

Laboratory aspects of psychopharmacology 1: General psychopharmacology

Introduction

Almost all medications used in the treatment of psychiatric disorders have been reported to have metabolic side-effects, although many of these are rare (frequencies <1%) and idiosyncratic. In many cases, adverse effects may arise early in treatment and may be reversed by discontinuation or substitution of the putative offending agent.

A small number of agents are associated with either commonly occurring or potentially fatal adverse effects on laboratory parameters, and are discussed in detail in Chapter 3. For other agents not amenable to therapeutic drug monitoring, this chapter summarizes the current reported metabolic changes with suggested laboratory monitoring.

For each agent, the following information will be provided:

- indications
- laboratory-related cautions
- laboratory-related side-effects, i.e. those conditions that are amenable to laboratory investigation and monitoring. Note that pregnancy is a caution for all psychotropics
- laboratory monitoring
- therapeutic drug monitoring.

Antidepressants

There are a number of antidepressant agents in current use which may induce alterations in laboratory parameters.

While many of these laboratory changes are of no clinical significance, others are important and may require withdrawal and cessation of the offending agent. As always, clinical assessment is important in determining potential changes in management.

Duloxetine

Indications

* psychiatric: treatment of major depressive disorder
* other: treatment of stress incontinence in women; treatment of neuro-pathic pain in diabetes mellitus.

Laboratory-related cautions   Hepatic impairment, renal impairment.

Laboratory-related side-effects

Table Laboratory-related side-effects of duloxetine			
System	*Event*	*Laboratory tests*	*Notes*
Gastrointestinal	Abnormal LFT	LFT	Hepatitis, jaundice rare, elevated liver enzymes (ALP, ALT, AST) reported
Haematological	Anaemia, leukopaenia, leukocytosis, thrombocytopaenia	FBC; haematinics (anaemia)	Rare, and idiosyncratic effects which usually occur in the first few months of treatment; effects are usually reversible upon cessation of drug
Metabolic	Hyponatraemia, syndrome of inappropriate antidiuretic hormone secretion (SIADH)	U&E	
	Serotonin syndrome	See Chapter 3	
	Hypolycaemia	Blood glucose, HbA1c	Rare and idiosyncratic effect

Laboratory monitoring   Routine laboratory tests: no specific monitoring required; baseline blood tests as per condition being treated.

Therapeutic drug monitoring   None.

Flupentixol

See Antipsychotics below.

Maprotiline

Indications   Depressive illnesses, especially when sedative effect is desired.

Laboratory-related cautions   As for amitriptyline.

Laboratory-related side-effects   In general, the side-effect profile is similar to that of amitriptyline; liver toxicity and haematological abnormalities occur most commonly.

Of note, the literature contains a single report of reversible cutaneous vasculitis in an 83-year-old female thought to be due to maprotiline treatment[1] (symptoms resolved after cessation of the medication) and two reports describing hepatotoxicity[2,3]

Note: although the diagnosis of cutaneous vasculitis is primarily clinical, useful laboratory parameters may include ESR and ANCA (antineutrophil cytoplasmic antibodies), which will reflect disease severity and response to treatment.

Routine laboratory monitoring   No specific monitoring required; baseline blood tests as per condition being treated.

Therapeutic drug monitoring   None. A therapeutic blood reference range for maprotiline has been reported (200–600 ng/ml); this has yet to be fully validated and routine monitoring is therefore not recommended.

Mianserin

Indications   Depressive illnesses, especially when sedative effect is desired.

Laboratory-related cautions   As for amitriptyline; if leukopaenia, agranulocytosis, or aplastic anaemia present, use of mianserin is contraindicated.

Laboratory-related side-effects

Table Laboratory-related adverse effects of mianserin			
System	*Event*	*Laboratory investigation*	*Notes*
Cardiovascular	Hypokalaemia	U&E	Elderly with previous history of cardiovascular system disorders may be especially susceptible
Endocrine	SIADH/ hyponatraemia	See Chapter 3	Rare effect, more likely in early stages of treatment
Gastrointestinal	Jaundice/abnormal liver function	LFT	Effects reversible on reduction/cessation of dose
Haematological	Agranulocytosis Granulocytopaenia/ leukopaenia	FBC	More common in elderly, no sex difference, most likely within first 3 months of treatment
	Aplastic anaemia		One case reported[4]

Routine laboratory monitoring Baseline FBC then repeat FBC recommended every **4 weeks** for first **3 months** with subsequent clinical/ laboratory monitoring if signs of infection (fever, sore throat, stomatitis, etc.) develop.

Therapeutic drug monitoring None. A therapeutic blood reference range for mianserin has been reported (15–70 ng/ml); this has yet to be fully validated and routine monitoring is therefore not recommended.

Mirtazepine

Indication Treatment of depressive illness.

Laboratory-related cautions Hepatic impairment (contraindicated if jaundice develops), renal impairment (contraindicated in severe impairment), diabetes mellitus, blood dyscrasias, especially leukopaenia, agranulocytosis, or aplastic anaemia.

General Psychopharmacology

Laboratory-related side-effects

Table	Laboratory-related adverse effects of mirtazepine		
System	**Event**	**Laboratory investigation**	**Notes**
Endocrine	Hyponatraemia (SIADH)	Urine/plasma osmolality	Urine osmolality usually greater than plasma osmolality; dilutional hyponatraemia present (plasma osmolality low)
		Urine sodium	Urinary sodium persistently elevated (>50 mmol/l)
		U&E	*Note*: U&E may be normal
Gastrointestinal	Jaundice/raised liver enzymes	LFT	Rare event; reversible upon withdrawal of drug
Haematological	Anaemia, agranulocytosis, leukopaenia, pancytopaenia, thrombocytopaenia	FBC	Rare, reversible on withdrawal of drug
Metabolic	Hypercholesterolaemia	Lipid panel	Incidence may be as high as 15%

Routine laboratory monitoring   In addition to baseline blood tests as per condition being treated, FBC should be monitored if patient develops signs of infection such as stomatitis, fever, or sore throat. If blood dyscrasia is suspected, mirtazepine treatment should be stopped. Monitoring of cholesterol/triglycerides may be appropriate in individuals at greater risk; monitoring will be guided by clinical presentation.

Therapeutic drug monitoring   None. A therapeutic blood reference range for mirtazepine has been reported (40–80 ng/ml); this has yet to be fully validated and routine monitoring is therefore not recommended.

Moclobemide

Indications

- depressive illness
- anxiety disorders (especially social phobia)
- facilitation of smoking cessation.

General Psychopharmacology

Laboratory-related cautions Diabetes mellitus, phaeochromocytoma (absolute contraindication), hepatic impairment (absolute contraindication in severe impairment), thyrotoxicosis (may precipitate a hypertensive reaction).

Laboratory-related side-effects

Table Moclobemide and laboratory-related side-effects			
System	*Event*	*Laboratory investigation*	*Notes*
Endocrine	Thyrotoxicosis	TFT	Possibility of hypertensive reaction
	Phaeochromocytoma	24-hour urinary vanillylmandelic acid, free catecholamines, adrenocorticotropic hormone (ACTH)	Possible potentiation of tyramine pressor effects leading to hypertensive crisis; free catacholamines less commonly measured; ACTH measurement may indicate an ectopic ACTH syndrome; note that the following may result in a false positive urinary vanillylmandelic acid: foods (bananas, vanilla), labetalol, methyldopa
Gastrointestinal	Raised liver enzymes	LFT	Raised AST/ALT occasionally reported

Routine laboratory monitoring No specific monitoring required; baseline blood tests as per condition being treated.

Therapeutic drug monitoring None. A therapeutic blood reference range for moclobemide has been reported (300–1000 ng/ml); this has yet to be fully validated and routine monitoring is therefore not recommended.

Monoamine oxidase inhibitors

Examples include phenelzine, isocarboxazid, and tranylcypromine.

Indications (phenelzine)

- depressive illnesses, especially in patients refractory to treatment with other agents
- anxiety disorders, especially panic disorder, phobic disorders such as social phobia, as adjuncts in post-traumatic stress disorder; may be of utility in 'atypical' depressive states
- hyperactivity states (may be of utility in attention-deficit hyperactivity disorder although side-effect profile and interactions limit use)
- treatment of orthostatic hypotension (when used together with a sympathomimetic; the use of MAOIs in this context is not recommended).

Laboratory-related cautions Hepatic dysfunction (contraindicated in severe impairment), phaechromocytoma (absolute contraindication), haematological abnormalities (blood dyscrasias), hyperthyroidism (increased sensitivity to pressor amines), diabetes mellitus (possible altered glucose metabolism).

Note: patients should be warned not to eat tyramine-containing foods when taking MAOIs in order to avoid a hypertensive crisis ('cheese reaction'). Foods to be avoided include: matured cheese; matured/cured meats; meat, poultry, or fish that is 'off'; broad (fava) bean pods; yeast extract (e.g. Marmite™); sauerkraut; soy sauce and soy bean condiments.

Laboratory-related side-effects

Table Laboratory-related adverse effects of monoamine oxidase inhibitors

System	Event	Laboratory investigation	Notes
Endocrine	Hyperglycaemia or hypoglycaemia	Random blood glucose, glycated haemoglobin (HbA1c)	Idiosyncratic effect; use of MAOIs best avoided in diabetic patients
	Hyperprolactinaemia	Prolactin levels	May be manifest as galactorrhoea
	Dilutional hyponatraemia (secondary to enhanced vasopressin release and increased antidiuretic hormone)	U&E	May be more common in elderly patients; rarely hypernatraemia may occur (especially with phenelzine and tranlcypromine), as may SIADH

Table Laboratory-related adverse effects of monoamine oxidase inhibitors (Cont.)

System	Event	Laboratory investigation	Notes
Gastrointestinal	Jaundice Hepatitis Fulminant hepatic failure/hepatocellular necrosis	LFT	Rare event, may be related to hypersensitivity reactions; iproniazid especially implicated in hepatitis; fulminant hepatic failure secondary to phenelzine has been reported[5]
Haematological	Agranulocytosis, anaemia, thrombocytopaenia	FBC	Rare events
	Leukopaenia		Rare event, may be especially associated with tranylcypromine
Skin/allergy	Serotonin syndrome	See Chapter 3	

Routine laboratory monitoring   No specific monitoring required; baseline blood tests as per condition being treated.

Therapeutic drug monitoring   None. A therapeutic blood reference range for tranylcypromine has been reported (0–50 ng/ml); this has yet to be fully validated and routine monitoring is therefore not recommended.

Reboxetine

Indication   Treatment of depressive illness.

Laboratory-related cautions   Renal impairment (contraindicated in severe impairment), hepatic impairment (contraindicated in severe impairment).

Laboratory-related side-effects

Table	Laboratory-related adverse effects of reboxetine		
System	**Event**	**Laboratory investigation**	**Notes**
Endocrine	Hyponatraemia (SIADH)	Urine/plasma osmolality	Urine osmolality usually greater than plasma osmolality; dilutional hyponatraemia present (plasma osmolality low)
		Urine sodium	Urinary sodium persistently elevated (>50 mmol/l)
		U&E	*Note*: U&E may be normal
Metabolic	Hypokalaemia	U&E	Especially in elderly after prolonged administration

Routine laboratory monitoring   No specific monitoring required; baseline blood tests as per condition being treated.

Therapeutic drug monitoring   None. A therapeutic blood reference range for reboxetine has been reported (10–100 ng/ml); this has yet to be fully validated and routine monitoring is therefore not recommended.

Selective serotonin reuptake inhibitors

Indications (fluoxetine)

- Psychiatric indications:

  ○ depressive illness
  ○ anxiety disorders (especially fluvoxamine and fluoxetine in obsessive–compulsive disorder; other disorders which may respond to SSRIs include panic disorder, social phobia, post-traumatic stress disorder (PTSD), and trichotillomania)
  ○ eating disorders (anorexia nervosa and bulimia nervosa: fluoxetine may be useful)
  ○ hypochondriasis (may be helpful in patients with comorbid hypochondriasis and depression).

- Other reported indications:

  ○ alcohol dependence (may help to reduce alcohol intake)
  ○ abnormal behaviour (impulsiveness, aggression, paraphilas)
  ○ epilepsy (one case report of anticonvulsant effect of fluoxetine[6] – *note*: fluoxetine and other SSRIs can lower seizure threshold and should be used with caution in epilepsy)
  ○ pain (fluoxetine and fluvoxamine may be helpful in chronic headache; fluoxetine may be of benefit in fibromyalgia)

General Psychopharmacology

109

- hyperactivity (fluoxetine reported to be a useful adjunct to methylphenidate or metamphetamine treatment of attention-deficit hyperactivity disorder)
- hypotension (may be helpful in refractory hypotension; fluoxetine especially may be of benefit in refractory orthostatic hypotension)
- parkinsonism (controversial effect of fluoxetine in patients with Parkinson's disease who experience levodopa-induced dyskinesia)
- pathological crying/laughing (fluoxetine reported to be helpful)
- peripheral vascular disease (fluoxetine may be of benefit in Reynaud's syndrome)
- premenstrual syndrome (low dose fluoxetine reported to be effective in symptom control)
- sexual dysfunction (delay of premature ejaculation with paroxetine and sertraline).

Laboratory-related cautions Hepatic dysfunction (liver failure is an absolute contraindication), renal failure (severe renal dysfunction is an absolute contraindication), diabetes mellitus, history of bleeding disorders.

Laboratory-related side-effects

Table Laboratory-related adverse effects of SSRIs			
System	*Event*	*Laboratory investigation*	*Notes*
Endocrine	SIADH	Urine and plasma osmolality	Urine osmolality usually greater than plasma osmolality; dilutional hyponatraemia present (plasma osmolality low)
		Urine sodium	Urinary sodium persistently elevated (>50 mmol/l)
		U&E	U&E may be normal but hyponatraemia may occur; fluoxetine and paroxetine especially implicated; effect appears to be greater in early stages of treatment and the elderly may be more susceptible; baseline levels in adults <20 µg/l, <10 µg/l in men
	Hyperprolactinaemia	Prolactin levels	Effects may be related to higher doses and may manifest as sexual side-effects
Gastrointestinal	Hepatitis	LFT	Rare; paroxetine and sertraline implicated
	Liver failure	LFT, prothrombin time	Sertraline implicated; laboratory tests not diagnostic but will help to confirm the clinical diagnosis
	Pancreatitis	Serum amylase, urine amylase, serum lipase	Pancreatitis is rare and idiosyncratic Serum amylase >4× normal is diagnostic; urine amylase >5× normal may be helpful; serum lipase >2× normal is diagnostic and may be a useful marker of disease progression

General Psychopharmacology

111

Table Laboratory-related adverse effects of SSRIs (Cont.)

System	Event	Laboratory investigation	Notes
		C-reactive protein (CRP) Others: white cell count (WCC), glucose, urea, PO_2, albumin, calcium, lactate dehydrogenase (LDH), AST/ALT	Glasgow Prognostic Score (>3=acute pancreatitis; the more factors, the worse the prognosis): WCC >15000/ mm^3, glucose >10 mmol/l, urea >16 mmol/l, PO_2 <8 kPa, albumin <32 g/l, calcium <2.0 mmol/l, LDH >600 IU/l, AST/ALT >200 U/l
Haematological	Abnormal bleeding Aplastic anaemia Haemolytic anaemia Pancytopaenia Thrombocytopaenia	FBC	Thrombocytopaenia reported with sertraline. Fluoxetine has rarely been associated with disseminated intravascular coagulation
	Leukocytosis/ leukopaenia	FBC	Rare event reported with citalopram
	Platelet dysfunction	FBC, clotting screen	Citalopram, fluoxetine, fluvoxamine, paroxetine, and sertraline rarely implicated in causing abnormal platelet aggregation
Miscellaneous	Neuroleptic malignant syndrome	See Chapter 3	Rare event; fluoxetine implicated
	Serotinin syndrome	See Chapter 3	Rare event; sertraline and citalopram especially implicated
Respiratory	Eosinophilic pneumonia	FBC	Eosinophil count >1×10^9/ml; rare event
Skin/allergy	Vasculitis	ESR may be helpful	Rare event, may be heralded by a skin rash

Routine laboratory monitoring   No specific monitoring required; baseline blood tests as per condition being treated. *Note*: paroxetine is associated with increased incidence of extrapyramidal effects and withdrawal syndrome.

Therapeutic drug monitoring   None. Therapeutic blood reference ranges for a number of SSRIs have been reported; these have yet to be fully validated and routine monitoring is therefore not recommended.

Table Therapeutic drug monitoring of SSRIs	
Agent	*Reported reference range (ng/ml)*
Citalopram	30–130
Escitalopram	15–80
Fluoxetine	100–800
Fluvoxamine	150–300
Paroxetine	70–120
Sertraline	10–50

Trazodone

Indications

- depressive illness, especially when sedative effect is desired
- anxiety states (especially chronic generalized anxiety with depression)
- agitation, aggression, and disruptive behaviour; may be helpful in the management of disturbed behaviour in some patients with dementia
- sexual dysfunction (treatment of erectile dysfunction, especially as trazodone treatment may be associated with priapism)
- as adjunct in treatment of symptoms secondary to withdrawal from cocaine and benzodiazepines.

Laboratory-related cautions   As for amitriptyline.

Laboratory-related side-effects

System	Event	Laboratory investigation	Notes
Table Laboratory-related adverse effects of trazodone			
Endocrine	SIADH/hyponatraemia	Rare event, see Chapter 3	
Gastrointestinal	Abnormal liver enzymes Intrahepatic cholestasis/hepatitis Chronic active hepatitis Fatal hepatic necrosis	LFT	Rare events, liver function may return to normal after discontinuing the drug
Haematological	Agranulocytosis, anaemia, leukocytosis, neutropaenia, thrombocytopaenia	FBC	Rare events

Routine laboratory monitoring No specific monitoring required; baseline blood tests as per condition being treated.

Therapeutic drug monitoring A therapeutic blood reference range for trazodone has been reported (800–1600 ng/ml); this has yet to be fully validated and routine monitoring is therefore not recommended.

Tricyclic antidepressants

Examples include secondary (desipramine, nortriptyline, protriptyline) and tertiary TCAs (amitriptyline, clomipramine, doxepin, imipramine, trimipramine).

Indications (amitriptyline)

- Psychiatric indications:
  - depression
  - eating disorders (anorexia and bulimia nervosa)
  - anxiety/panic disorders (especially with coexistent depression)
  - as an adjunct in schizophrenia (post-psychosis depression)
  - as second-line agents in hyperactivity syndromes.

- Other reported indications:

  - alcohol dependence (desipramine in depression secondary to alcohol dependence)
  - treatment of neurological symptoms following ciguatera poisoning (ciguatoxin is found in certain fish in the Caribbean and Asia)
  - cocaine dependence (desipramine in depression secondary to cocaine withdrawal)
  - pain (certain types of chronic headache, neurogenic pain, post-herpetic neuralgia, and migraine)
  - hiccup
  - interstitial cystitis (amitriptyline or imipramine in combination with hexamine hippurate)
  - irritable bowel syndrome
  - nocturnal enuresis (amitriptyline, nortriptyline, and clomipramine) and urinary incontinence
  - narcoleptic syndrome (cataplexy and narcolepsy-associated sleep paralysis; clomipramine and imipramine most widely utilized)
  - pathological crying (following head trauma or with certain frontal lobe insults; amitriptyline or nortriptyline may be of utility)
  - premenstrual syndrome (clomipramine for premenstrual irritability and depression)
  - sexual dysfunction (clomipramine has been used to treat impotence and ejaculatory failure)
  - skin disorders (doxepin has been used for chronic urticaria and pruritus)
  - smoking cessation (may help to alleviate withdrawal syndrome)
  - stuttering (clomipramine).

Laboratory-related cautions Acute porphyria, hepatic disease (contraindicated in severe liver disease), renal impairment, thyroid disease, phaeochromocytoma.

Laboratory-related side-effects

Table	Laboratory-related adverse effects of TCAs		
System	**Event**	**Laboratory investigation**	**Notes**
Metabolic	Neuroleptic malignant syndrome	See Chapter 3	Amitriptyline, amoxapine, dothiepin, and clomipramine associated
	Serotonin syndrome	See Chapter 3	Rare event
Endocrine	Hyperprolactinaemia	Prolactin	Rare, may be associated with lofepramine, clomipramine, and imipramine
	SIADH leading to hyponatraemia	U&E	SIADH reported especially with dothiepin, lofepramine, and other TCAs
	Alteration of blood glucose levels	Random blood glucose; HbA1c	Levels may rise or fall
Gastrointestinal	Nausea/vomiting	U&E	Rarely of clinical significance; may occur with all TCAs
	Raised liver enzymes	LFT	Hepatotoxicity has been reported especially with lofepramine; effects may be reversible upon discontinuation of the drug
Haematological	Agranulocytosis	FBC	Rare, may be associated particularly with imipramine in first 4–8 weeks of treatment; elderly patients are possibly more sensitive. Note that all TCAs may cause agranulocytosis
	Eosinophilia	FBC	Amitriptyline, nortriptyline, and imipramine especially implicated

Table	Laboratory-related adverse effects of TCAs (Cont.)		
System	**Event**	**Laboratory investigation**	**Notes**
	Neutropaenia	FBC	Rare, idiosyncratric side-effect; imipramine and nortriptyline implicated
	Thrombocytopaenia	FBC	Amitriptyline, clomipramine, imipramine, and nortriptyline especially implicated
	Aplastic anaemia	FBC	Rare, associated with dothiepin
Renal	Haematuria	U&E, urinalysis	One case implicating amitriptyline reported[7]
Skin/allergy	Toxic epidermal necrolysis leading to fluid imbalance, septicaemia, pneumonia	Seek expert guidance	Amoxapine implicated

Laboratory monitoring

- routine laboratory tests: no specific monitoring required; baseline blood tests as per condition being treated
- therapeutic drug monitoring: not normally undertaken; blood reference ranges have been reported for some agents, but these have yet to be fully validated and routine monitoring is therefore not recommended.

Table	Therapeutic drug monitoring of TCAs
Agent	**Reference range (ng/ml)**
Amitriptyline	80–250
Amoxapine	20–100
8-Hydroxyamoxapine	150–400
Desipramine	75–350
Doxepin	150–250
Imipramine	150–250
Nortriptyline	50–150
Protriptyline	70–250

Tryptophan

Indications

- depressive illness (usually as adjunct to other antidepressants in severe, chronic, and disabling depression refractory to other treatments; in the UK use of tryptophan is restricted to hospital specialists)
- as a dietary supplement (controversial and not recommended)
- treatment of insomnia (use described in obstructive sleep apnoea; controversial and not recommended).

Laboratory-related cautions Haemotological changes, especially raised eosinophil counts.

Laboratory-related side-effects

Table	Laboratory-related adverse effects of tryptophan		
System	Event	Laboratory investigation	Notes
Haematological	Eosinophila	FBC	Eosinophil count $>1 \times 10^9$/l; may not be initially abnormal
Musculoskeletal	Eosinophilia–myalgia syndrome	FBC	Mainly a clinical diagnosis but raised eosinophil count may suggest diagnosis
		Creatine kinase	May be increased
		Aldolase	May be increased
		PO_2	May be increased

Routine laboratory tests Close monitoring of eosinophil count/general haematological indices (FBC) required. Clinical monitoring of muscle symptomatology (fatigue, muscle pain) required. Patients and prescribers are required to be registered with the OPTICS (Optimax® Information and Clinical Support Unit, Merck Pharmaceuticals).

Therapeutic drug monitoring None.

Venlafaxine

Indications Treatment of depressive illness.

Laboratory-related cautions Hepatic impairment, renal impairment, electrolyte disturbance, history of bleeding disorders.

Laboratory-related side-effects

System	Event	Laboratory investigation	Notes
Table Laboratory-related adverse effects of venlafaxine			
Endocrine	Hyponatraemia (SIADH)	Urine/plasma osmolality	Urine osmolality usually greater than plasma osmolality; dilutional hyponatraemia present (plasma osmolality low)
		Urine sodium	Urinary sodium persistently elevated (>50 mmol/l)
		U&E	U&E may be normal; effect appears to be greater in early stages of treatment and the elderly may be more susceptible
	Galactorrhoea (hyperprolactinaemia)	Prolactin	Rare; baseline levels in adults <20 µg/l, <10 µg/l in men
Gastrointestinal	Raised liver enzymes	LFT	Mild elevations, not normally clinically significant; hepatitis reported but rare
Haematological	Anaemia, leukocytosis or leukopaenia	FBC	Rare events
	Bleeding disorders/ thrombocytopaenia	FBC, clotting	Ecchymoses common; frank haemorrhage rare
Metabolic	Raised serum cholesterol	Fasting cholesterol/ triglycerides	Rare association
	Serotonin syndrome	See Chapter 3	Rare association

General Psychopharmacology

Routine laboratory monitoring No specific monitoring required; baseline blood tests as per condition being treated.

Therapeutic drug monitoring None. *Note*: although there is a published reference range for venlafaxine (25–400 µg/l) this has yet to be validated and therefore monitoring of plasma levels is not routinely recommended.

Antipsychotics

Phenothiazines and related agents

Benperidol
Indications

- psychotic illness
- control of antisocial sexual deviant behaviour.

Laboratory-related cautions Hepatic impairment, renal impairment, myasthenia gravis, blood dyscrasias, phaeochromocytoma (contraindicated).

Laboratory-related side-effects

Table Laboratory-related adverse effects of benperidol			
System	**Event**	**Laboratory investigation**	**Notes**
Endocrine	Hyperprolactinaemia	Prolactin levels	May manifest as changes in sexual dysfunction
Gastrointestinal	Jaundice/abnormal liver function	LFT	Rare, idiosyncratic effects; liver enzymes and bilirubin may be increased
Haematological	Blood dyscrasias	FBC	Rare events
Metabolic	Neuroleptic malignant syndrome	See Chapter 3	Rare event
	Increased uric acid	Plasma urate	

Routine laboratory monitoring Regular monitoring of FBC and LFT advised by manufacturer for long-term treatment; frequency will depend on clinical presentation/baseline blood tests as per condition being treated.

Therapeutic drug monitoring None. Although a therapeutic reference range has been reported (2–10 ng/ml), this has yet to be fully validated and routine monitoring is therefore not recommended.

Chlorpromazine
Psychiatric indications

- psychotic illness including schizophrenia
- severe anxiety (short-term treatment)
- violent or dangerous impulsive behaviour
- acute mania.

Other reported indications

- as possible adjunct in treatment of alcohol withdrawal
- treatment of movement disorders (chorea and dystonias, especially in those refractory to other treatments)
- treatment of eclampsia and pre-eclampsia in early stages of pregnancy
- treatment of migraine
- treatment of intractable hiccup
- symptomatic treatment of Lesch–Nyhan syndrome
- treatment of nausea and vomiting
- treatment of opioid dependence in neonates
- treatment of postherpetic neuralgia
- treatment of taste disorders such as ageusia, hypogeusia, and phanto-geusia.

Laboratory-related cautions Bone-marrow suppression (contraindication), phaeochromocytoma (contraindication), prolactin-dependent tumours (contraindication), hepatic impairment, renal impairment, diabetes mellitus, hypothyroidism, myasthenia gravis.

Laboratory-related side-effects

Table	Laboratory-related adverse effects of chlorpromazine		
System	**Event**	**Laboratory investigation**	**Notes**
Endocrine	Hyperglycaemia/ altered glucose tolerance	Fasting blood glucose, HbA1c	Rare effects, may be associated with longer-term usage
	Hyperprolactinaemia	Prolactin	May manifest with sexual side-effects
	Hyponatraemia (SIADH)	Urine/plasma osmolality	Rare event[8] Urine osmolality usually greater than plasma osmolality Dilutional hyponatraemia present (plasma osmolality low)
		Urine sodium	Urinary sodium persistently elevated (>50 mmol/l)
		U&E	U&E may be normal
Gastrointestinal	Hepatotoxicity, including hepatocanalicular cholestasis/jaundice	LFT	Rare, idiosyncratic effects
Haematological	Agranulocytosis Aplastic anaemia Eosinophilia Haemolytic anaemia Leukocytosis or leukopaenia Neutropaenia Thrombocytopaenia	FBC	Usually occur within 4–10 weeks of starting; mild leukopaenia may be present in a third of patients on prolonged high dose treatment
Metabolic	Hypercholesterolaemia and/or decreased HDL	Lipid screen	Extremely rare effect – few data at present
	Neuroleptic malignant syndrome	See Chapter 3	Rare event

Routine laboratory monitoring No specific monitoring required; baseline blood tests as per condition being treated. Note: may rarely cause a postive pregnancy test.

Therapeutic drug monitoring None. Although a therapeutic reference range has been reported (50–300 ng/ml), this has yet to be fully validated and routine monitoring is therefore not routinely recommended.

Flupentixol
Indications

- treatment of psychotic illnesses (including schizophrenia) especially when negative symptoms predominate
- treatment of depression (not a first-line agent).

Laboratory-related cautions As for chlorpromazine.

Note: in addition to the laboratory effects noted above, flupentixol has been shown to be porphyrogenic in animals and is therefore not recommended in patients with acute porphyria.

Laboratory-related side-effects As for chlorpromazine.

Laboratory monitoring

- routine laboratory tests: no specific monitoring required; baseline blood tests as per condition being treated
- therapeutic drug monitoring: none; although a therapeutic reference range has been reported (>2 ng/ml), this has yet to be fully validated and routine monitoring is therefore not recommended.

Fluphenazine
Indications

- treatment of schizophrenia and other psychotic illnesses
- treatment of chorea
- treatment of Tourette's syndrome.

Laboratory-related cautions As for chlorpromazine.

Laboratory-related side-effects As for chlorpromazine; on rare occasions fluphenazine may also cause a pancytopaenia.

Note: fluphenazine has been rarely reported to cause reversible liver toxicity (jaundice, hyperbilirubinaemia, raised liver enzymes) which responds to medication withdrawal and substitution.

General Psychopharmacology

Laboratory monitoring

- routine laboratory tests: no specific monitoring required; baseline blood tests as per condition being treated
- therapeutic drug monitoring: none; although a therapeutic reference range has been reported (0.2–4 ng/ml), this has yet to be fully validated and routine monitoring is therefore not recommended.

Haloperidol
Indications

- Psychiatric indications:

  - treatment of schizophrenia and other psychotic disorders
  - treatment of acute mania
  - treatment of acute behavioural disturbances.

- Other reported indications:

  - movement disorders (ballism, chorea, dystonia, especially in severe cases or cases refractory to other treatments)
  - intractable sneezing
  - treatment of stuttering
  - treatment of taste disorders, especially phantogeusia
  - treatment of Tourette's syndrome.

Laboratory-related cautions As for chlorpromazine; *note*: severe extrapyramidal side-effects may occur in patients with hyperthyroidism and use of haloperidol should be avoided in acute porphyria.

Laboratory-related side-effects

System	Event	Laboratory investigation	Notes
Table Laboratory-related adverse effects of haloperidol			
Endocrine	Hyperprolactinaemia	Serum prolactin	Amenorrhoea, galactorrhoea, gynaecomastia may be signs
	Hyperglycaemia or hypoglycaemia	Blood glucose/ urinalysis	Rare events
	Hyponatraemia (SIADH)	See Chapter 3	
Gastrointestinal	Liver dysfunction	LFT	Rare effects, potentially reversible upon discontinuation of the drug. Cholestatic or obstructive jaundice may occur.
Haematological	Leukocytosis, leukopaenia, eosinophilia, monocytosis	FBC	Rare and transient effects
	Porphyria	See Chapter 6	Rare, idiosyncratic effect
Metabolic	Neuroleptic malignant syndrome	See Chapter 3	Rare, idiosyncratic effect
	Electrolyte abnormalities: hypokalaemia, hypocalcaemia, hypomagnesaemia	U&E, calcium, magnesium	Rare events

Routine laboratory monitoring   No specific monitoring required; baseline blood tests as per condition being treated.

Therapeutic drug monitoring   None. Although a therapeutic reference range has been reported (5–20 ng/ml), this has yet to be fully validated and routine monitoring is therefore not recommended.

Levomepromazine
Indications

• treatment of schizophrenia
• treatment of pain, restlessness, and distress in palliative care.

Laboratory-related cautions As for chlorpromazine.

Laboratory-related side-effects As for chlorpromazine. *Note*: occasionally raised inflammatory markers, especially ESR, may be seen.

Routine laboratory tests No specific monitoring required; baseline blood tests as per condition being treated.

Therapeutic drug monitoring None. Although a therapeutic reference range has been reported (15–60 ng/ml), this has yet to be fully validated and routine monitoring is therefore not recommended.

Pericyazine
Indications

- treatment of schizophrenia and other psychotic illnesses
- treatment of disturbed behaviour
- treatment of severe anxiety.

Laboratory-related cautions As for chlorpromazine.

Laboratory-related side-effects As for chlorpromazine.

Routine laboratory tests No specific monitoring required; baseline blood tests as per condition being treated.

Therapeutic drug monitoring None. Although a therapeutic reference range has been reported (15–60 ng/ml), this has yet to be fully validated and routine monitoring is therefore not recommended.

Perphenazine
Indications

- treatment of schizophrenia and others psychotic illnesses
- treatment of severe nausea and vomiting
- treatment of vertigo and labyrinthine disorders.

Laboratory-related cautions As for chlorpromazine.

Laboratory-related side-effects As for chlorpromazine.

Routine laboratory tests No specific monitoring required; baseline blood tests as per condition being treated.

Therapeutic drug monitoring None. Although a therapeutic reference range has been reported (0.8–1.2 nmol/l), this has yet to be fully validated and routine monitoring is therefore not recommended.

Pimozide
Indications

- treatment of schizophrenia and other psychotic illnesses
- treatment of monosymptomatic hypochondriacal delusions (e.g. of parasitosis or of having venereal disease)
- treatment of movement disorders (chorea, Huntington's chorea, and dystonia, especially in cases refractory to treatment)
- treatment of taste disorders, especially phantogeusia
- treatment of Tourette's syndrome.

Laboratory-related cautions As for chlorpromazine; also, use should be avoided in certain conditions, e.g. those with prolonged QT interval or those which cause electrolyte disturbances; effects of polypharmacy must be considered before beginning pimozide.

Laboratory-related side-effects As for chlorpromazine; *note*: pimozide is associated with hypokalaemia which may lead to cardiac disturbances.

Routine laboratory monitoring No specific monitoring required (minimum of an annual electrocardiogram (ECG) recommended); baseline blood tests as per condition being treated.

Therapeutic drug monitoring None. Although a therapeutic reference range has been reported (15–20 ng/ml), this has yet to be fully validated and routine monitoring is therefore not recommended.

Pipotiazine
Indications Maintenance treatment (as depot injection) of schizophrenia and other psychotic illnesses.

Laboratory-related cautions As for chlorpromazine.

Laboratory-related side-effects As for chlorpromazine.

Routine laboratory tests No specific monitoring required; baseline blood tests as per condition being treated.

Therapeutic drug monitoring None.

Prochlorperazine
Indications

- Psychiatric indications:

  - treatment of schizophrenia and other psychotic illnesses
  - adjunct treatment of acute anxiety
  - treatment of acute mania.

- Other reported indications:

  ○ treatment of headaches, especially migraine
  ○ treatment of nausea and vomiting, especially drug-induced and migraine-associated emesis
  ○ symptomatic relief of vertigo, especially when associated with Ménière's disease or labyrinthitis.

Laboratory-related cautions   As for chlorpromazine.

Laboratory-related side-effects   As for chlorpromazine.

Routine laboratory tests   No specific monitoring required; baseline blood tests as per condition being treated.

Therapeutic drug monitoring   None.

Promazine
Indications

- treatment of psychotic illness, including schizophrenia
- treatment of disturbed behaviour (short-term only)
- treatment of nausea and vomiting (especially in labour or postoperatively)
- treatment of intractable hiccup.

Laboratory-related cautions   As for chlorpromazine.

Laboratory-related side-effects   As for chlorpromazine.

Note: haemolytic anaemia is a rare and idiosyncratic side-effect. FBC should be monitored as per clinical presentation.

Routine laboratory monitoring   No specific monitoring required; baseline blood tests as per condition being treated.

Therapeutic drug monitoring   None.

Sulpiride
Indications

- treatment of schizophrenia and other psychotic disorders
- treatment of Tourette's syndrome
- treatment of anxiety, especially that associated with psychosis or anxiety refractory to other treatments
- as an adjunct treatment of vertigo
- treatment of Huntington's chorea (controversial)
- treatment of gastrointestinal disorders such as peptic ulcer disease and irritable colon (rare indications).

Laboratory-related cautions   As for chlorpromazine.

Laboratory-related side-effects   As for chlorpromazine.

Routine laboratory monitoring   No specific monitoring required; baseline blood tests as per condition being treated.

Therapeutic drug monitoring   None. Although a therapeutic reference range has been reported (200–1000 ng/ml), this has yet to be fully validated and routine monitoring is therefore not recommended.

Thioridazine
Indications

- treatment of schizophrenia and other psychotic illnesses
- treatment of acute manic states
- short-term treatment of acute anxiety
- short-term treatment of behavioural disturbances
- treatment of movement disorders, especially choreiform movements and behavioural problems in Huntington's chorea
- treatment of taste disorders, especially phantogeusia.

Laboratory-related cautions   As for chlorpromazine.

Laboratory-related side-effects   As for chlorpromazine.

Note: thioridazine is especially associated with exacerbation of porphyria. In overdose it has been associated with rhabdomyolysis. In a single published case report[9] a 22-year-old male prescribed thioridazine (100 mg nocte) took an overdose of 9.4 g. Within 24 hours he presented with muscle weakness, limb tenderness, and symmetrical swelling. Laboratory investigation revealed a serum creatine kinase of 32,620 IU/l, serum AST of 532 IU/l, and serum creatinine of 167 μmol/l. His urine contained myoglobin. He received a stomach washout and activated charcoal, and within a week biochemical values returned to normal and the muscle tenderness and weakness disappeared.

Routine laboratory monitoring   No specific monitoring required; baseline blood tests as per condition being treated.

Therapeutic drug monitoring   None. Although a therapeutic reference range has been reported (1.0–1.5 μg/ml), this has yet to be fully validated and routine monitoring is therefore not recommended.

Trifluoperazine
Indications

- treatment of schizophrenia and other psychotic illnesses
- short-term treatment of acute anxiety
- short-term treatment of behavioural disturbances
- Treatment of nausea and vomiting, especially postoperatively.

Laboratory-related cautions   As for chlorpromazine.

Laboratory-related side-effects   As for chlorpromazine.

Note: Hyperpyrexia, pancytopaenia, and thrombocytopaenia may be rare effects, occurring especially at high doses (>6 mg daily).

Routine laboratory tests   No specific monitoring required; baseline blood tests as per condition being treated.

Therapeutic drug monitoring   None.

Zuclopenthixol
Indications

- treatment of schizophrenia and other psychotic illnesses
- adjunct treatment of mania.

Laboratory-related cautions   As for chlorpromazine; use should be avoided in porphyria.

Laboratory-related side-effects   As for chlorpromazine.

Routine laboratory monitoring   No specific monitoring required; baseline blood tests as per condition being treated.

Therapeutic drug monitoring   None. Although a therapeutic reference range has been reported (4–50 ng/ml), this has yet to be fully validated and routine monitoring is therefore not recommended.

Atypicals

Amisulpride
Indications

- treatment of schizophrenia and other psychotic illnesses
- as augmentation agent in treatment of depression (rarely used).

Laboratory-related cautions   As for chlorpromazine; use should be avoided in porphyria.

Laboratory-related side-effects   As for chlorpromazine.

Routine laboratory monitoring   No specific monitoring required; baseline blood tests as per condition being treated.

Therapeutic drug monitoring   None. Although a therapeutic reference range has been reported (100–400 ng/ml), this has yet to be fully validated and routine monitoring is therefore not recommended.

Aripiprazole
Indication   Treatment of schizophrenia.

Laboratory-related cautions   Hepatic insufficiency, renal insufficiency.

Laboratory-related side-effects

Table Laboratory-related adverse effects of aripiprazole			
System	**Event**	**Laboratory investigation**	**Notes**
Endocrine	Hyperprolactinaemia	Prolactin levels	Rare event; manufacturer reports no medically important difference in serum prolactin levels compared to placebo
Haematology	Anaemia	FBC, haematinics if indicated	Rare event
Metabolic	Hypercholesterolaemia/ hypertriglyceridaemia	Lipid panel	Rare events, aripiprazole appears to be associated with a low risk of hypercholesterolaemia
	Hyperglycaemia	Fasting blood glucose, HbA1c	Rare event; one published case report suggesting aripiprazole is associated with diabetic ketoacidosis[10]
	Neuroleptic malignant syndrome	See Chapter 3	Rare, idiosyncratic event

Routine laboratory monitoring   No specific monitoring required; baseline blood tests as per condition being treated.

Therapeutic drug monitoring   None.

Clozapine
See Chapter 5.

Olanzapine
See Chapter 5.

Paliperidone
Indications   Treatment of schizophrenia.

Laboratory-related cautions Hepatic impairment, renal impairment.

Laboratory-related side-effects Hyperglycaemia (rare), raised prolactin.

Routine laboratory tests No specific monitoring required; baseline blood tests as per condition being treated.

Therapeutic drug monitoring None.

Quetiapine
Indication Treatment of schizophrenia.

Laboratory-related cautions As for chlorpromazine.

Laboratory-related side-effects As for chlorpromazine; additional, specific effects are listed below.

Table Laboratory-related adverse effects of quetiapine

System	Event	Laboratory investigation	Notes
Endocrine	Hypothyroidism (reduced plasma thyroid hormone concentrations)	TFT	Incidence approximately 0.4%
	Hyperprolactinaemia	Prolactin levels	May manifest with sexual side-effects
Gastrointestinal	Liver failure	LFT	Case report in the literature[11] describing raised enzyme levels
Haematological	Leukocytosis, leukopaenia, eosinophilia, agranulocytosis	FBC	Rare and transient effects
Metabolic	Hypercholesterolaemia/ hypertriglyceridaemia	Lipid panel	Idiosyncratic effect, some studies report significant (< 10%) rises in cholesterol and triglycerides following quetiapine
	Hyperglycaemia	Blood glucose, HbA1c	May rarely progress to diabetes mellitus

Routine laboratory monitoring No specific monitoring required; baseline blood tests as per condition being treated.

Therapeutic drug monitoring None. Although a therapeutic reference range has been reported (70–170 ng/ml), this has yet to be fully validated and routine monitoring is therefore not recommended.

Risperidone
Indications

- treatment of schizophrenia and other psychotic illnesses
- treatment of acute mania
- treatment of obsessive–compulsive disorder (rarely used)
- treatment of behavioural disturbance in dementia
- treatment of movement disorders (dystonia refractory to other treatments)
- treatment of Parkinsonism (controversial)
- treatment of Tourette's syndrome.

Laboratory-related cautions As for chlorpromazine.

Laboratory-related side-effects As for chlorpromazine; *note*: risperidone is not thought to be associated with agranulocytosis or eosinophilia.

Routine laboratory tests No specific monitoring required; baseline blood tests as per condition being treated. NICE recommends 3-monthly glucose and lipid profile and TFT annually.

Therapeutic drug monitoring None. Although a therapeutic reference range has been reported (20–60 ng/ml), this has yet to be fully validated and routine monitoring is therefore not recommended.

Sertindole
Indication Treatment of schizophrenia.

Laboratory-related cautions As for chlorpromazine.

Note: due to prolongation of QT interval with associated arrhythmia and increased risk of sudden death, sertindole is only available on a named patient basis in the UK.

Laboratory-related side-effects As for chlorpromazine.

Note: should not be given to patients with hypokalaemia or hypomagnesaemia (risk of cardiac arrhythmias/sudden deaths).

Routine laboratory monitoring U&E and magnesium levels recommended prior to treatment, baseline and repeat ECG throughout course of treatment recommended.

Therapeutic drug monitoring None.

Zotepine
Indications Treatment of schizophrenia and other psychotic illnesses.

General
Psychopharmacology

133

Laboratory-related cautions As for chlorpromazine; additionally, should not be used in acute gout or nephrolithiasis.

Laboratory-related side-effects As for chlorpromazine; additional effects include the following.

System	Event	Laboratory investigation	Notes
Table Laboratory-related adverse effects of zotepine			
Gastrointestinal	Liver failure	LFT	Rare, idiosyncratic effect
Haematological	Raised ESR	ESR	Rare and transient effects
	Anaemia, eosinophilia, leukocytosis, leukopaenia, thrombocytopaenia	FBC	
Metabolic	Hyperglycaemia or hypoglycaemia	Blood glucose, urinalysis	
	Hyperlipidaemia	Lipid panel	
	Hyperuricaemia	Serum urate	
Renal	Increased serum creatinine	U&E	

Routine laboratory monitoring U&E and occasionally magnesium (low magnesium may contribute to prolonged QT interval) should be measured before treatment and monitored when increasing dose; regular ECG monitoring required (baseline and upon dose increase) due to possible prolonging effects of quetiapine on QT interval.

Therapeutic drug monitoring None. Although a therapeutic reference range has been reported (12–120 ng/ml), this has yet to be fully validated and routine monitoring is therefore not recommended.

Anxiolytics and hypnotics

Anxiolytics

Benzodiazepines
Indications (diazepam)

- Psychiatric indications:

  - short-term treatment of anxiety disorders
  - as diagnostic aid in conversion and dissociative disorders
  - treatment of agitated behaviour
  - as adjuncts in the treatment of schizophrenia
  - control of panic attacks (not routinely recommended).

- Other reported indications:

  - treatment of cardiac arrythmias
  - treatment of dyspnoea
  - treatment of eclampsia (rarely used)
  - treatment of epilepsy and other seizure disorders, especially status epilepticus
  - as adjunct in the treatment of extrapyramidal movement disorders and dystonias
  - treatment of irritable bowel syndrome (controversial)
  - treatment of muscle spasm (such as in stiff-man syndrome, spasticity, and some forms of poisoning such as tetanus)
  - as adjuncts to treatment of nausea and vomiting, especially in cancer chemotherapy
  - treatment of acute parasomnias
  - treatment of premenstrual syndrome (short-term, limited to luteal phase of cycle)
  - treatment of vertigo
  - treatment of withdrawal symptoms (alcohol and opioid withdrawal)
  - use as premedication in anaesthesia.

Laboratory-related cautions respiratory disease, hepatic impairment, renal impairment, porphyria.

Laboratory-related side-effects

Table Laboratory-related adverse effects of benzodiazepines			
System	**Event**	**Laboratory investigation**	**Notes**
Endocrine	Galactorrhoea	Prolactin levels	Associated with normal prolactin levels
	Gynaecomastia		Raised serum oestradiol levels may be seen
	Hypertestosteronaemia	Testosterone levels	Raised testosterone levels have been reported in men taking diazepam 10–20 mg daily for 2 weeks
	Hyponatraemia (SIADH)	See Chapter 3	Rare idiosyncratic effect; elderly may be more susceptible
Gastrointestinal	Cholestatic jaundice, focal hepatic necrosis	LFT	Rare, idiosyncratic effects: single case reports of each of these effects
Haematological	Agranulocytosis	FBC	Chlordiazepoxide and diazepam implicated
	Anaemia		Chlordiazepoxide, clonazepam, clorazepate, and diazepam implicated
	Eosinophilia		May be associated with clonazepam
	Leukopaenia		Clonazepam, lorazepam, and oxazepam implicated
	Pancytopaenia		Rare, idiosyncratic events; one case in the literature of pancytopaenia with lorazepam[12] may also be associated with diazepam
	Thrombocytopaenia		Chlordiazepoxide, clonazepam, and diazepam implicated

General Psychopharmacology

Table Laboratory-related adverse effects of benzodiazepines (Cont.)			
System	Event	Laboratory investigation	Notes
Metabolic	Hyponatraemia	U&E	Rare event
	Porphyria	See Chapter 6	Alprazolam, chlordiazepoxide, nitrazepam, and possibly oxazepam associated
Musculoskeletal	Rhabdomyolysis	Serum creatine kinase, aspartate transaminase, myoglobin (urine)	Event secondary to hyponatraemia; total of five cases reported thus far with diazepam

Routine laboratory monitoring No specific monitoring required; baseline blood tests as per condition being treated.

Therapeutic drug monitoring None. Although therapeutic reference ranges have been reported for a number of benzodiazepines (see Table below), these have yet to be fully validated and routine monitoring is therefore not recommended.

Table Therapeutic drug monitoring of benzodiazepines	
Agent	Reported reference range (ng/ml)
Alprazolam	20–40
Clonazepam	20–40
Diazepam (and metabolites)	300–400
Lorazepam	10–15
Midazolam	6–15

Buspirone
Indications

- short-term treatment of anxiety disorders
- treatment of bruxism (one case report)
- treatment of cerebellar ataxia

- treatment of behavioural disorders in dementia
- treatment of dyskinesias (controversial)
- treatment of Tourette's syndrome
- treatment of alcohol withdrawal (controversial)
- treatment of non-ulcer (functional) dyspepsia (via relaxation of the gastric fundus – use in this context has yet to be fully validated).

Laboratory-related cautions   Hepatic insufficiency, renal insufficiency.

Laboratory-related side-effects   No specific laboratory-related effects reported.

Routine laboratory monitoring   No specific monitoring required; baseline blood tests as per condition being treated. *Note*: buspirone may interfere with laboratory tests for urinary catecholamines.

Therapeutic drug monitoring   None.

Beta blockers
Indications (propranolol)

- Psychiatric indications:
  - short-term reduction of somatic symptoms associated with anxiety.

- Other reported indications:

  - treatment of hypertension
  - treatment of portal hypertension
  - treatment of symptoms secondary to phaeochromocytoma
  - treatment of symptoms related to angina
  - treatment of cardiac arrhythmias
  - treatment of hypertrophic subaortic stenosis
  - treatment of hyperthyroidism (thyrotoxicosis)
  - treatment of essential tremor
  - treatment of migraine (prophylaxis)
  - treatment of obstructive cardiomyopathy.

Laboratory-related cautions   History of respiratory disease (asthma, chronic obstructive pulmonary disease (COPD), bronchospasm), metabolic acidosis, phaechromocytoma (beta-blockers not to be given without appropriate alpha-blockers), hyperthyroidism (beta-blockers may mask symptoms), hypoglycaemia (beta-blockers may mask symptoms), myasthenia gravis (beta-blockers may *unmask* symptoms).

Laboratory-related side-effects

Table	Laboratory-related adverse effects of beta-blockers		
System	*Event*	*Laboratory investigation*	*Notes*
Endocrine	Hyper-/ hypoglycaemia	Blood glucose, urinalysis, HbA1c	Hypoglycaemia more common, especially in patients with severe renal dysfunction; effects more likely in diabetic patients
Haematological	Purpura (non-thrombocytic)	FBC, clotting screen	Rare, transient events; may be reversible upon discontinuation of the drug
	Agranulocytosis Eosinophilia	FBC	Rare and usually transient effects, may be reversible upon discontinuation of the drug
Metabolic	Raised levels of very-low-density lipoprotein (VLDL) and triglyceride, reduced level of high-density lipoprotein (HDL)	Lipid screen	Effects may be less with β1 selective agents (pindolol not reported to have adverse effects)
	Hyperkalaemia	U&E	Rare and idiosyncratic effect

Routine laboratory tests   No specific monitoring required; baseline blood tests as per condition being treated.

Therapeutic drug monitoring   None.

Meprobamate
Indications

- treatment of anxiety disorders
- short-term treatment of insomnia
- management of muscle spasm (rarely used).

Laboratory-related cautions   Hepatic impairment, renal impairment, impaired respiratory function, porphyria.

Laboratory-related side-effects As for benzodiazepines; additional adverse laboratory effects are listed below.

Table Laboratory-related adverse effects of meprobamate			
System	*Event*	*Laboratory investigation*	*Notes*
Haematological	Aplastic anaemia Agranulocytosis Eosinophilia Leukopaenia Thrombocytopaenia	FBC, clotting screen	Rare events, may be reversible upon discontinuation of the drug
Metabolic	Porphyria	See Chapter 6	Rare, idiosyncratic effect

Routine laboratory monitoring No specific monitoring required; baseline blood tests as per condition being treated.

Therapeutic drug monitoring None. Although a therapeutic reference range has been reported (6–12 μg/ml), this has yet to be fully validated and routine monitoring is therefore not recommended.

Barbiturates
Indications (amylobarbitone)

- treatment of severe, intractable insomnia (only in patients already taking barbiturates)
- to induce coma (and thereby protect the brain) in patients with cerebral ischaemia secondary to various conditions including hepatic encephalopathy, Reye's syndrome, and head injury
- in the evaluation of temporal lobe epilepsy (to test memory prior to surgery)
- use in anaesthesia (thiopentone)
- treatment of epilepsy (phenobarbital).

Laboratory-related cautions Respiratory insufficiency (contraindication), hepatic insufficiency (contraindication if severe), renal insufficiency, acute porphyia (contraindication).

Laboratory-related side-effects

Table Laboratory-related adverse effects of barbiturates

System	Event	Laboratory investigation	Notes
Gastrointestinal	Hepatitis/cholestasis	LFT	Rare, idiosyncratic effects
Haematological	Megaloblastic anaemia, agranulocytosis, and thrombocytopaenia	FBC	
Metabolic	Porphyria	See Chapter 6	
	Oliguria	U&E	Rare effect

Routine laboratory tests No specific monitoring required; baseline blood tests as per condition being treated.

Therapeutic drug monitoring None.

Pregabalin
Pregabalin is an antiepileptic which has recently been licensed for the treatment of generalized anxiety disorder – see below for more details.

Hypnotics

Benzodiazepines
See above.

'Z' agents: zaleplon, zolpidem, zopiclone
Indications

- short-term management of insomnia
- use as diagnostic aid in catatonia (zolpidem)
- possible role in treatment of Parkinson's disease (zolpidem).

Laboratory-related cautions Hepatic impairment, renal impairment, severe respiratory insufficiency (contraindication).

Laboratory-related side-effects As for benzodiazepines.

Routine laboratory tests No specific monitoring required; baseline blood tests as per condition being treated.

Therapeutic drug monitoring None. Although therapeutic reference ranges have been reported (zopiclone 60–75 ng/ml; zolpidem 90–325 ng/ml), these have yet to be fully validated and routine monitoring is therefore not recommended.

General Psychopharmacology

141

Chloral hydrate
Indications

- short-term treatment of insomnia; previously thought to be agent of choice in children undergoing invasive procedures but use not recommended due to carcinogenicity concerns
- external use as rubefascient (counter-irritant).

Laboratory-related cautions   Hepatic impairment, renal impairment, respiratory impairment, gastritis, porphyria.

Laboratory-related side-effects

Table Laboratory-related adverse effects of chloral hydrate			
System	**Event**	**Laboratory investigation**	**Notes**
Gastrointestinal	Jaundice/liver damage	LFT, clotting screen	May worsen hepatic encephalopathy; hyperbilirubinaemia in neonates reported
Haematological	Eosinophilia/ leukocytosis	FBC	Rare, idiosyncratic effect
	Increased prothrombin time	Clotting screen	Rare, possibly reversible effect
	Lymphopaenia/ neutropaenia secondary to bone narrow suppression	FBC	Rare effect
Renal	Ketonuria	Urinalysis	Rare event
	Renal damage leading to albuminuria	U&E	Possible, rare consequence of long-term use

Routine laboratory tests   No specific monitoring required; baseline blood tests as per condition being treated. In addition to baseline blood tests as per condition being treated, FBC should be monitored if patient develops signs of infection such as stomatitis, fever, or sore throat. If blood dyscrasia is suspected, chloral hydrate treatment should be stopped.

Therapeutic drug monitoring   None.

Triclofos
Indication   Short-term sedation.

Laboratory-related cautions   See chloral hydrate.

142

General Psychopharmacology

Laboratory-related side-effects See chloral hydrate; fewer gastrointestinal disturbances reported as compared to chloral hydrate.

Routine laboratory tests No specific monitoring required; baseline blood tests as per condition being treated.

Therapeutic drug monitoring None.

Clomethiazole
Indications

- short-term treatment of severe insomnia (especially in the elderly)
- treatment of alcohol withdrawal symptoms
- treatment of status epilepticus
- treatment of eclampsia
- use as regional anaesthetic
- seizure prophylaxis in porphyria
- treatment of stroke (possible neuroprotective effects)
- treatment of opioid withdrawal.

Laboratory-related cautions Respiratory impairment (hypoxia), hepatic impairment (sedation may mask hepatic coma), renal impairment.

Laboratory-related side-effects

Table Laboratory-related adverse effects of clomethiazole			
System	*Event*	*Laboratory investigation*	*Notes*
Gastrointestinal	Hyperbilirubinaemia	LFT	Rare, reversible effect
	Alteration in liver enzymes	LFT	Rare, idiosyncratic effect

Routine laboratory tests No specific monitoring required; baseline blood tests as per condition being treated.

Therapeutic drug monitoring None. Although a therapeutic reference range has been reported (100–5000 ng/ml), this has yet to be fully validated and routine monitoring is therefore not recommended.

Antihistamines (e.g. promethazine)
Indications

- symptomatic relief of symptoms secondary to allergy (itching, rhinitis, conjunctivitis, angioedema)
- treatment of nausea and vomiting
- treatment of symptoms of Ménière's disease
- use as sedative in surgical procedures and for night-time sedation
- use in eclampsia and pre-eclampsia as part of a 'lytic' cocktail.

Laboratory-related cautions Hepatic impairment, renal impairment, hypokalaemia/other metabolic abnormalities.

Laboratory-related side-effects

Table Laboratory-related adverse effects of promethazine

System	Event	Laboratory investigation	Notes
Gastrointestinal	Jaundice/ hyperbilirubinaemia	LFT	Rare, idiosyncratic effects
Haematological	Agranulocytosis Aplastic anaemia Eosinophilia Haemolytic anaemia Leukopaenia Thrombocytopaenia Thrombocytopaenic purpura Porphyria	FBC, clotting screen, porphyria screen (see Chapter 6), haematinics	
Metabolic	Hyperglycaemia or hypoglycaemia	Blood glucose, HbA1c	Rare event

Routine laboratory tests No specific monitoring required; baseline blood tests as per condition being treated.

Therapeutic drug monitoring None.

Mood stabilizers/anticonvulsants

Carbamazepine
See Chapter 5.

Valproic acid
See Chapter 5.

Lamotrigine
See Chapter 5.

Lithium
See Chapter 5.

Pregabalin

Indications

- treatment of neuropathic pain
- as adjunct in treatment of epilepsy (partial seizures)
- treatment of generalized anxiety disorder.

Laboratory-related cautions Diabetes mellitus, renal impairment.

Laboratory-related side-effects

Table Laboratory-related adverse effects of pregabalin			
System	*Event*	*Laboratory investigation*	*Notes*
Gastrointestinal	Abnormal liver enzymes (raised ALT, AST)	LFT	Pregabalin has recently been marketed in the UK as a treatment for generalized anxiety disorder; effects on laboratory parameters are reported by manufacturer to be rare (<1%)
	Pancreatitis	Amylase, lipase	
Haematological	Neutropaenia Leukopaenia Thrombocytopaenia	FBC	
Metabolic	Hyperkalaemia	U&E	
	Hypoglycaemia	Blood glucose, HbA1c, urinalysis	
Renal	Renal failure	U&E, creatinine	
	Rhabdomyolysis	Enzymes: alanine transferase, amylase, aspartate transferase, creatine kinase, lactate dehydrogenase U&E/creatinine (rise in urea/ creatinine may herald renal failure) Hyperkalaemia may be present Calcium (hypocalcaemia may be present)	

Routine laboratory tests No specific monitoring required; baseline blood tests as per condition being treated.

Therapeutic drug monitoring None.

Miscellaneous agents

Antidementia drugs

Note: NICE has published guidelines for dementia (http://www.nice.org.uk/
nicemedia/pdf/word/CG042NICEGuideline.doc), but does not make specific
recommendations regarding laboratory monitoring of any of the antidementia
drugs.

Donepezil
Indication Treatment of dementia (mild to moderate) in Alzheimer's
disease.

Laboratory-related cautions Hepatic impairment, hyperthyroidism, renal
impairment.

Laboratory-related side-effects

Table Laboratory-related side-effects of donepezil			
System	*Event*	*Laboratory investigation*	*Notes*
Endocrine	Hyperglycaemia, diabetes mellitus	Fasting glucose, urinalysis, HbA1c	Rare and idiosyncratic effects
Gastrointestinal	Hepatitis, jaundice	LFT (especially raised ALP and AST)	Neuroleptic malignant syndrome and pancreatitis are thought to be extremely rare effects
	Pancreatitis	Amylase, lipase	
Haematological	Anaemia, eosinophilia, erythrocytopaenia, thrombocytopaenia	FBC; haematinics for anaemia	
Metabolic	Neuroleptic malignant syndrome	See Chapter 3	
	Hyperglycaemia	Blood glucose, HbA1c	
	Hyponatraemia	U&E	
	Raised enzyme levels: creatine kinase, increased lactate dehydrogenase	Measurement of specific enzymes	

Routine laboratory monitoring No specific monitoring required; baseline
blood tests as per condition being treated.

146

Therapeutic drug monitoring   None.

Galantamine

Indications   Treatment of dementia (mild to moderate) in Alzheimer's disease; it has also been used to treat neuromuscular disorders and to antagonize muscle relaxation following administration of neuromuscular blocking agents.

Laboratory-related cautions   Hepatic impairment.

Laboratory-related side-effects

Table Laboratory-related side-effects of galantamine			
System	*Event*	*Laboratory investigation*	*Notes*
Haematological	Anaemia, thrombocytopaenia	FBC; haematinics for anaemia	Rare, idiosyncratic effects
Metabolic	Diabetes mellitus	Fasting glucose, urinalysis, HbA1c	
	Raised alkaline phosphatase	Enzyme measurement	

Routine laboratory monitoring   No specific monitoring required; baseline blood tests as per condition being treated.

Therapeutic drug monitoring   None.

Memantine

Indications   Treatment of dementia (moderate to severe) in Alzheimer's disease; it has also been used in the treatment of coma and cerebral spasticity.

Laboratory-related cautions   Renal impairment.

Laboratory-related side-effects

Table	Laboratory-related side-effects of memantine		
System	*Event*	*Laboratory investigation*	*Notes*
Haematological	Anaemia	FBC; haematinics	Anaemia may commonly occur
	Leukopaenia Thrombocytopaenia	FBC	Rare, idiosyncratic effects
Metabolic	Hyperlipidaemia	Lipid screen	
	Hyponatraemia	U&E	
	Increased alkaline phosphatase	LFT including alkaline phosphatase	
Gastrointestinal	Abnormal liver function	LFTs (especially raised ALP)	

Routine laboratory monitoring   No specific monitoring required; baseline blood tests as per condition being treated.

Therapeutic drug monitoring   None.

Rivastigmine
Indication   Treatment of dementia (mild to moderate) in Alzheimer's disease.

Laboratory-related cautions   Hepatic impairment, renal impairment.

Laboratory-related side-effects

Table Laboratory-related side-effects of rivastigmine			
System	**Event**	**Laboratory investigation**	**Notes**
Endocrine	Hypothyroidism	TFT	Rare, idiosyncratic events
Gastrointestinal	Pancreatitis	Amylase, lipase	
Haematological	Anaemia	FBC; haematinics for anaemia	Anaemia is frequently reported
	Leukocytosis Thrombocytopaenia		Rare, idiosyncratic events
Metabolic	Diabetes mellitus	Fasting glucose, urinalysis, HbA1c	
	Gout	Raised serum urate	
	Hypercholesterolaemia	Lipid screen	
	Hyperglycaemia or hypoglycaemia	Fasting glucose, urinalysis, HbA1c	
	Hyperlipidaemia	Lipid screen	
	Hypokalaemia	U&E, creatinine	Hypokalaemia frequently reported
	Hyponatraemia		Rare, idiosyncratic event

Routine laboratory monitoring No specific monitoring required; baseline blood tests as per condition being treated.

Therapeutic drug monitoring None.

Antimuscarinics

Benztropine
Indications Treatment of idiopathic parkinsonism and alleviation of extrapyramidal side-effects secondary to antipsychotics.

Laboratory-related cautions Thyrotoxicosis, electrolyte disturbance (e.g. with diarrhoea).

Laboratory-related side-effects None reported; may rarely provoke hyperthermia in susceptible individuals, especially when the ambient temperature is high.

Routine laboratory monitoring None required; most effects of antimuscarinics are clinical, and laboratory monitoring is not generally required, except to rule out other differential diagnoses such as malignant hyperthermia or a toxic psychosis secondary to antimuscarinic treatment.

Therapeutic drug monitoring None.

Hyoscine
Indications Treatment of idiopathic parkinsonsism and alleviation of extrapyramidal side-effects secondary to antipsychotics. *Note*: hyoscine can rarely induce a toxic psychosis.

Laboratory-related cautions Impaired hepatic and renal function; porphyria (hyoscine is unsafe for use in porphyria).

Laboratory-related side-effects None reported.

Routine laboratory monitoring None; laboratory monitoring is not generally required, except where there is suspicion of antimuscarinic toxicity.

Therapeutic drug monitoring None.

Orphenadrine
Indications Treatment of idiopathic parkinsonism and alleviation of extrapyramidal side-effects secondary to antipsychotics.

Laboratory-related cautions Porphyria.

Laboratory-related side-effects None reported; may rarely provoke hyperthermia in susceptible individuals, especially when the ambient temperature is high.

Routine laboratory monitoring None; most effects of antimuscarinics are clinical, and laboratory monitoring is not generally required, except to rule out other differential diagnoses such as malignant hyperthermia or a toxic psychosis secondary to antimuscarinic treatment.

Therapeutic drug monitoring None.

Procyclidine
Indications Treatment of idiopathic parkinsonism and alleviation of extrapyramidal side-effects secondary to antipsychotics.

Laboratory-related cautions Porphyria.

Laboratory-related side-effects None reported; may rarely provoke hyperthermia in susceptible individuals, especially when the ambient temperature is high.

Routine laboratory monitoring None; most effects of antimuscarinics are clinical, and laboratory monitoring is not generally required, except to rule out other differential diagnoses such as malignant hyperthermia or a toxic psychosis secondary to antimuscarinic treatment.

Therapeutic drug monitoring None.

CNS stimulants

Dexamphetamine
Indications

- treatment of narcolepsy
- treatment of hyperactivity disorders in children refractory to other treatment
- treatment of obesity (use not currently recommended)
- treatment of epilepsy (use not currently recommended).

Laboratory-related cautions Hyperthyroidism (contraindication), renal impairment, diabetes mellitus (when used in treatment of obesity), acute porphyria.

Laboratory-related side-effects

Table	Laboratory-related adverse effects of dexamphetamine		
System	*Event*	*Laboratory investigation*	*Notes*
Cardiac	Dilated cardiomyopathy	Creatine phosphokinase	May be elevated in acute myocarditis
Endocrine	Hyperthyroxinaemia	Thyroxine levels	Rare, may be associated with heavy amphetamine abuse
Gastrointestinal	Hepatic dysfunction (hepatitis and acute hepatic necrosis)	LFT	May occur in heavy users or in overdose
	Ischaemic colitis	FBC (to check for leukocytosis)	Rare event
	Disseminated intravascular coagulation (DIC)	FBC, coagulation studies, fibrin/ fibrin degradation products	Rare events, may occur with abuse
	Idiopathic thrombocytopaenic purpura	FBC, clotting screen	

Table Laboratory-related adverse effects of dexamphetamine (Cont.)

System	Event	Laboratory investigation	Notes
Musculoskeletal	Rhabdomyolysis	Serum creatine kinase, aspartate transaminase, urine myoglobin	Myoglobin may be detected in urine
Renal	Renal failure	Creatinine, U&E, myoglobin in suspected rhabdomyolysis	May be secondary to dehydration or rhabdomyolysis

Note: three laboratory syndromes have been described in individuals abusing amphetamines.

Table Laboratory syndromes related to dexamphetamine abuse

Syndrome	Clinical and laboratory events	Laboratory investigation	Notes
Syndrome 1	Circulatory collapse Fever Leukaemoid reaction DIC Rhabdomyolysis Diffuse myalgias Muscle tenderness	ESR, FBC, U&E, serum creatine kinase, aspartate transaminase, urine myoglobin	WCC may be >40
Syndrome 2	Rhabdomyolysis Myoglobinuric renal failure		Extremely rare events
Syndrome 3	Acute interstitial nephritis Acute renal failure		

Routine laboratory tests No specific monitoring required; baseline blood tests as per condition being treated.

Therapeutic drug monitoring None.

Modafinil
Indication Treatment of narcolepsy.

Laboratory-related cautions Hepatic impairment, renal impairment.

Laboratory-related side-effects

Table	Laboratory-related adverse effects of modafinil		
System	**Event**	**Laboratory investigation**	**Notes**
Endocrine	Hyperglycaemia	Blood glucose, urinalysis, HbA1c	Rare, idiosyncratic event
Gastrointestinal	Increased alkaline phosphatase	LFT	Dose-related effect
	Increased GGT	LFT	Rare event, not clinically significant
Haematological	Eosinophilia Leukopaenia	FBC	Rare, idiosyncratic events
	Decreased prothrombin time	Clotting screen	
Metabolic	Albuminuria	LFT	
	Hypercholesterolaemia	Lipid screen	

Routine laboratory tests   No specific monitoring required; baseline blood tests as per condition being treated.

Therapeutic drug monitoring   None.

Drugs used in substance dependence

Acamprosate
Indication   To prevent relapse in alcoholics weaned off alcohol.

Laboratory-related cautions   Hepatic impairment, renal impairment.

Laboratory-related side-effects

Table	Laboratory-related adverse effects of acamprosate		
System	**Event**	**Laboratory investigation**	**Notes**
Metabolic	Hypercalcaemia	Serum calcium levels	Rare event, may occur in chronic overdose
Renal	Acute renal failure	U&E	Rare, idiosyncratic effect observed in three patients only; may be reversible on stopping the drug

Routine laboratory tests No specific monitoring required; baseline blood tests as per condition being treated.

Therapeutic drug monitoring None. Although a therapeutic reference range has been reported (300–400 ng/ml), this has yet to be fully validated and routine monitoring is therefore not recommended.

Acetylcysteine
See also Chapter 2 – 'Suicide/deliberate self-harm'.

Indication Used in the treatment of paracetamol overdose.

Laboratory-related cautions Hypersensitivity to any ingredient; *note*: patients with liver dysfunction secondary to chronic alcohol abuse or use of enzyme-inducing medications may experience hepatotoxicity at lower paracetamol levels than other patient groups.

Laboratory-related side-effects

Table Laboratory-related adverse effects of acetylcysteine			
System	*Event*	*Laboratory investigation*	*Notes*
Gastrointestinal	Deterioration of hepatic function (non-specific)	LFT	Rare, idiosyncratic events
Haematological	Thrombocytopaenia	FBC	
Metabolic	Acidosis, cyanosis	Blood gases	
	Hypokalaemia	U&E	Rare event, may be related to paracetamol toxicity rather than to acetylcysteine *per se*

Routine laboratory monitoring No specific monitoring required; baseline blood tests as per condition being treated.

Therapeutic drug monitoring None.

Disulfiram
Indication Adjunct in treatment of chronic alcoholism.

Laboratory-related cautions Diabetes mellitus, hepatic impairment, hypothyroidism, renal impairment.

Laboratory-related side-effects

Table	Laboratory-related adverse effects of disulfiram		
System	*Event*	*Laboratory investigation*	*Notes*
Gastrointestinal	Fatal hepatic coma	LFT	Extremely rare event (seven reports in literature)
	Hepatitis Hepatic cell damage		Symptoms usually begin within 10 days and 6 months of starting therapy; liver enzymes may not return to normal for several months
Haematological	Blood dyscrasias	FBC	Rare, idiosyncratic events
Metabolic	Disulfiram–alcohol reaction: mild=no laboratory changes; severe=possibility of cardiac and respiratory collapse	None except in severe, life-threatening reaction (see Chapter 3)	Subjectively unpleasant reactions due to acetaldehyde accumulation. When severe can be life-threatening

Routine laboratory monitoring   No specific monitoring required (*note*: in the USA, FBC recommended every 6 months); baseline blood tests as per condition being treated.

Therapeutic drug monitoring   None. Although a therapeutic reference range has been reported, levels above 5.0 mg/l are reported to be toxic. There is as yet no fully validated plasma reference range for disulfiram, and routine monitoring is therefore not recommended.

Buprenorphine
Indications

- treatment of opioid dependence
- treatment of moderate to severe pain
- as an adjunct in anaesthesia.

Laboratory-related cautions   Hepatic impairment, hypothyroidism.

Table	Laboratory-related adverse effects of buprenorphine		
System	*Event*	*Laboratory investigation*	*Notes*
Immunology	Local, allergic/ inflammatory reactions (erythema, pruritus)	Inflammatory markers (CRP, ESR)	Medication should be stopped if it is suspected or implicated Laboratory tests not usually required but may be useful for monitoring purposes

Routine laboratory monitoring   No specific monitoring required; baseline blood tests as per condition being treated.

Therapeutic drug monitoring   None.

Bupropion
Indications   Treatment of depressive disorders; use as adjunct to smoking cessation.

Laboratory-related cautions   Hepatic impairment, renal impairment.

Laboratory-related side-effects

Table	Laboratory-related adverse effects of bupropion		
System	*Event*	*Laboratory investigation*	*Notes*
Endocrine	Hyperglycaemia or hypoglycaemia	Fasting glucose, urinalysis, possibly HbA1c	Rarely reported effects
	SIADH	U&E, urinalysis	
Gastrointestinal	Hepatitis	LFT	
Haematological	Anaemia Leukocytosis or leukopaenia Pancytopaenia	FBC; possibly haematinics for anaemia	
	Prothrombin time	INR	Rare effect, may be raised or lowered especially with coadministration of warfarin
	Thrombocytopaenia	FBC	Rarely reported

Routine laboratory monitoring   No specific monitoring required; baseline blood tests as per condition being treated.

Therapeutic drug monitoring   None. Although a therapeutic reference range has been reported (<100 ng/ml), this has yet to be fully validated and routine monitoring is therefore not recommended.

Flumazenil
Indications   A benzodiazepine antagonist used to reverse the effects of benzodiazepines such as when used for sedation or following overdose. Also reverses the effects of zaleplon, zolpidem, and zopiclone.

Laboratory-related cautions   As for benzodiazepines.

Laboratory-related side-effects   None reported.

Routine laboratory monitoring   No specific monitoring required; baseline blood tests as per condition being treated.

Therapeutic drug monitoring   None.

Lofexidine
Indication   Used in the management of opioid withdrawal symptoms.

Laboratory-related cautions   Renal impairment.

Laboratory-related side-effects   None reported.

Routine laboratory monitoring   No specific monitoring required; baseline blood tests as per condition being treated.

Therapeutic drug monitoring   None.

Methadone
Indications   Adjunct in treatment of opioid withdrawal; use in palliative medicine to control cough symptoms in terminal lung cancer.

Laboratory-related cautions   Acute alcoholism, adrenocortical insufficiency, hepatic impairment, hypothyroidism, renal impairment.

Laboratory-related side-effects

Table Laboratory-related adverse effects of methadone			
System	**Event**	**Laboratory investigation**	**Notes**
Endocrine	Hyperglycaemia	Fasting glucose, urinalysis	Effects especially in individuals with diabetes mellitus (type I or II)
	Hypoadrenalism	U&E, morning cortisol, or short synacthen test	Biochemical changes in hypoadrenalism may include hypoglycaemia, hyponatraemia, hyperkalaemia, and low morning (09.00) cortisol levels (especially <50 nmol/l)
Gastrointestinal	Raised enzyme levels	Amylase, lactate dehydrogenase, LFT	Rare effects, with possibly raised amylase, ALT, and/or AST. Raised lactate dehydrogenase is rare
Haematological	Thrombocytopaenia	FBC	Rare, idiosyncratic effect may be increased in patients with chronic hepatitis
Musculoskeletal	Rhabdomyolysis progressing to renal failure	Enzymes: alanine transferase, amylase, aspartate transferase, creatine kinase, lactate dehydrogenase U&E/creatinine (rise in urea/creatinine may herald renal failure) Hyperkalaemia may be present Calcium (hypocalcaemia may be present)	May especially occur in overdose
Metabolic	Hypokalaemia	U&E	Rare event
	Hypomagnesaemia	Serum magnesium	May manifest as cardiac arrhythmia

158

Routine laboratory monitoring No specific monitoring required; baseline blood tests as per condition being treated.

Therapeutic drug monitoring None.

Naloxone
Indications

- reversal of opioid toxicity (coma, respiratory depression)
- diagnosis of opioid tolerance/overdose (controversial)
- as an adjunct in treatment of septic shock (to increase blood pressure).

Laboratory-related cautions As for opioids.

Laboratory-related side-effects None reported.

Routine laboratory monitoring No specific monitoring required; baseline blood tests as per condition being treated.

Therapeutic drug monitoring None.

Naltrexone
Indications An adjunct in treatment of opioid withdrawal (to help prevent relapse); may also have similar use as adjunct in treatment of alcohol dependence.

Laboratory-related cautions Hepatic impairment, renal impairment.

Laboratory-related side-effects

Table	Laboratory-related adverse effects of naltrexone		
System	**Event**	**Laboratory investigation**	**Notes**
Gastrointestinal	Liver toxicity: abnormal liver function tests, hepatitis, jaundice	LFT	Rare, reversible effects; abnormal LFT may be especially apparent in obese subjects (especially raised AST)
Haematological	Thrombocytopaenia	FBC	Rare, idiosyncratic effect. Reversible upon stopping offending agent

Routine laboratory monitoring No specific monitoring required; baseline blood tests as per condition being treated.

Therapeutic drug monitoring None.

Nicotine
Indication   As an adjunct in smoking cessation.

Laboratory-related cautions   Diabetes mellitus, hepatic impairment, hyperthyroidism, phaeochromocytoma, renal impairment.

Laboratory-related side-effects   None reported.

Routine laboratory monitoring   No specific monitoring required; baseline blood tests as per condition being treated.

Therapeutic drug monitoring   None.

Pabrinex® (parenteral thiamine complex)
See also Chapter 8 – 'Vitamins'

Indications   Treatment of vitamin depletion due to inadequate intake or malabsorption as may occur in such states as alcoholism, haemodialysis (chronic intermittent), postoperatively, acute infections, and some psychotic states (such as post-electroconvulsive therapy (ECT) or drug intoxication).

Laboratory-related cautions   History of anaphylaxis or allergy to any of the components (ascorbic acid, nicotinamide, pyridoxine hydrochloride, riboflavin, thiamine hydrochloride).

Laboratory-related side-effects   None reported.

Routine laboratory monitoring   No specific monitoring required; baseline blood tests as per condition being treated.

Therapeutic drug monitoring   None.

Omega-3 triglycerides

There are two forms of omega-3 compounds available in the UK: Omacor® contains omega-3 ethyl esters, eicosapentaenoic acid, and decosahexanoic acid; Maxepa® contains concentrated fish oils, eicosapentaenoic acid, docosa-hexanoic acid, vitamin A, and vitamin D.

Indications

* augmentation of clozapine (after 3–6 months of poor efficacy with clozapine)
* possible use as first-line or adjunct treatment in some patients with schizophrenia
* as adjunct to treatment of refractory depression
* as adjunct in treatment of hypertriglyceridaemia.

Laboratory-related cautions Anticoagulant treatment, bleeding disorders, diabetes mellitus (omega-3 triglycerides), liver impairment (omega-3 ethyl esters).

Laboratory-related side-effects Rare; no side effects reported for omega-3 triglycerides; for omega-3 ethyl esters hepatic disorders, hyperglycaemia, and leukocytosis very rarely reported.

Routine laboratory monitoring None for omega-3 triglycerides; for omega-3 ethyl esters monitoring of LFT recommended.

Therapeutic drug monitoring None.

Psychotropics associated with abnormal glucose metabolism

Note: a number of agents may cause either hyper- or hypoglycaemia, including beta-blockers, tricyclic antidepressants, and zotepine. For further details see individual agents, above.

Agents associated with hyperglycaemia
Note: effects may be idiosyncratic and are especially associated with atypical antipsychotics.

Aripiprazole, beta-blockers, bupropion, chlorpromazine, clozepine, donepezil, galantamine, lithium, MAOIs, methadone, modafinil, opioids, pregabalin, quetiapine, rivastigmine, zotepine.

Agents associated with hypoglycaemia
Alcohol, beta-blockers, duloxetine, haloperidol, MAOIs, pregabalin, zotepine; may also be seen with agents associated with metabolic syndrome.

Summary of haematological effects of psychotropics

The following entries summarize those psychotropics associated with specific haematological syndromes. *Note*: many of these are idiosyncratic and rare, and may manifest with non-specific clinical symptoms. Those agents with the highest risk of adverse laboratory-related effects may be amenable to therapeutic drug monitoring (see Chapter 5). For biochemical effects and additional details regarding haematological effects, see the appropriate entries in Part Two.

Psychotropics associated with agranulocytosis

Amitriptyline, amoxapine, barbiturates, beta-blockers, carbamazepine, chlordiazepoxide, chlorpromazine, clomipramine, clozapine, diazepam, fluphenazine, haloperidol, meprobamate, minaserin, mirtazepine, nortriptyline, olanzaopine, promethazine, quetiapine, TCAs (especially imipramine), tranylcypromine, frazodone, valproate. May be a feature of severe disulphiram–alcohol reaction.

Psychotropics associated with anaemia

Aripiprazole, barbiturates, buproprion, carbamazepine, chlordiazepoxide, chlorpromazine, citalopram, clonazepam, diazepam, donepazil, galantamine, lamotrigine, MAOIs, memantine, meprobamate, mianserin, mirtazepine, nefazodone, promethazine, rivastigmine, sertraline, tranylcypromine, trazodone, valproate, venlafaxine, zotepine.

Psychotropics associated with increased APTT

Buproprion, phenothiazines, especially chlorpromazine.

Note: Buproprion and modanifil may rarely be associated with a decreased APTT.

Psychotropics associated with basophilia

Tricyclic antidepressants, especially desipramine.

Note: there are currently no psychotropics thought to be associated with a basopaenia.

Psychotropics associated with eosinophilia

Amitriptyline, beta-blockers (when used for anxiety), carbamazepine, chloral hydrate, chlorpromazine, clonazepam, clozapine, donepazil, fluphenazine, haloperidol, imipramine, meprobamate, modafinil, nortriptyline, olanzapine, promethazine, quetiapine, SSRIs, tryptophan, valproate, zotepine; may be associated with severe disulphuram–alcohol reaction.

For agents associated with eosinopaenia see below, 'Psychotropics associated with pancytopaenia'.

Psychotropics associated with decreased erythrocyte counts

Carbamazepine, donepazil, phenytoin, chlordiazepoxide, chlorpromazine, meprobamate, trifluoperazine.

Note: there are currently no psychotropics thought to be associated with *increased* erythrocyte counts.

Psychotropics associated with a raised ESR

Clozapine, levomepromazine, maprotiline, SSRIs, zotepine.

Note: there are currently no psychotropics thought to be associated with a *decreased* ESR.

Psychotropics associated with decreased haemoglobin

Carbamazepine, phenytoin, chlordiazepoxide, chlorpromazine, meprobamate, trifluoperazine.

Note: there are currently no psychotropics thought to be associated with *increased* haemoglobin.

Psychotropics associated with impaired platelet aggregation

Chlordiazepoxide, citalopram, diazepam, fluoxetine, fluvoxamine, paroxetine, sertraline.

Psychotropics associated with leukocytosis

Bupropion, carbamazepine*, chlorpromazine, citalopram, clozapine*, duloxetine, fluphenazine, haloperidol, lithium, olanzapine, quetiapine, risperidone, rivastigmine, trazodone, venlafaxine, zotepine; leukocytosis may also be associated with anticonvulsant hypersensitivity syndrome, neuroleptic malignant syndrome, and serotonin syndrome.

*Usually associated with leukopaenia.

Psychotropics associated with leukopaenia

Amitriptyline, amoxapine, bupropion, carbamazepine, chlorpromazine, citalopram, clomipramine, clonazepam, clozapine, duloxetine, fluphenazine, gabapentin, haloperidol, lamotrigine, lorazepam, MAOIs, memantine, meprobamate, mianserin, mirtazepine, modafinil, nefazodone, olanzapine, oxazepam, pregabalin, promethazine, quetiapine, risperidone, tranylcypromine, valproate, venlafaxine, zotepine.

Psychotropic associated with lymphopaenia

Chloral hydrate.

Psychotropics associated with monocytosis

Chloral hydrate, haloperidol.

Note: there are currently no psychotropics thought to be associated with monocytopaenia.

Psychotropics associated with neutropaenia

Amitriptyline, chloral hydrate, chlorpromazine, citalopram, clomipramine, clonazepam, clozapine, desipramine, fluphenazine, haloperidol, imipramine, lorazepam, mirtazepine, nefazodone, nortriptyline, olanzapine, prochlorperazine, promazine, quetiapine, risperidone, thioridazine, tranylcypromine, trazodone, valproate, venlafaxine, ziprasidone.

Psychotropics associated with pancytopaenia

Bupropion, carbamazepine, clomipramine, diazepam, fluphenazine, lamotrigine, lorazepam, mirtazepine, valproate.

Psychotropics associated with thrombocytopaenia

Acetylcysteine, amitriptyline, barbiturates, bupropion, carbamazepine, clomipramine, chlordiazepoxide, chlorpromazine, clonazepam, clozapine, diazepam, donepazil, duloxetine, fluphenazine, imipramine, galantemine, lamotrigine, MAOIs, memantine, meprobamate, methodone, mirtazepine, naltrexone, olanzapine, pregabalin, promethazine, risperidone, rivastigmine, sertraline, tranylcypromine, trazodone, valproate, zotepine; thrombocytopaenia may also be associated with the disulfiram–alcohol syndrome.

Psychotropics associated with thrombocytosis

Lithium, naltrexone.

Psychotropics associated with hepatotoxicity

Note: almost all psychotropics may be associated with non-specfic, abnormal LFT, as may certain medication-associated syndromes (anticonvulsant–hypersensitivity syndrome, disulfiram–alcohol syndrome, neuroleptic malignant syndrome, and serotonin syndrome) and substances of abuse (alcohol, amphetamines, caffeine, ketamine, opioids, and volatile solvents).

Agents specifically associated with cholestasis

Amitriptyline, benzodiazepines, carbamazepine, imipramine, phenothiazines.

Agents specifically associated with hepatocellular injury

Amitriptyline, carbamazepine, disulfiram, ethanol, imipramine, MAOIs, phenobarbital, phenytoin, valproate.

Psychotropics associated with nephrotoxicity

A large number of psychotropics have been reported to have effects on renal function, with impaired renal function influencing all aspects of drug metabolism, especially excretion.

Below is a list of the agents reported to be associated with impaired renal function; for further details see the relevant entry for each individual agent in Chapters 4 and 5.

Hyponatraemia is the most common effect, and may result from various causes, including hyperglycaemia, severe hyperlipidaemia, SIADH, or water intoxication (as, for example, in psychogenic polydypsia).

Table Psychotropics associated with nephrotoxicity

Class	Agent	Renal effects	Relevant laboratory tests	Notes
Anticonvulsants/ mood stabilizers	Carbamazepine	Acute renal failure	FBC, phosphate, U&E, urinalysis	Rare event, may manifest with tubular necrosis or tubulointerstitial nephritis
		Hyponatraemia Proteinuria		
	Lamotrigine	None reported		
	Lithium	Hypokalaemia	U&E	Lithium is recognized to be highly nephrotoxic, with polyuria/polydipsia a common symptom. Close monitoring of patients receiving lithium is therefore vital
		Nephrogenic diabetes insipidus	U&E Plasma and urine osmolality	
		Nephropathy	U&E, urinalysis	
		Raised levels of ADH	See Chapter 3	
	Valproic acid	Nephropathy Renal failure	FBC, phosphate, U&E	Renal damage may be related to chronic use at high doses
		Fanconi's syndrome	Blood gases, plasma lactate, U&E	Fanconi's syndrome is characterized by injury to the proximal renal tubule
Antidementia drugs	Donepezil	Glycosuria	Blood glucose, urinalysis	May be secondary to diabetes mellitus
		Hyponatraemia	U&E	See Chapter 3
	Galantamine	Glycosuria	Blood glucose, urinalysis	May be secondary to diabetes mellitus
	Memantine	Hyponatraemia	U&E	See Chapter 3

	Rivastigmine	Glycosuria	Blood glucose, urinalysis	May be secondary to diabetes mellitus
		Hypokalaemia Hyponatraemia	U&E	Rare effects
Antidepressants	Duloxetine Flupentixol	Hyponatraemia/SIADH	See Chapter 3	
	Maprotiline Mianserin Mirtazepine	Hypokalaemia	U&E	Rare effect
		Hyponatraemia/SIADH	See Chapter 3	
	Moclobemide	None reported		
	MAOIs	Hyponatraemia/SIADH	See Chapter 3	
	Reboxetine	Hyponatraemia/SIADH		
		Hypokalaemia	U&E	Rare effect
	SSRIs Trazodone TCAs	Hyponatraemia/SIADH	See Chapter 3	
	Tryptophan	None reported		
	Venlafaxine	Hyponatraemia/SIADH	See Chapter 3	
Antimuscarinics	Benztropine Hyoscine Orphenadrine Procyclidine	None reported		
Antipsychotics: atypicals	Amisulpride	Hyponatraemia/SIADH	See Chapter 3	
	Aripiprazole	None reported		
	Clozapine	Glycosuria	Blood glucose, urinalysis	May be secondary to diabetes mellitus
		Interstitial nephritis	U&E, urinalysis	Rare effect

Table Psychotropics associated with nephrotoxicity (Cont.)

Class	Agent	Renal effects	Relevant laboratory tests	Notes
	Olanzapine	None reported		
	Quetiapine Risperidone Sertindole	Hyponatraemia/SIADH	See Chapter 3	
	Zotepine	Increased serum creatinine	U&E	Rare effect
Antipsychotics: phenothiazines and related agents	Benperidol	None reported		
	Chlorpromazine Flupentixol Fluphenazine Haloperidol Levomepromazine Pericyazine Perphenazine	Hyponatraemia/SIADH	See Chapter 3	
	Pimozide	Hypokalaemia	U&E	Rare effect
	Pipotiazine Prochlorperazine Promazine Sulpiride	Hyponatraemia/SIADH	See Chapter 3	
	Thioridazine	Myoglobinuria	Serum creatine kinase, aspartate transaminase, myoglobin (urine)	Rare event, may be a consequence of rhabdomyolysis in overdose
	Trifluoperazine Zuclopenthixol	Hyponatraemia/SIADH	See Chapter 3	
Anxiolytics	Benzodiazepines	Hyponatraemia/SIADH		
		Myoglobinuria	Serum creatine kinase, aspartate transaminase, myoglobin (urine)	Rare event, may be a consequence of rhabdomyolysis in overdose

Buspirone Beta-blockers	None reported		
Meprobamate	Hyponatraemia/SIADH	See Chapter 3	
	Proteinuria	U&E, urinalysis	May be seen with drug-induced porphyria
Barbiturates	Hyponatraemia/SIADH	See Chapter 3	
	Proteinuria	U&E, urinalysis	May be seen with drug-induced porphyria
CNS stimulants — Dexamphetamine	Renal failure	FBC, phosphate, U&E	May be manifest in overdose
	Rhabdomyolysis	Serum creatine kinase, aspartate transaminase, myoglobin (urine)	
Modafinil	None reported		
Drugs used in substance dependence — Acamprosate	Acute renal failure	FBC, phosphate, U&E	
Disulfiram Buprenorphine	None reported		
Bupropion	Hyponatraemia/SIADH	See Chapter 3	
Lofexidine	None reported		
Methadone	Hypokalaemia Hyponatraemia	U&E	May be secondary to hypo-adrenalism
	Myoglobinuria	Serum creatine kinase, aspartate transaminase, myoglobin (urine)	May be secondary to rhabdomyolysis
Naltrexone Nicotine	None reported		

Table Psychotropics associated with nephrotoxicity (Cont.)

Class	Agent	Renal effects	Relevant laboratory tests	Notes
Hypnotics	Antihistamines	Proteinuria	U&E, urinalysis	May be seen with drug-induced porphyria
	Chloral hydrate	Albuminuria Ketonuria	U&E, urinalysis	Rare events, may be a result of non-specific renal toxicity
	Clomethiazole	None reported		
	Triclofos	Albuminuria	U&E, urinalysis	Rare event following non-specific renal toxicity
	Zaleplon Zolpidem Zopiclone	Hyponatraemia/SIADH	See Chapter 3	

Psychotropics specifically associated with thyroid dysfunction

Agents associated with hyperthyroidism
Dexamphetamine, moclobemide.

Agents associated with hypothyroidism
Aripiprazole, carbamazepine, lithium, rivastigmine.

Psychotropics associated with pancreatitis

Clozapine, donepazil, olanzapine, pregabalin, rivastigmine, SSRIs (rare), valproate.

Psychotropics associated with raised cholesterol/hyperlipidaemia

Aripiprazole, beta-blockers, chlorpromazine, clozapine, memantine, mirtazapine, modafinil, olanzapine, quetiapine, rivastigmine, venlafazine, zotepine.

References

1. Oakley AM, Hodge L. Cutaneous vasculitis from maprotiline. Aust NZ J Med 1985; 15: 256–7.
2. Moldawsky RJ. Hepatotoxicity associated with maprotiline therapy: case report. J Clin Psychiatry 1984; 45: 178–9.
3. Weinstein RP, Gosselin JY. Case report of hepatotoxicity associated with maprotiline. Can J Psychiatry 1988; 33: 233–4.
4. Durrant S, Read D. Fatal aplastic anaemia associated with mianserin. Br Med J (Clin Res Ed) 1982; 285: 437.
5. Gomez-Gil E, Salmeron JM, Mas A. Phenelzine-induced fulminant hepatic failure. Ann Intern Med 1996; 124: 692–3.
6. Favale E, Rubino V, Mainardi P, Lunardi G, Albano C. Anticonvulsant effect of fluoxetine in humans. Neurology 1995; 45: 1926–7.
7. Gillman MA, Sandyk R. Hematuria following tricyclic therapy. Am J Psychiatry 1984; 141: 463–4.
8. Chan TY. Drug-induced syndrome of inappropriate antidiuretic hormone secretion. Causes, diagnosis and management. Drugs Aging 1997; 11: 27–44.
9. Nankivell BJ, Bhandari PK, Koller LJ. Rhabdomyolysis induced by thioridazine. BMJ 1994; 309: 378.
10. Church CO, Stevens DL, Fugate SE. Diabetic ketoacidosis associated with aripiprazole. Diabet Med 2005; 22: 1440–3.
11. El Hajj I, Sharara AI, Rockey DC. Subfulminant liver failure associated with quetiapine. Eur J Gastroenterol Hepatol 2004; 16: 1415–18.
12. El-Sayed S, Symonds RP. Lorazepam induced pancytopenia. Br Med J (Clin Res Ed) 1988; 296: 1332.

General
Psychopharmacology

Further Reading

ABPI Medicines Compendium 2007. London: Datapharm Communications, 2007.

Bazaire S. Psychotropic Drug Directory 2007. Aberdeen, UK: HealthComm, 2007.

British National Formulary 55 (March 2008). London: British Medical Association and Royal Pharmaceutical Society of Great Britain, 2008.

Hall RL, Smith AG, Edwards JG. Haematological safety of antipsychotic drugs. Expert Opin Drug Saf 2003; 2: 395–9.

Jacobs DS, DeMott WR, Grady HJ et al. Laboratory Test Handbook, 4th edn. Hudson, OH: Lexi-Comp, 1996.

Lacy CF, Armstrong LL, Goldman MP, Lance LL. Drug Information Handbook with International Trade Name Index, 11th edn. Hudson, Ohio: Lexi-Comp, 2007.

Newcomer JW. Second-generation (atypical) antipsychotics and metabolic effects: a comprehensive literature review. CNS Drugs 2005; 19 (Suppl 1): 1–93.

Newcomer JW. Metabolic considerations in the use of antipsychotic medications: a review of recent evidence. J Clin Psychiatry 2007; 68 (Suppl 1): 20–7.

Oyesanmi O, Kunkel EJ, Monti DA, Field HL. Hematologic side effects of psychotropics. Psychosomatics 1999; 40: 414–21.

Pies RW. Handbook of Essential Psychopharmacology. Washington, DC: American Psychiatric Press, 1998.

Taylor D, Paton C, Kerwin R. The Maudsley Prescribing Guidelines, 9th edn. London: Informa, 2007.

Young DS. Effects of Drugs on Laboratory Tests, 5th edn. Washington, DC: AACC Press, 2001.

Young DS, Friedman RB. Effects of Disease on Laboratory Tests, 4th edn. Washington, DC: AACC Press, 2001.

chapter 5

Laboratory aspects of psychopharmacology 2: Therapeutic drug monitoring

Important facts

Therapeutic drug monitoring (TDM) in psychiatry has three main applications: (1) in individualizing therapy; (2) in diagnosing potential toxicity; and (3) for measuring compliance.

There are comparatively few psychotropic medications for which therapeutic drug monitoring is currently performed.

Table Psychotropics for which therapeutic drug monitoring may be indicated

Indication	Agent
In individualizing therapy	Carbamazepine Clozapine Lithium
In diagnosing potential toxicity	Carbamazepine Clozapine Lithium Olanzapine* Valproate
For measuring compliance	Carbamazepine Clozapine Lamotrigine* Lithium Olanzapine* Valproate
*TDM not routinely performed.	

Note: although TDM has been mooted for a number of other psychotropics (see 'Other agents' at end of chapter), appropriate reference ranges have yet to be validated for these agents and TDM is therefore not currently recommended for these agents.

All patients being considered for TDM must have the following performed: full psychiatric, medical, and drug history in addition to a full physical examination, appropriate baseline laboratory investigations (see individual agents for specific details), and general baseline parameters including weight, height, blood pressure, and pulse/temperature/respiratory rate.

Current or future pregnancy requires specialist advice.

Note: the UK NICE has published guidelines for TDM of selected medications; this advice is summarized below.

Table NICE recommended reviews in medicated patients following initial screening			
Time	*Medication*	*Laboratory parameter*	*Notes*
3-Monthly	Lithium	Lithium levels	Three times over 6 weeks following initiation of treatment and 3-monthly thereafter
	Olanzapine Quetiapine Risperidone	Glucose Lipid profile	Olanzapine is associated with increased risk of metabolic syndrome (see Chapter 5); NICE suggests that antipsychotic levels be done 1 week after initiation and 1 week after dose change until levels are stable and then 3-monthly
6-Monthly	Carbamazepine	Carbamazepine levels	NICE suggests that these be done 6-monthly
		FBC LFT U&E	Other laboratory tests may be required depending on clinical presentation
	Lithium	U&E	U&E may be needed more frequently if patient deteriorates or is on angiotensin converting enzyme (ACE) inhibitors, diuretics, or non-steroidal anti-inflammatory drugs (NSAIDs)
		TFT	Thyroid function, for individuals with rapid-cycling bipolar disorder; thyroid antibodies may be measured if TFT are abnormal
	Sodium valproate	FBC LFT	NICE suggests that these be done 'over the first 6 months'
Annually	All patients	Blood glucose TFT	Other laboratory tests may be required depending on clinical presentation
	Lithium	Glucose	
	Olanzapine	Glucose Lipid profile	
	Sodium valproate	Glucose	

Therapeutic drug monitoring

For each agent the following information will be provided:

- important facts
- laboratory-related cautions
- important laboratory-related drug interactions
- laboratory monitoring
- blood concentrations.

Carbamazepine

Important facts

Carbamazepine is an anticonvulsant agent, which is also licensed for prophylaxis of bipolar affective disorder in patients non-responsive to lithium. Its various uses are summarized below.

Table   Clinical uses of carbamazepine
1. Treatment of epilepsy (partial and secondary generalized tonic–clonic seizures as well as some generalized seizures
2. Prophylaxis of bipolar affective disorder in patients non-responsive to lithium
3. Augmentation of antidepressants in refractory depression
4. Treatment of trigeminal neuralgia
5. Treatment of aggressive behaviour in patients with schizophrenia
6. Treatment (as last resort) of various other psychiatric disorders such as panic disorder and borderline personality disorder
7. Management of alcohol withdrawal symptoms

The main side-effect for which TDM is indicated is agranulocytosis (risk estimated at 1 in 20 000) although it can also be useful to monitor carbamazepine-associated alterations of liver enzymes (usually not clinically significant).

Other side-effects

Carbamazepine has a large number of side-effects which are amenable to laboratory monitoring. These include the following.

Table	Laboratory-related adverse effects of carbamazepine		
System	*Event*	*Laboratory investigation*	*Notes*
Endocrine	Galactorrhoea, gynaecomastia, impaired fertility	Prolactin	Rare events
	Thyroid dysfunction	TFT	Slight decrease in total or free T4 or elevation of thyroid stimulating hormone (TSH), important for patients receiving thyroid treatment
Gastrointestinal	Cholestatic jaundice, hepatitis	LFT	Rare events although can be fatal
	Pancreatitis	Serum amylase, lipase	Rare event
Haematological	Agranulocytosis, aplastic anaemia, bone marrow suppression, eosinophilia, leukocytosis, leukopaenia, pancytopaenia, pure red cell aplasia, thrombocytopaenia	FBC, blood smear	Rare events, leukopaenia common (up to about 7% of patients) especially in first 3 months of treatment but usually benign; eosinophilia and thrombocytopaenia have been reported in up to 2% of patients, but are usually mild and transient
	Acute intermittent porphyria	Porphyria screen	Rare event
	Folic acid deficiency	FBC, serum folate levels	Extremely rare event; mechanism unclear, effects may be less than those of other antiepileptics such as phenytoin

Table	Laboratory-related adverse effects of carbamazepine (Cont.)		
System	**Event**	**Laboratory investigation**	**Notes**
Metabolic	Hyponatraemia/ SIADH	U&E	Rare event
	Osteomalacia and other bone disturbances	Bone profile	Rare events; may manifest with raised alkaline phosphatase and reduction in 25-hydroxycholecalciferol
	Azotaemia	U&E, blood ammonia	Rare event
Renal	Proteinuria, acute renal failure	U&E, urinalysis	Rare events, may be manifest at higher doses and with polypharmacy

Laboratory-related cautions

- hepatic impairment (which causes impaired metabolism of carbamazepine)
- renal impairment (use of carbamazepine requires caution due to increased risk of renal toxicity)
- haematological disorders (especially history of haematological reactions to other medications).

Therapeutic drug monitoring

Important laboratory-related drug interactions

A large number of agents have been reported either to increase the risk of agranulocytosis (to be avoided) or affect carbamazepine levels (use with caution or avoid) and are summarized below.

Table Important laboratory-related drug interactions with carbamazepine

Agents likely to cause agranulocytosis	Azapropazone, carbamazepine, chloramphenicol, clozapine, cytotoxics, mianserin, sulphonamides; depot antipsychotics such as flupentixol, fluphenazine, haloperidol, penicillamine, pipotiazine, zuclopenthixol
Agents which may cause an increase in carbamazepine levels	Acetazolamide, amprenavir, cimetidine, clarithromycin, danazol, fluoxetine, fluvoxamine, ritonavir
Agents which may cause a decrease in carbamazepine levels	Isotretinoin, rifabutin, St John's wort, phenobarbital, phenytoin, primadone
Agents associated with increased risk of hyponatraemia	All diuretics

Laboratory monitoring

NICE guidelines

The following are recommended by NICE.

Table NICE recommended reviews in medicated patients following initial screening

Time	Medication	Laboratory parameter	Notes
6-Monthly	Carbamazepine	Carbamazepine levels	NICE suggests that these be done 6-monthly
		FBC LFT U&E	Other laboratory tests may be required depending on clinical presentation

Additional advice (non-NICE)

Prior to commencing carbamazepine, all patients should have a full psychiatric, medical, and drug history taken, undergo a thorough physical examination, and as a minimum have the following baseline laboratory measurements performed.

Table Baseline laboratory measurements for patients initiating carbamazepine	
Clinical biochemistry	U&E, creatinine, LFT
Haematology	Full blood count
Immunology	No special investigations required
Microbiology	No special investigations required

Additional, further monitoring is suggested as follows.

Table Additional laboratory monitoring with carbamazepine	
Regular monitoring in initial stages of treatment, especially with dosage titration	U&E, FBC, LFT*
6-Monthly	U&E, LFT
Other	None specific; other parameters as based on clinical suspicion
*Note: See below for advice regarding altered liver function tests with carbamazepine.	

Alterations in LFT have been reported in 5–15% of patients receiving carbamazepine and are usually benign.

A raised GGT by itself (up to twice normal) is frequently reported and is rarely clinically significant.

However, a raised ALP and GGT may suggest a hypersensitivity reaction, which may then lead to severe hypersensitivity reaction/hepatitis characterized by a low white cell count together with the raised ALP and GGT. Management strategies can include stopping the medication, reducing the dosage/re-challenging at a lower dose, or substituting a different agent.

Blood concentrations

Monitoring of plasma levels can be used to optimize treatment, monitor for possible toxicity, and check compliance; an accepted reference range in bipolar disorder is 7–12 mg/l (4–12 mg/l in epilepsy).

Blood should be collected for trough levels (i.e. just before the dose) in a plain tube. It should be noted that the time to steady-state is approximately 14 days, and as carbamazepine induces its own metabolism, levels may vary widely within a dosage interval.

Levels should be repeated 2–4 weeks after a dose alteration to ensure that they are in the therapeutic range. A starting dose of 100–200 mg daily in 1–2 divided doses is suggested, aiming to reach a maximum daily dose between 800 and 1200 mg (in divided doses).

Clozapine

Important facts

Clozapine is an 'atypical' antipsychotic which is used in the treatment of schizophrenia in patients who either have not responded to two full courses of other antipsychotics (one of which should be an 'atypical') or are intolerant of conventional antipsychotic agents (e.g. suffer from severe extrapyramidal side-effects or severe tardive dyskinesia).

Although currently unlicensed for other uses, it has been reported to have utility in the treatment of other disorders such as psychosis related to Huntington's chorea and Parkinson's disease, as well as treatment-resistant mania.

It has a number of rare, idiosyncratic but potentially life-threatening side-effects which necessitate laboratory monitoring; these include the following.

Table Important life-threatening side-effects of clozapine	
Agranulocytosis	Incidence around 0.8%, risk of fatal agranulocytosis estimated at 1 in 5000; women/older age may be risk factors
Pulmonary embolism	Rare, risk estimated at 1 in 2000–6000; may be more likely in early stages of treatment (first 3 months)
Myocarditis/ cardiomyopathy	Risk variable (from 1 in 1300 up to 1 in 67000) and may be more likely in early stages of treatment (first 2–3 months)
Seizures	Incidence around 3%, risk is dose-related and may require use of prophylactic valproate (see, for example, reference 1)

Note: the occurrence of seizures is not necessarily grounds for discontinuing clozapine; specialist advice should be sought.

Other side-effects

Clozapine has a large number of side-effects which are amenable to laboratory measurement. These include the following.

Table Clozapine side-effects which may require laboratory monitoring

System	Condition	Notes
Endocrine	Diabetes mellitus	Increasingly recognized association between clozapine and glucose intolerance/diabetes mellitus. Regular monitoring of blood glucose advised
Gastrointestinal	Cholestatic jaundice Fulminant hepatic necrosis Hepatitis	Rare events
	Pancreatitis	Rare event, may be associated with higher doses/overdose
Haematological	Agranulocytosis Eosinophilia Leukocytosis Leukopaenia Neutropaenia Thrombocytopaenia	Agranulocytosis occurs in about 1% of patients, regular monitoring of FBC mandatory *Note*: in rare cases clozapine has been associated with a 'morning pseudoneutropaenia' with lower levels of circulating neutrophil found with morning blood sampling. As neutrophil counts may show circadian rhythms, repeating the FBC at a later time of day may be instructive
Metabolic	Hypertriglyceridaemia	Rare event but regular monitoring recommended due to increased risk of cardiovascular and other complications
	Neuroleptic malignant syndrome	Rare event, may present with lower rises in creatine kinase than other atypicals
	SIADH (with increased plasma and urine osmolality)	Rare events
Renal	Interstitial nephritis	

Laboratory-related cautions

- renal impairment (slow titration suggested, plasma levels may be useful; contraindicated in acute renal disease)
- hepatic impairment (slow titration suggested as guided by plasma determinations; contraindicated in acute hepatic disorders)
- pregnancy.

Important laboratory-related drug interactions

A large number of agents have been reported either to increase the risk of agranulocytosis (to be avoided) or affect clozapine levels (use with caution or avoid) and are summarized below.

Table	Important laboratory-related drug interactions with clozapine
Agents likely to cause agranulocytosis	Azapropazone, carbamazepine, chloramphenicol, cytotoxics, mianserin, sulphonamides; depot antipsychotics such as flupentixol, fluphenazine, haloperidol, penicillamine, pipotiazine, zuclopenthixol
Agents which may cause **increased** plasma clozapine levels	Amprenavir, cimetidine, erythromycin, fluoxetine, fluvoxamine, ritonavir, sertraline, venlafaxine
Agent which may cause **decreased** plasma clozapine levels	Phenytoin

Laboratory monitoring

NICE advice   NICE does not provide any specific laboratory-related advice regarding clozapine.

Prior to commencing clozapine, all patients should have a full psychiatric, medical, and drug history taken, undergo a thorough physical examination, and as a minimum have the following baseline laboratory measurements performed.

Table Baseline laboratory measurements for patients initiating clozapine

Clinical biochemistry	U&E, creatinine, LFT, glucose, glycated haemoglobin (HbA1c), lipid panel (fasting),* prolactin
Haematology	Full blood count
Immunology	No special investigations required
Microbiology	No special investigations required

*Especially advised when specific risk factors present, e.g. obesity, history of cardiovascular disease, diabetes mellitus, hypercholesterolaemia, etc.

As the main severe side-effect is agranulocytosis, weekly full blood counts are required for the first 18 weeks, then 2-weekly until 1 year; if blood counts remain stable, then 4-weekly thereafter (including 4 weeks post-discontinuation).

In the UK there is a 'traffic light' system of monitoring FBC.

Result	Interpretation	Action
Green	Within normal limits	Continue dosing/routine monitoring
Amber	Reduced white cell count (WCC)	Senior advice required re continued dosing/ repeat test (twice weekly) until green
Red	WCC <3.0×10^9/l or neutrophil count <1.5×10^9/l	Stop treatment and monitor blood daily/seek senior advice

Regular laboratory monitoring of laboratory parameters is suggested below.

Table Additional laboratory monitoring with clozapine

Regular monitoring	FBC
3-Monthly	HbA1c, lipid panel
6-Monthly	U&E, LFT, lipid panel*
Other	Creatine phosphokinase (CPK) (if NMS suspected); other parameters as based on clinical suspicion (see Table below)

*Especially advised when specific risk factors present.

Additional monitoring is indicated by clinical suspicion of specific adverse effects.

Table Other laboratory investigations for side-effects of clozapine

System	Condition	Laboratory investigation
Cardiac	Myocarditis	Raised cardiac enzymes (creatine kinase-MB, α-hydroxybutyrate dehydrogenase, troponin T measured in some laboratories) Raised ESR
	Cardiomyopathy	No specific laboratory investigations
Endocrine	Diabetes mellitus	Raised fasting blood sugar (especially >10 mmol/l in whole blood, >12 mmol/l in capillary plasma); oral glucose tolerance test (OGTT) may be required HbA1c
Gastrointestinal	Colitis	None specific, ESR C-reactive protein (CRP) suggested for monitoring purposes
	Cholestatic jaundice Fulminant hepatic necrosis Hepatitis	LFT, clotting screen
	Pancreatitis	Pancreatic amylase
Haematological	Eosinophilia Leukocytosis Leukopaenia Thrombocytopaenia Thrombocytosis	FBC
Metabolic	Hypertriglyceridaemia	Plasma lipids
Renal	Interstitial nephritis	U&E Creatinine

Blood concentrations

Monitoring of plasma levels can be used to optimize treatment, monitor for possible toxicity, and check compliance; an accepted reference range is 350–500 µg/l.

Blood should be collected for trough levels (i.e. just before the dose) in a plain tube. It should be noted that the time to steady-state is approximately

3 days, and levels may be lower in males, especially those who are younger and smoke.

Reported clozapine levels may also include a measurement of norclozapine (*N*-desmethylclozapine) levels. Norclozapine is a major, pharmacologically active metabolite of clozapine but as yet there is no accepted reference range. The metabolic ratio of clozapine to norclozapine (reference value=1.32) may be a useful marker of compliance, with high ratios suggestive of over-dose and lower ratios suggestive of poor compliance.[2,3]

A recent publication[3] has suggested that pre-dose (trough) clozapine levels may be individualized through the use of nomograms.

These nomograms suggest that levels are influenced by factors such as smoking and body fat, which may therefore alter plasma levels and increase the likelihood of serious side-effects in susceptible individuals. Additionally, these nomograms may be useful in assessing treatment compliance.

Although most clozapine-related side-effects may not necessarily require cessation of treatment, any suspicion of adverse effects must be investigated immediately, with specialist advice sought where appropriate.

It is suggested that clozapine be commenced at a dose of 12.5 mg on day one, then 12.5 mg twice a day with slow titration upwards if the patient is able to tolerate this (beware hypotensive effects).

Although the average daily dose in the UK is approximately 450 mg/day, there is wide variation in individual patient response, with effective daily doses ranging between 150 and 900 mg/day.

Criteria for discontinuation

- if leukocyte count falls below 3.0×10^9/l or absolute neutrophil count falls below 1.5×10^9/l
- if patients report influenza-like illness (may herald agranulocytosis)
- if myocarditis/cardiomyopathy is suggested (may present clinically with arrhythmia, especially tachycardia)
- In the UK there is a traffic light system for monitoring risk of clozapine-associated agranulocytosis via FBC/neutrophil counts.

Colour	Action
Green	Continue treatment and follow routine monitoring guidelines
Amber	Continue treatment but continue monitoring FBC at least twice weekly until green or red result
Red	Stop treatment, daily FBC

Lamotrigine

Important facts

Lamotrigine is an anticonvulsant agent, which also has activity in mania, although it is not currently used as a first-line agent and is often given as an adjunct to other mood stabilizers. Its main clinical uses are summarized below.

Table Clinical uses of lamotrigine
1. Treatment of epilepsy (partial and secondary generalized tonic–clonic seizures as well as partial and myoclonic seizures)
2. Treatment of mania/bipolar affective disorder (either as monotherapy or in combination with another mood stabilizer)
3. Augmentation of clozapine in refractory schizophrenia
4. Treatment of seizures associated with the Lennox–Gastaut syndrome (progressive epileptic syndrome in infancy, associated with generalized brain damage with absences, myoclonic jerks, drop attacks)

It has a number of severe, dose-related side-effects including hypersensitivity reactions (skin rash, Stevens–Johnson syndrome), blood disorders (bone-marrow failure), and neurological symptoms; TDM is mainly performed to check treatment compliance.

Other side-effects

Lamotrigine has a number of side-effects which are amenable to laboratory measurement. These include the following.

Table Lamotrigine side-effects which are amenable to laboratory monitoring			
System	**Event**	**Laboratory tests**	**Notes**
Gastrointestinal	Hepatic dysfunction	LFT	Rare events
Haematological	Anaemia Leukopaenia Pancytopaenia Pure red cell aplasia Thromobocytopaenia Clotting disorders	FBC, clotting screen	

Therapeutic drug monitoring

Laboratory-related cautions

- hepatic impairment
- renal impairment
- pregnancy.

Important laboratory-related drug interactions

A number of agents have been reported to affect lamotrigine levels (use with caution or avoid) and are summarized below.

Table Important laboratory-related drug interactions with lamotrigine

Implicated agent	Effect	Notes
Valproate	May cause *increase* in lamotrigine plasma levels	Valproate inhibits metabolism of lamotrigine
Carbamazepine	May cause *decrease* in plasma lamotrigine levels	Increased neurotoxicity has been reported with carbamazepine and lamotrigine
Phenobarbital Phenytoin Primidone		Phenobarbital and phenytoin increase elimination of lamotrigine

Laboratory monitoring

There are currently no NICE guidelines for laboratory monitoring of lamotrigine.

Prior to commencing lamotrigine, all patients should have a full psychiatric, medical, and drug history taken, undergo a thorough physical examination, and as a minimum have the following baseline laboratory measurements performed.

Table Baseline laboratory measurements for patients initiating lamotrigine

Clinical biochemistry	U&E, creatinine, LFT
Haematology	Full blood count, clotting screen
Immunology	No special investigations required
Microbiology	No special investigations required

Regular laboratory monitoring of laboratory parameters is suggested below.

Table	Additional laboratory monitoring with lamotrigine
Regular monitoring with dose titration	U&E, LFT, FBC, clotting
3–6-Monthly	U&E, LFT
Other	None specific; other parameters as based on clinical suspicion

Blood concentrations

Monitoring of serum levels can be used to assess possible toxicity and check compliance; although there is currently no firmly established reference range, ranges of 2–4 μg/ml and 10–60 μmol/l have been reported.

Blood should be collected for trough levels (i.e. just before the dose) in a plain tube. It should be noted that the time to steady-state is approximately 5 days.

It is suggested that doses be titrated slowly and closely monitored, with a target dose range of 50–200 mg/day. A suggested regimen for lamotrigine monotherapy is 25 mg daily for 14 days, then increased as required by 25-mg increments every 14 days with close monitoring of clinical and laboratory parameters.

Lithium

Important facts

Lithium is a monovalent cation which has the following clinical uses.

Table	Clinical uses of lithium
1. Prophylaxis and treatment of bipolar affective disorder
2. Prophylaxis of recurrent depression, especially as an adjunct in refractory depression
3. As an adjunct to antipsychotics in the treatment of schizoaffective disorder
4. In the treatment of aggressive or self-mutilating behaviour
5. In the treatment of steroid-induced psychosis

Therapeutic drug monitoring

Lithium has a narrow therapeutic index and has a number of important adverse effects in overdose, which may be fatal; these include neurological effects (tremor, ataxia, nystagmus, convulsions, confusion, slurred speech, coma) as well as renal impairment.

Other side-effects

Early side-effects of lithium are dose-related and include gastrointestinal side-effects (nausea, vomiting, diarrhoea), tremor (may manifest as intention tremor), and dry mouth.

Later side-effects amenable to laboratory measurement are more numerous and appear at higher plasma concentrations (especially >2.0 mmol/l).

Table Later side-effects of lithium which may affect laboratory parameters

System	Condition	Laboratory tests
Endocrine	Hypothyroidism/ hyperthyroidism	TFT
	Hyperparathyroidism	See Chapter 6
	Nephrogenic diabetes insipidus	U&E
	Raised levels of antidiuretic hormone (ADH)	See Chapter 3
Haematology	Leukocytosis Thrombocytosis	FBC
Metabolic	Hypercalcaemia (may cause cardiac arrhythmias)	Calcium
	Hypokalaema (may cause cardiac arrhythmias)	U&E
	Hyperglycaemia	Blood glucose, HbA1c
	Diabetes insipidus	Calcium, plasma osmolality (increased), serum sodium (decreased), U&E, urine osmolality (decreased); a water deprivation test may be needed (specialist guidance required)
Renal	Nephropathy Renal failure	eGFR, U&E, urinalysis
	SLE	Autoantibody screen
	Myasthenia gravis	Acetylcholine receptor antibodies, Tensilon® (edrophonium) test

Laboratory-related cautions

- renal impairment – avoid
- conditions with sodium imbalance (e.g. Addison's disease, diuretic treatment, low salt diet)
- hypothyroidism
- diarrhoea/vomiting (discontinue or reduce dose)
- other: myasthenia gravis, pregnancy.

Important laboratory-related drug interactions

There are a large number of agents which interact with lithium which are best avoided or used with caution where possible.

Table Important laboratory-related drug interactions with lithium	
Increased plasma lithium concentration/reduced excretion	ACE inhibitors, NSAIDs (azapropazone, diclofenac, ibuprofen, indometacin, mefenamic acid, naproxen, parecoxib, piroxicam, rofecoxib, valdecoxib; ketoralac – avoid); angiotensin II receptor antagonists; loop diuretics, thiazides, potassium-sparing diuretics
Reduced plasma lithium concentration/increased excretion	Sodium bicarbonate, acetazolamide, theophylline
Increased risk of hypothyroidism	Amiodarone
Increased neurotoxicity (*may not increase plasma concentration of lithium*)	Carbamazepine, diltiazem, metronidazole, methyldopa, phenytoin, SSRIs, verapamil

Laboratory monitoring

NICE guidelines
NICE recommends the following laboratory monitoring for lithium.

Table NICE recommended reviews in medicated patients following initial screening

Time	Medication	Laboratory parameter	Notes
3-Monthly	Lithium	Lithium levels	Three times over 6 weeks following initiation of treatment and 3-monthly thereafter
		U&E	U&E may be needed more frequently if patient deteriorates or is on ACE inhibitors, diuretics, or NSAIDs
		TFT	Thyroid function, for individuals with rapid-cycling bipolar disorder; thyroid antibodies may be measured if TFT are abnormal
		Glucose	As based on clinical presentation

Additional advice (non-NICE)
Prior to commencing lithium, the following baseline tests should be performed.

Table Baseline laboratory measurements for patients initiating lithium

Clinical biochemistry	eGFR, U&E, calcium, creatinine, TFT
Haematology	Full blood count
Immunology	No special investigations required
Microbiology	No special investigations required

Additional, regular laboratory monitoring of laboratory parameters is suggested below.

Table Additional laboratory monitoring with lithium

After 7 days	Plasma lithium levels then **weekly** until the required level is reached (between 0.6 and 1.0 mmol/l)
3-Monthly	U&E, plasma lithium levels
6–12–Monthly	eGFR, U&E, calcium, TFT
Other	CPK (if NMS suspected) Calcium if hyperparathyroidism suspected U&E if patient dehydrated/vomiting/having diarrhoea Other parameters as based on clinical suspicion

Blood concentrations

Monitoring of serum levels can be used to monitor for possible toxicity and to check compliance; an accepted reference range is 0.6–1.0 mmol/l.

Severe toxicity may occur at levels >1.5 mmol/l and death may occur at higher levels (>2.0 mmol/l), although toxicity has also been reported at only mildly elevated serum concentrations.

Blood should be collected for peak levels (i.e. 12 hours post-dose) in a plain tube (*note*: not lithium heparin tubes). It should be noted that the time to steady-state is approximately 5 days, and there is some individual variation in levels, although the above reference range is well established.

Lithium doses should be adjusted so that serum levels fall within the above range. Starting at a daily dose of 400 mg is suggested, with weekly monitoring of levels until the target serum concentration is reached and stabilized.

If toxicity/overdose suspected (serum levels >1.5 mmol/l or clinical suspicion of overdose with lower measured levels), treatment should be stopped and supportive measures implemented.

Olanzapine

Important facts

Olanzapine is an atypical antipsychotic, which has the following indications.

Table Clinical uses of olanzapine
1. As a first-line agent for the treatment of new-onset schizophrenia
2. For management of an acute psychotic episode
3. For individuals who are intolerant of conventional antipsychotics
4. For individuals whose symptoms were previously inadequately controlled
5. In the control of acute manic episodes

Laboratory-related cautions

- renal impairment (slow titration suggested, plasma levels may be useful)
- hepatic impairment (slow titration suggested as guided by plasma determinations)
- diabetes mellitus (may exacerbate condition or cause ketoacidosis)
- haematological disorders (myeloproliferative disorders, leukopaenia, hypereosinophilia, bone-marrow depression)
- pregnancy (expert advice required).

Therapeutic drug monitoring

Laboratory monitoring

NICE guidelines
NICE recommends the following laboratory monitoring of olanzapine.

Table NICE recommended reviews in medicated patients following initial screening

Time	Medication	Laboratory parameter	Notes
3-Monthly	Olanzapine	Glucose Lipid profile	Olanzapine is associated with increased risk of metabolic syndrome (see Chapter 3); NICE suggests that antipsychotic levels be done 1 week after initiation and 1 week after dose change until levels are stable and then 3-monthly

Additional advice (non-NICE)
Prior to initiating olanzapine, the following baseline laboratory tests should be undertaken.

Table Baseline laboratory measurements for patients initiating olanzapine

Clinical biochemistry	U&E, creatinine, LFT, glucose, HbA1c, prolactin
Haematology	Full blood count
Immunology	No specific investigations required
Microbiology	No specific investigations required

Additional, regular laboratory monitoring is suggested below.

Table Additional laboratory monitoring with olanzapine

3-Monthly	HbA1c, LFT
6-Monthly	U&E, LFT
Other	CPK (if NMS suspected) Prolactin if symptoms suspected Other parameters as based on clinical suspicion (see Table below)

Olanzapine has a number of other, recognized side-effects for which laboratory monitoring may be indicated.

Table Side-effects of olanzapine amenable to laboratory measurement

System	Event	Laboratory tests
Endocrine	Hyperprolactinaemia	Prolactin levels
Gastrointestinal	Hepatitis	LFT
	Pancreatitis	Serum amylase
Haematological	Blood dyscrasias (agranulocytosis, eosinophilia, neutropaenia, leukopaenia, and thrombocytopaenia)	FBC
Metabolic	Hyper- or hypoglycaemia	Blood glucose, HbA1c
	Triglyceridaemia	Lipid screen
	Neuroleptic malignant syndrome	See Chapter 3
Other	Raised creatine kinase concentration	Enzyme levels

Note: there is an increased risk of stroke, especially in elderly patients with dementia. An appropriate history with special emphasis on risk factors (hypertension, diabetes mellitus, smoking, atrial fibrillation, thromboembolic disorders) should therefore be taken in all patients.

Blood concentrations

Monitoring of serum levels can be used to check for possible toxicity and to assess compliance; an accepted reference range is 20–40 µg/l.

Severe toxicity may occur at levels >100 µg/l and death may occur at higher levels (>160 µg/l).

Blood should be collected for peak levels (i.e. 12 hours post-dose) in a plain tube. It should be noted that the time to steady-state is approximately 7 days, and there is substantial variation in serum levels, which may be lower in males.

Although olanzapine has a number of side-effects which can alter laboratory parameters, these are rare and may not require the cessation of treatment; specialist advice should be sought where there is clinical suspicion of olanzapine-related adverse events. A starting dose of 10 mg/day is suggested, increasing to 15 or 20 mg daily as required.

Valproate

Important facts

Valproate is an antiepileptic which, in its semisodium valproate form, has utility in the treatment of mania; its various clinical uses are summarized below.

Table Clinical uses of valproate
1. Use in all forms of epilepsy (tonic–clonic seizures in primary generalized epilepsy, absences (generalized, atypical), atonic, tonic, and partial seizures)   2. Acute treatment of mania (not prophylaxis)   3. As an adjunct in treatment of aggressive behaviour in dementia, mental retardation, and organic brain syndromes

It has a number of important side-effects which necessitate laboratory monitoring.

Table Side-effects of valproate amenable to laboratory measurement

System	Event	Laboratory tests
Gastrointestinal	Hepatotoxicity (abnormal liver enzymes, increased prothrombin time, jaundice)	LFT
	Pancreatitis (rare)	Serum amylase
Haematological	Anaemia	FBC
	Decreased fibrinogen	Clotting screen
	Impaired platelet aggregation	FBC, clotting screen
	Leukopaenia Pancytopaenia	FBC
	Red cell aplasia/hypoplasia	FBC, blood film
	Thrombocytopaenia	FBC, clotting screen

Other side-effects

In addition to the above, valproate has a number of other side-effects amenable to laboratory measurement; investigation should be always guided by clinical suspicions based on the presence of appropriate physical signs and symptoms.

Therapeutic drug monitoring

Table	Valproate side-effects that may require laboratory monitoring	
System	**Event**	**Laboratory tests**
Constitutional	Nausea/vomiting (secondary to possible gastric irritation)	U&E
	Vasculitis	Autoantibody screen, ESR
Endocrine	Hyperandrogenism	Urine steroid profiling
Gastrointestinal	Abnormal LFTs	Usually raised ALT, AST, and bilirubin
	Pancreatitis	Amylase, lipase
Hematologic	Agranulocytosis, anaemia (aplastic), bone marrow suppression, eosinophilia, hypofibrinogenaemia, leukopaeia, lymphocytosis, macrocytosis, pancytopaenia, thrombocytopaenia	FBC, blood smear; plasma fibrinogen levels
Metabolic	Hyperammonaemia	LFT, blood ammonium levels (use arterial blood, test not usually performed); normal range 10–$47\,\mu mol/l$ (lithium heparin or EDTA tube). May cause encephalopathy or coma
Renal	Fanconi's syndrome (renal tubular acidosis, aminoaciduria, tubular proteinaemia)	U&E, urinalysis (pH, proteinuria)

Therapeutic drug monitoring

Laboratory-related cautions

- hepatic impairment
- porphyria
- renal impairment
- pregnancy.

Important laboratory-related drug interactions

A number of agents interact with valproate to alter plasma levels or cause other effects.

Table	Important laboratory-related interactions with valproate
Agents which may increase plasma valproate levels	Cimetidine Erythromycin Fluoxetine* Topiramate
Agents which may decrease plasma valproate levels	Carbamazepine Cholestyramine (decreased absorption) Ertapenem Fluoxetine* Meropenem Phenobarbital Phenytoin Primidone
Agents which may increase risk of neutrophilia with valproate	Olanzapine

*Inconsistent effects.

Laboratory monitoring

NICE guidelines
NICE recommends the following laboratory monitoring for valproate.

Table	NICE recommended reviews in medicated patients following initial screening		
Time	*Medication*	*Laboratory parameter*	*Notes*
6-Monthly	Sodium valproate	TFT	Thyroid function, for individuals with rapid-cycling bipolar disorder; thyroid antibodies may be measured if TFT are abnormal
		FBC LFT Glucose	NICE suggests that these be done 'over the first 6 months'

Additional advice (non-NICE)
Prior to commencing valproate, the following baseline laboratory measurements should be performed.

Table Baseline laboratory investigations for patients initiating valproate

Domain	Laboratory investigations
Clinical biochemistry	U&E Creatinine LFT Clotting screen (including prothrombin time)
Haematology	FBC
Immunology	No specific investigations required
Microbiology	

Regular laboratory monitoring of laboratory parameters is guided by clinical suspicion but basic guidelines are suggested below.

Table Additional suggested laboratory monitoring with valproate

3–6-Monthly	U&E Creatinine LFT FBC
6-Monthly	FBC LFT
Others	As based on clinical suspicion/need

Blood concentrations

Therapeutic blood monitoring of valproate is useful for determining treatment compliance and in investigating potential toxicity; an accepted target range for both epilepsy and bipolar disorder is 50–100 mg/l.

Blood should be collected for trough levels (i.e. just before the dose) in a plain tube. It should be noted that the time to steady state is 2–3 days.

It is suggested that slow dose titration is undertaken, starting from a daily dose of 750 mg (as semisodium) or 500 mg (as sodium valproate slow release) in divided doses and increased up to a maximum of 2.5 g daily as guided by clinical presentation and plasma levels. The usual daily maintenance dose range is 1–2 g.

Therapeutic drug monitoring

Other agents

A number of other psychotropics have been mooted as suitable for TDM; however, currently their blood measurement is not routinely undertaken, despite a number of these having reported reference ranges. These ranges may be helpful for monitoring compliance/toxicity in rare, specific instances only.

The following Table lists those psychotropics with reported therapeutic reference ranges.

Table Psychotropics for which blood reference ranges have been reported

Class of agent	Drug	Reference range (ng/ml unless otherwise specified)
Antidepressants	Amitriptyline	80–250
	Amoxapine	20–100
	Citalopram	30–130
	Desipramine	75–350
	Doxepin	150–250
	Escitalopram	15–80
	Fluoxetine	100–800
	Fluvoxamine	150–300
	8-Hydroxyamoxapine	150–400
	Imipramine	150–250
	Maprotiline	200–600
	Mianserin	15–70
	Mirtazepine	40–80
	Moclobemide	300–1000
	Nortriptyline	50–150
	Paroxetine	70–120
	Protriptyline	70–250
	Reboxetine	10–100
	Sertraline	10–50
	Tranylcypromine	0–50
	Trazodone	800–1600

Table Psychotropics for which blood reference ranges have been reported (Cont.)

Class of agent	Drug	Reference range (ng/ml unless otherwise specified)
	Trimipramine	150–350
	Venlafaxine	25–400 µg/l
	Viloxazine	20–500
Antipsychotics	Amisulpride	100–400
	Benperidol	2–10
	Chlorpromazine	50–300
	Clozapine	350–500
	Flupentixol	>2
	Fluphenazine	0.2–4.0
	Haloperidol	5–20
	Levomepromazine	15–60
	Olanzapine	20–80
	Perazine	100–230
	Pericyazine	15–60
	Perphenazine	0.8–1.2 nmol/l
	Pimozide	15–20
	Quetiapine	70–170
	Risperidone	20–60
	Sulpiride	200–1000
	Thioridazine	1.0–1.5 µg/ml
	Ziprasidone	50–120
	Zotepine	12–120
	Zuclopentixol	4–50
Benzodiazepines	Alprazolam	20–40
	Chlordiazepoxide	0.7–1.0 µg/ml
	Clonazepam	10–50
	Diazepam	0.2–1.0 µg/ml
	Flurazepam	0–4
	Lorazepam	10–15
	Midazolam	6–15

Class of agent	Drug	Reference range (ng/ml unless otherwise specified)
	Nordiazepam	0.1–0.5 µg/ml
	Oxazepam	0.2–1.4 µg/ml
'Z' drugs	Zolpidem	90–325
	Zopiclone	60–75
Others	Acamprosate	30–75
	Bupropion	<100
	Clomethiazol	100–5000
	Meprobamate	6–12 µg/ml

Table Psychotropics for which blood reference ranges have been reported (Cont.)

References

1. Foster R, Olajide D. A case of clozapine-induced tonic-clonic seizures managed with valproate: implications for clinical care. J Psychopharmacol 2005; 19: 93–6.
2. Flanagan RJ, Amin A, Seinen W. Effect of post-mortem changes on peripheral and central whole blood and tissue clozapine and norclozapine concentrations in the domestic pig (Sus scrofa). Forensic Sci Int 2003; 132: 9–17.
3. Rostami-Hodjegan A, Amin AM, Spencer EP et al. Influence of dose, cigarette smoking, age, sex, and metabolic activity on plasma clozapine concentrations: a predictive model and nomograms to aid clozapine dose adjustment and to assess compliance in individual patients. J Clin Psychopharmacol 2004; 24: 70–8.

Therapeutic drug monitoring

Further reading

General

Bazaire S. Psychotropic Drug Directory 2007. Aberdeen, UK: HealthComm, 2007.

British National Formulary 55 (March 2008). London: British Medical Association and Royal Pharmaceutical Society of Great Britain, 2008.

Jacobs DS, DeMott WR, Grady HJ et al. Laboratory Test Handbook, 4th edn. Hudson, OH: Lexi-Comp, 1996.

Pies RW. Handbook of Essential Psychopharmacology. Washington, DC: American Psychiatric Press, 1998.

Taylor D, Paton C, Kerwin R. The Maudsley Prescribing Guidelines, 9th edn. London: Informa, 2007.

Young DS. Effects of Drugs on Laboratory Tests, 5th edn. Washington, DC: AACC Press, 2001.

Young DS, Friedman RB. Effects of Disease on Laboratory Tests, 4th edn. Washington, DC: AACC Press, 2001.

TDM of antipsychotics

Hiemke C, Dragicevic A, Grunder G et al. Therapeutic monitoring of new antipsychotic drugs. Ther Drug Monit 2004; 26: 156–60.

Carbamazepine

Taylor D, Duncan D. Doses of carbamazepine and valproate in bipolar affective disorder. Psychiatr Bull 1997; 21: 221–3.

Clozapine

Raggi MA, Mandrioli R, Sabbioni C, Pucci V. Atypical antipsychotics: pharmacokinetics, therapeutic drug monitoring and pharmacological interactions. Curr Med Chem 2004; 11: 279–96.

Lamotrigine

Goldsmith DR, Wagstaff AJ, Ibbotson T, Perry CM. Lamotrigine: a review of its use in bipolar disorder. Drugs 2003; 63: 2029–50.

Johannessen SI, Battino D, Berry DJ et al. Therapeutic drug monitoring of the newer antiepileptic drugs. Ther Drug Monit 2003; 25: 347–63.

Lithium

Schweyen DH, Sporka MC, Burnakis TG. Evaluation of serum lithium concentration determinations. Am J Hosp Pharm 1991; 48: 1536–7.

Olanzapine

Perry PJ. Therapeutic drug monitoring of atypical antipsychotics. CNS Drugs 2000; 13: 167–71.

Robertson MD, McMullin MM. Olanzapine concentrations in clinical and post-mortem blood specimens – when does therapeutic become toxic? J Forensic Sci 2000; 42: 418–21.

Valproate

Taylor D, Duncan D. Doses of carbamazepine and valproate in bipolar affective disorder. Psychiatr Bull 1997; 21: 221–3.

Other Agents

Baumann P, Hiemke C, Ulrich S et al. The AGNP-TDM expert group concensus guidelines: therapeutic drug monitoring in psychiatry. Pharmacopsychiatry 2004; 37: 243–65.

Jacobs DS, DeMott WR, Grady HJ et al. Laboratory Test Handbook, 4th edn. Hudson, OH: Lexi-Comp, 1996.

Therapeutic drug monitoring

Laboratory aspects of important organic disorders with psychiatric sequelae

This chapter will consider only the disorders listed below. For additional disorders the reader is advised to consult appropriate specialist sources of information:

- Addison's syndrome
- Cushing's syndrome
- diabetes mellitus
- hyperparathyroidism
- hyperthyroidism
- hypoparathyroidism
- hypopituitarism
- hypothyroidism
- iron-deficiency anaemia
- metachromatic leukodystrophy
- multiple sclerosis
- neuroacanthocytosis
- phaeochromocytoma
- porphyria
- systemic lupus erythematosus
- water intoxication
- Wernike–Korsakoff syndrome
- Wilson's disease.

For each condition the following information will be provided:

- definition
- psychiatric symptoms
- clinical symptoms
- clinical signs
- laboratory investigations – basic and additional.

Organic disorders

Addison's syndrome

Definition   A primary disorder of the adrenal gland resulting in inadequate production of adrenocorticoids.

Psychiatric symptoms   Observed in at least two-thirds of patients, and can include the following:

- non-specific manifestations: apathy, anxiety, cognitive impairment, fatigue, irritability, low mood, negativity, social withdrawal
- specific psychiatric disorders which may occur as a result of the illness, especially in Addisonian 'crisis': delirium, depression, psychosis; other disorders such as conversion disorders or hypochondriasis may be attributed to these patients.

Clinical symptoms (often of insidious onset)   Abdominal pain, anorexia, diarrhoea, dizziness, hypotension, joint and muscle pains (non-specific), menstrual disturbances, salt-craving, vomiting, weakness, weight loss.

Clinical signs   Increased pigmentation (especially axillae, mouth, mucous membranes, nipples, pressure areas, sun-exposed areas, skin creases), postural hypotension, vitiligo.

Laboratory investigations

Basic investigations   Basic, routine investigations should include calcium, FBC, glucose, U&E; the synacthen test should also be performed. There are a wide variety of possible changes in laboratory parameters in Addison's disease, with the major changes reported below.

Table	Possible laboratory findings in adrenal insufficiency	
System	**Laboratory parameter**	**Notes**
Metabolic	Calcium	Hypercalcaemia may be present
	Magnesium	May be increased
	Phosphate	Hypophosphataemia may be present
	Potassium	Hyperkalaemia present in about 65% of cases, although not usually in pituitary insufficiency
	Protein	May be increased due to haemoconcentration
	Sodium	Hyponatraemia present in approximately 90% of cases, and may be due to SIADH in pituitary insufficiency

Possible laboratory findings in adrenal insufficiency (Cont.)

System	Laboratory parameter	Notes
Endocrine	Adrenocorticotropic hormone (ACTH)	Diagnosis based on 'short' synacthen test: 250 µg of synacthen is injected and plasma cortisol is measured at time 0, 30, and 60 minutes post-dose. Peak levels less than 550 nmol/l suggest adrenal insuffiency. A 'long' synacthen test can be used to distinguish between primary and secondary adrenal failure
	Cortisol	Plasma and urinary free cortisol are usually low to normal
	Glucose	Hypoglycaemia may be found in as many as 50% of individuals with chronic adrenal insufficiency
	Prolactin	Levels may be increased
Haematological	Eosinophils	Eosinophilia usually present and helps to support the diagnosis
	ESR	Usually raised
	Haemoglobin	May be reduced
	Lymphocytes	Lymphocytosis may be present
	Neutrophils	Neutropaenia common
Immunology	Adrenal cortex antibodies	Found in about 70% of patients with idiopathic Addison's; destruction of the adrenal cortex may be secondary to tuberculosis, fungal infection, or lymphoma
Renal function	Creatinine	May be increased due to renal impairment (pre-renal)
	eGFR	May be decreased due to fluid depletion
	Urea	Blood urea concentration is usually increased

Organic disorders

Additional investigations

System	Laboratory parameter	Notes
Table Additional laboratory investigations and adrenal insufficiency		
Endocrine	Insulin-hypoglycaemia (insulin tolerance) test	In normal subjects insulin-induced hypoglycaemia will induce rises in ACTH and cortisol levels
	Mineralocorticoids	Normally there is a deficiency in primary hypoadrenalism, with low or low normal aldosterone levels
	Renin	Plasma renin activity usually elevated in primary hypoadrenalism
Immunology	Antibodies to 21-hydroxylase	Antibodies against 21-hydroxylase may suggest this as a cause

Cushing's syndrome

Definition Cushing's syndrome is a general term for adrenal glucocorticoid excess. Cushing's disease refers to the syndrome when it is due to a pituitary basophil adenoma.

Psychiatric symptoms At leat 50% will experience moderate to severe depressive symptoms while others will experience psychotic symptoms. Euphoria and manic presentations are rare and cognitive changes (poor concentration, memory impairment) may also occur.

Clinical symptoms Decreased libido in men, diabetes mellitus, hypertension, increased appetite, menstrual irregularities, proximal muscle weakness and wasting, osteoporosis, poor wound healing, sleep disturbances.

Clinical signs Acne, bruising, central obesity and fat redistribution, hyperglycaemia, increased disposition to infection, mild hirsutism in women, 'moon' facies, peripheral oedema, plethora, striae, thin skin, water retention.

Laboratory investigation

Basic investigations Blood: FBC, glucose; U&E; cortisol (serum and urine – see Table below).

Organic disorders

208

Table	Cushing's syndrome and laboratory parameters	
System	**Laboratory parameter**	**Notes**
Endocrine	Cortisol	Circadian secretion of cortisol lost in Cushing's (in normal subjects cortisol peaks first thing in the morning and is lowest at midnight). Levels affected by stress, hence ideally free cortisol should be measured Urinary free cortisol measured as cortisol/creatinine ratio in urine collected over a 24-hour period may be helpful Measurement of urinary 6β-hydroxycortisol may aid diagnosis Dexamethasone suppression tests are diagnostic: dexamethasone (1 mg) is given at midnight and plasma cortisol is measured at 08.00 or 09.00. In normal subjects there will be suppression of cortisol which is lost in Cushing's. The longer 48-hour test involves administration of dexamethasone 0.5 mg 6-hourly for 48 hours with the last dose 6 hours before the final blood sample. *Note*: depressive disorders and excessive alcohol intake may result in false positives
	Glucose	Hyperglycaemia often present. Glucose intolerance common, with diabetes present in approximately one-third of patients
	Insulin tolerance test	Insulin-induced hypoglycaemia in normal subjects causes a rise in cortisol levels but not normally in subjects with Cushing's syndrome (although 20% of these patients may show rises). Test may be used to distinguish between severe endogenous depression and Cushing's
Haematology	Eosinophils	Eosinopaenia may be present
	Erythrocytes	Polycythaemia may be present
	Neutrophils	Neutrophilia may be present
Clinical biochemistry	Alkaline phosphatase	May be increased
	Calcium	May be increased (increase especially associated with osteoporosis)
	Cholesterol	Slight increases may be seen (rarely clinically significant)
	Potassium	Hypokalaemia generally uncommon in patients with Cushing's; more common in ectopic ACTH syndrome
	Triglycerides	Hypertriglyceridaemia common

Organic disorders

209

Possible additional (second-line) investigations

Table Additional laboratory investigations in adrenal insufficiency

System	Laboratory parameter	Notes
Endocrine	ACTH	Plasma concentrations of ACTH in subjects with Cushing's syndrome whose blood is taken between 09.00 and 09.30 are generally significantly higher than levels in normal subjects
	Cortisol	High dose dexamethasone-suppression test involves giving 2 mg dexamethasone 6-hourly for 48 hours and measuring plasma cortisol at 0 and 48 hours An alternative is to give 8 mg dexamethasone at 23.00 and measure plasma cortisol at 08.00 subsequently for 2 days. More than 50% suppression of plasma cortisol as compared to the initial measurement suggests Cushing's rather than ectopic ACTH secretion There is also a 5-hour dexamethasone infusion test of 1 mg/hour
	Corticotropin releasing factor (CRF) test	In normal subjects, CRF produces a rise in ACTH and cortisol but causes an exaggerated response in Cushing's
	Metyrapone test	Metyrapone blocks the conversion pathway of 11-deoxycortisol to cortisol which lowers cortisol and increases plasma ACTH. This test is not often used

Diabetes mellitus

Definition A multisystem disorder associated with persistent and chronic hyperglycaemia due to a defect of insulin secretion and/or action.

A variety of subtypes have been identified, including:

- insulin-dependent diabetes (IDDM) (type Ia and Ib)
- non-insulin-dependent diabetes (NIDDM)
- diabetes secondary to other disorders (e.g. secondary to pancreatic diseases such as chronic pancreatitis or following surgery)
- diabetes associated with other hormonal states (e.g. corticosteroid excess, glucagonomas, thyrotoxicosis, phaeochromocytoma, acromegaly)
- drug-induced diabetes (secondary to, e.g. antipsychotics, diuretics, or salbutamol)
- insulin receptor abnormalities (e.g. autoantibodies to the receptor, congenital lipodystrophy, acanthosis nigricans)
- associated with genetic syndromes, e.g. Down's syndrome, Friedrich's ataxia, Huntington's chorea, porphyria.

Psychiatric symptoms A wide range of possible presentations has been identified, including anxiety, delirium, depression, eating disorders, hypochondriasis, and psychosis. In many cases it is unclear whther the psychiatric symptoms result directly from an organic syndrome or are secondary to this. It is thought that patients with poor diabetic control are more likely to have psychiatric conditions.

Early clinical symptoms and signs Balanitis, cramps in calves or feet, excessive thirst, increased urine volume, lassitude, pruritus vulvae, tingling sensation in fingers, weight loss.

Later clinical symptoms and signs Arteriosclerosis, cataracts, high-risk pregnancy, increased susceptibility to infections, myocardial disease, nephropathy, neuropathy, peripheral vascular disease, retinopathy.

Laboratory investigation

The UK NICE has published guidelines for diabetes mellitus (http://guidance. nice.org.uk/download.aspx?o=220927) and recommends the following laboratory tests.

For diagnosis Blood glucose (if classical symptoms present); if classical symptoms not present, the two glucose measurements. Measurement of glycated haemoglobin (HbA1c) may support the diagnosis. Other tests, such as autoantibodes or C-peptide, should *not* be routinely measured.

Organic disorders

Basic investigations in a psychiatric setting may include FBC, glucose (fasting), HbA1c, U&E, urine dipstick. *Note*: diabetes is a complex illness with a great many metabolic sequelae, some of which are summarized below.

Table	Laboratory parameters and diabetes mellitus	
System	**Laboratory parameter/ condition**	**Notes**
Endocrine	Blood glucose	Ideally, a fasting, venous plasma sample should be used; *note*: whole blood values are about 10% lower than plasma, fasting capillary values are about 7% higher than venous values. Values will be affected by nutritional status, and may be raised by infection, presence of inflammation, psychological state (increased in 'stress'), and medications such as beta-blockers, glucocorticoids, and thiazide diuretics
	C-peptide	A subunit of proinsulin; measurement may differentiate between endogenously and exogenously produced insulin as well as in the investigation of hypoglycaemia. Blood reference range approximately 0.5–2.0 ng/ml
	Insulin	Measurement may be used in patients with fasting hypoglycaemia in order to diagnose insulin-secreting tumours; blood reference range approximately 6–27 μIU/ml
	Proinsulin	A prohormone and major storage form of insulin; measurement may be useful for diagnosing islet cell tumours or multiple endocrine neoplasia (MEN type 1); blood reference range approximately 0–9.4 pmol/l
Gastrointestinal	Pancreatic amylase	Is often raised in diabetic ketoacidosis even without pancreatitis
Haematology	Basophils	May be increased
	HbA1c	Provides a measure of the average glucose level over the past 60 days or so; will be affected by conditions that shorten red cell life span, e.g. anaemia, B12, folate deficiency, infection, porphyria
	Leukocytes	Leukocytosis common, especially in diabetic ketoacidosis; impaired neutrophil function may result secondary to hyperosmolarity and the elevated white cell count (WCC) may occur in the absence of infection
	Platelets	May be increased

System	Laboratory parameter/ condition	Notes
Clinical biochemistry	Albumin	May be decreased
	Alkaline phosphatase	May be increased
	Calcium	May be decreased
	Chloride	May be decreased
	Dehydration	May herald hyperglycaemic ketoacidotic coma or hyperglycaemic hyperosmolar non-ketotic coma. Both are medical emergencies and will require careful rehydration and close potassium monitoring in the former
	Hypoglycaemia	Hypoglycaemia may present with features of delirium with no acidosis. May be due to altered counter-regulatory hormones, e.g secondary to pituitary tumours; may be heralded by a decrease in insulin requirements
	Ketoacidosis	Possible changes include: glycosuria, hyperglycaemia, hyperkalaemia, hypertriglyceridaemia, hyponatraemia, increased creatinine, ketonaemia, uraemia; non-respiratory adidosis (low bicarbonate, high hydrogen, normal or lowered PCO_2). Ketones may occur in other conditions such as alcoholism or prolonged fasting, especially if glucose is normal
	Lactate	Hyperlactataemia is a rare but serious complication, especially when blood lactate >5 mmol/l
	Lipoproteins	IDDM: hypertriglyceridaemia as manifested by increased very-low-density lipoprotein (VLDL) and possibly chylomicronaemia NIDDM: hypertriglyceridaemia with usually normal low-density lipoprotein (LDL) and possibly decreased high-density lipoprotein (HDL); cholesterol may be increased
	Non-ketotic hyperglycaemia	Decreased bicarbonate, hyperglycaemia, hypernatraemia, high serum osmolality, increased urea and creatinine
	Potassium	May be normal or increased

Table Laboratory parameters and diabetes mellitus (Cont.)

Organic disorders

213

Table	Laboratory parameters and diabetes mellitus (Cont.)	
System	Laboratory parameter/ condition	Notes
Renal	Creatinine	Often raised, but ketone bodies may interfere with measurement, hence measurement may not accurately reflect renal function
	Glycosuria	Most commonly due to diabetes mellitus but also occurs in pregnancy and renal tubular disorders such as Fanconi's syndrome; may be affected by a number of agents, such as ascorbic acid, lactose, with very high concentrations of creatinine, and salicylic acid (in aspirin overdose)
	Nephropathy	Proteinuria (microalbuminuria is earliest measurable change); may lead to end-stage renal failure

Hyperparathyroidism

Definition Increased secretion of parathyroid hormone with resulting raised calcium levels. May be primary (usually due to adenoma), secondary (commonly due to vitamin D deficiency or chronic renal failure), tertiary (especially following renal transplantation, chronic renal failure, or chronic malabsorption), or due to ectopic secretion.

Psychiatric symptoms Cognitive impairment, confusion, delirium, depression, impaired concentration, lethargy; psychosis and even stupor/coma in severe cases (especially when calcium levels >3 mmol/l).

Clinical symptoms Anorexia, constipation, nausea, proximal muscle weakness.

Clinical signs Bone abnormalities visible on X-ray (e.g. 'brown tumours', subperiosteal erosions, osteoporosis), bradycardia, hypertension, polydipsia, polyuria, renal stones (up to 50% of patients), shortened QT interval, vomiting.

Medical associations Chronic pancreatitis, hypertension, malignancy (especially lung, pancreas, phaeochromocytoma), peptic ulceration.

Laboratory investigation

Note: there are currently no NICE guidelines for hyperparathyroidism.

Basic investigation Calcium, plasma parathyroid hormone – raised levels high compared to calcium.

215

System	Laboratory parameter/condition	Notes
Endocrine	Calcitriol	Raised plasma levels support the diagnosis
	Parathyroid hormone (PTH)	Levels may be normal but are usually raised (interpretation is related to calcium levels and may be difficult)
Haematology	ESR	May be normal or raised
	Haemoglobin	May be decreased
	Leukocytes	May be decreased
Immunology	Immunoglobulins	Increase in monoclonal immunoglobulins possible but non-specific
Metabolic	Alkaline phosphatase	Increased levels may be found (as bone marker)
	Calcium	Usually raised calcium levels with normal circulating PTH values; persistently raised calcium levels following thiazide diuretic administration may help to distinguish between primary hyperparathyroidism and idiopathic hypercalciuria. Increased tubular and intestinal reabsorption of calcium may be found
	Chloride	May be normal or increased
	Hydroxyproline	Increased urinary excretion supports the diagnosis
	Magnesium	May be normal or reduced
	Phosphate	Serum levels usually reduced due to decreased renal tubular absorption of phosphate
Renal	Amino acids	Aminoaciduria may occur
	Renal failure	Renal failure will influence the interpretation of calcitriol and hydroxyproline measurements
	U&E/creatinine	Increases may occur due to dehydration, polydipsia, polyuria, vomiting

Table Laboratory parameters and hyperparathyroidism

Organic disorders

Hyperthyroidism

Definition A clinical syndrome characterized by raised circulating thyroid hormone concentrations. Common causes include Graves' disease, toxic multinodular goitre, toxic solitary adenoma, and thyroiditis.

Psychiatric symptoms Anxiety, cognitive decline, delirium, depression, emotional lability, feeling of apprehension, irritability, nervousness, psychosis (rare).

Clinical symptoms Fatigue, heat intolerance, menstrual irregularities, weakness.

Clinical signs Agitation, atrial fibrillation, dermopathy (pretibial myxoedema, pruritus), diaphoresis, diarrhoea, dyspnoea, eye signs (exophthalmus, 'lid lag'), goitre, hair loss, palpitations, tachycardia, thyroid bruit, tremor, weight loss.

Laboratory investigation

Note: there are currently no NICE guidelines for hyperthyroidism.

Suggested basic laboratory investigations TFT, thyroid autoantobodies (especially in Hashimoto's thyroiditis – specialist advice needed).

A summary of possible changes in laboratory parameters in hyperthyroidism is given below.

Organic disorders

217

Table Laboratory parameters and hyperthyroidism

System	Laboratory parameter/condition	Notes
Clinical biochemistry	Albumin	May be increased
	Alkaline phosphatase	May be increased
	Creatinine	May be increased
	Glucose	May be increased
	Protein	May be decreased
	Urea	May be increased
Endocrine	Free triiodothyronine (fT3); free thyroxine (T4)	High levels found in hyperthyroidism; normal levels with low TSH can occur in the early stages of disease or in partially treated disease
	Thyroid releasing hormone (TRH)	200 µg of TRH are injected intravenously and TSH levels are measured pre-dose and then at 20 and 60 minutes post-dose. A normal response (an increase in TSH of 1–20 mU/l at 20 minutes and reversion to normal levels at 60 minutes) excludes thyroid disease. The test is now only used to investigate hypothalamic and pituitary conditions
	Thyroid stimulating hormone (TSH)	May be normal but is usually decreased
Haematology	Basophils	May be decreased
	Eosinophils	May be increased
	Haemoglobin	May be decreased
	MCH MCHC	May be decreased – mild hypochromic anaemia sometimes occurs
	MCV	May be raised occasionally or more frequently reduced in hyperthyroidism
	Monocytes	May be increased
	Neutrophils	May be decreased
	Serum/red cell folate	Raised levels may be significantly increased in hyperthyroidism
Immunology	Thyroid autoantibodies	Antibodies against TSH receptor may be raised in Graves'

Hypoparathyroidism

Definition   A clinical condition characterized by hypocalcaemia and hyper-phosphataemia due to decreased secretion or activity of parathyroid hormone. Common causes include surgery (thyroid, parathyroid, laryngeal) and the condition may be associated with autoimmune disorders (pernicious anaemia, Addison's) or infiltrative conditions (haemochromatosis, Wilson's, neoplasm).

Psychiatric symptoms   Anxiety, delirium (in severe cases), depression, emotional lability, intellectual decline (in long-standing untreated individuals), irritability, obsessions, phobias, social withdrawal.

Clinical symptoms   Abdominal cramps, laryngeal stridor, lethargy, paraes-thesiae.

Clinical signs   Carpopedal spasm, cataracts, Chvostek's sign (tapping of the facial nerve resulting in facial muscle contraction), convulsions (in severe cases, usually grand-mal), papilloedema (rare), skin changes (brittle, mal-formed nails, possibly with transverse grooves; dry, rough skin), parkinsonism (in long-standing untreated individuals), tetany, Trousseau's sign (carpal spasm following occlusion of the forearm arterial circulation).

Laboratory investigation (see also hypocalcaemia in Part Two)

Note: there are currently no NICE guidelines for hypoparathyroidism.

Suggested basic laboratory investigations   Alkaline phosphatase, PTH, phosphate.

Organic disorders

A summary of possible changes in laboratory parameters in hypoparathyroidism is given below.

Table	Laboratory investigations and hypoparathyroidism	
System	Laboratory parameter/condition	Notes
Endocrine	PTH	May be undetectable in plasma from patients with hypoparathyroidism
Metabolic	Alkaline phosphatase	Usually normal; may be raised in pseudohypoparathyroidism
	Calcium	Hypocalcaemia present
	Bicarbonate	May be decreased
	Magnesium	Deficiency (e.g. in malabsorption) may result in hypocalcaemia as magnesium is required for PTH secretion and activity
	Phosphate	Hyperphosphataemia may be present in the absence of renal failure, osteomalacia, or malabsorption state
Renal	Creatinine	Meaurement can rule out renal failure as a cause of raised calcium and phosphate
	Urinary calcium	24-hour collection usually reveals low excretion but fasting urinary excretion of calcium is usually normal

Hypopituitarism

Definition   A syndrome characterized by hypofunction of one or more pituitary hormones. Causes include infection (bacterial meningitis, encephalitis), infiltration (eosinophilic granuloma, sarcoidosis), vascular causes (bleeding, infarction), tumours, autoimmune (antibodies to pituicytes), trauma.

Psychiatric symptoms   May be non-specific and insidious, including amotivation, cognitive impairment, and dysphoria; delirium psychosis may occur in rapidly developing presentations.

Clinical symptoms   Cold insensitivity, confusion, loss of secondary sexual characteristics, malaise.

Clinical signs   Fever, hair loss, hypoglycaemia, hypotension, pale, waxy skin.

Laboratory investigation

Note: there are currently no NICE guidelines for hypopituitarism.

Suggested laboratory tests   FBC, prolactin, specific hormone tests (see below – specialist advice required), T4, U&E.

Organic disorders

221

A summary of possible changes in laboratory parameters in hypopituitarism is given below.

Table Laboratory investigations and hypopituitarism

System	Laboratory parameter/condition	Notes
Endocrine	'Combined test' of pituitary function	After fasting patient overnight basal blood is taken for analysis (glucose, cortisol, follicle stimulating hormone (FSH), luteinizing hormone (LH), TSH, fT3, thyroid hormone (TH), testosterone/oestradiol, prolactin). Following this stimulation testing involving administration of TSH, gonadotropin releasing hormone (GnRH), and insulin is undertaken with repeat blood sampling. Results are compared to normal responses
	Specific hormone levels and response tests	A number of these may be considered for specific hormones such as as the insulin tolerance test or arginine infusion test for growth hormone (GH) or water deprivation test for diabetes insipidus. Specialist advice should be sought. Note that anterior pituitary dysfunction is usually associated with decreased levels of various hormones, including aldosterone, androgens, angiotensin, cortisol, FSH, gonadotropin, GH, LH, progesterone, prolactin, renin, testosterone, TSH, T4
Haematology	Eosinophils	May be increased
	Erythrocytes	Normochromic, normocytic anaemia may be present
	Leukocytes	May be decreased
	Lymphocytes	May be increased
	Reticulocytes	May be decreased
Metabolic	Glucose	May be decreased
	Urea and electrolytes	May show dilutional hyponatraemia

Hypothyroidism

Definition A clinical syndrome resulting from decreased levels of circulating thyroid hormone. Common causes include autoimmune thyroiditis (Hashimoto's disease) and following treatments such as radioactive iodine or thyroid surgery. Other causes include iodine deficiency, radiation (treatment of malignancy), certain medications (e.g. lithium), and hypothalamic disorders. Signs and symptoms of disease may be insidious and may be unnoticed by patients and relatives.

Psychiatric symptoms Anhedonia, delirium (rare), dysphoria, irritability, mania, personality changes, psychomotor agitation or retardation, psychosis (rare, may occur in long-standing untreated individuals), slowing of cognitive function, sleep disturbance, suicidality.

Clinical symptoms Cold intolerance, constipation, cramps, deafness, fatigue, menstrual disturbances, muscle pain, weakness.

Clincial signs Bradycardia, cerebellar ataxia (rare), congestive cardiac failure, dry/cool skin, facial swelling, goitre, hair loss, hoarse voice, non-pitting oedema, slowed muscle reflexes (pseudomyotonia), slowed speech, tongue thickening, weight gain.

Laboratory investigation

Note: there are currently no NICE guidelines for hypothyroidism.

Suggested laboratory tests FBC, lipid panel, TFT.

Organic disorders

223

A summary of possible changes in laboratory parameters in hypothyroidism is given below.

Table Laboratory investigations and hypothyroidism

System	Laboratory parameter/condition	Notes
Endocrine	TSH	Usually increased in primary hypothyroidism although may be normal
	T4, T3	Usually raised
Haematology	Anaemia	Mild macrocytic or normochromic, normocytic anaemia may be present; megaloblastic anaemia suggests pernicious anaemia
	Basophils	May be increased
	ESR	May be increased
	Haemoglobin	May be decreased
	MCV	Levels may be raised in hypothyroidism
	Reticulocytes	May be decreased
Immunology	Antithyroid antibodies	Microsomal and thyroglobulin antibodies may suggest an autoimmune cause such as Hashimoto's thyroiditis
Clinical biochemistry	Albumin	May be increased
	Aspartate aminotransaminase	May be increased
	Calcium	May be increased
	Creatine kinase	May be increased
	Glucose	May be decreased
	Hypercholesterolaemia	Obesity may mimic hypothyroidism. Hypercholesterolaemia may be present and predispose to additional morbidity
	Lactate dehydrogenase	Levels may be raised in some cases
	Prolactin	Raised levels may occur
Renal	Urea and electrolytes	Hypothyroidism predisposes to hyponatraemia via inappropriate secretion of antidiuretic hormone (ADH)–sodium may be significantly decreased

Iron-deficiency anaemia

Definition A syndrome of iron deficiency defined by low haemoglobin, a microcytic, hypochromic blood film, and certain clinical symptoms (see below) which may be due to a diverse number of causes. These include:

- chronic blood loss, usually of gastrointestinal origin (e.g. angiodysplasia, carcinoma, peptic ulcer), but other sources of bleeding include uterine, haematuria, and rarely self-inflicted
- increased physiological demand (e.g. pregnancy)
- malabsorption (e.g. coeliac disease)
- medications (especially anticoagulants, non-steroidals, phenytoin, chloramphenicol)
- poor dietary intake of iron (rare in Western populations but possible in strict vegans, alcoholics, and the elderly).

Psychiatric symptoms Tiredness, lassitude, depression, pica (rare); may contribute to symptoms of chronic fatigue, somatization, other functional disorders, or personality disorders (e.g. those involving deliberate self-harm).

Clinical symptoms Dysphagia (may be due to Plummer–Vinson syndrome, also known as Paterson–Kelly syndrome, the association of iron-deficiency anaemia with dysphagia, splenomegaly, gastric achlorhydria and koilonychia; occurs mainly in pregnant women); sore tongue.

Clinical signs Face pallor, gastritis (may be asymptomatic), nail flattening/ koilonychia, tongue signs (angular stomatitis, glossitis, papillary atrophy).

Laboratory investigation

Note: there are currently no NICE guidelines for iron-deficiency anaemia.

Suggested laboratory investigations FBC; haematinics in some cases (specialist advice needed).

Organic disorders

Table Laboratory investigations and iron-deficiency anaemia

System	Laboratory parameter/condition	Notes
Clinical biochemistry	Cholesterol	May be decreased
	Erythrocytes	May be increased
Haematology	Ferritin (serum)	Levels will be low in iron-deficiency anaemia and usually raised in chronic inflammatory states and liver disease
	Free erythrocyte protoporphyrin*	Increased levels in early stages of iron-defiency anaemia but also other conditions, e.g. sideroblastic anaemia, lead poisoning
	Full blood count	A low haemoglobin will suggest anaemia
	Haemoglobin	Usually decreased
	Iron (serum)	Levels will be low in iron-deficiency anaemia but note that there may be fluctuation; levels also low in chronic disease states
	Leukocytes	May be decreased
	MCH MCHC MCV	Reduced in iron-defiency anaemia
	Serum transferrin receptor level*	Levels raised in iron-deficiency anaemia and haemolysis
	Total iron-binding capacity	Levels will be low in anaemia of chronic disease and raised in iron-deficiency anaemia
	Transferrin saturation	Levels usually >20%, will be low in iron-defiency anaemia; low levels may also be found in the elderly and in chronic disease states. Transferrin usually raised in haemochromatosis
	Zinc protoporphyrin*	Raised levels in iron-defiency anaemia in late stages

*Non-routine investigations.

Metachromatic leukodystrophy

Definition A lysosomal storage disease of various subtypes characterized by progressive motor and neurocognitive decline.

Psychiatric symptoms (adult onset form of metachromatic leuko-dystrophy (MLD) Behavioural changes, cognitive declines, dementia, disinhibition, impulsiveness, psychosis.

Clinical symptoms Behavioural changes, decreased attention span, intellectual decline, memory deficits, psychosis, seizures, speech abnormalities.

Clinical signs Gait abnormalities, hyperreflexia initially then hyporeflexia, optic atrophy, tremor, truncal ataxia.

Laboratory investigation

Note: there are currently no NICE guidelines for metachromatic leukodystrophy.

Suggested laboratory investigations Requires specialist advice.

A summary of possible changes in laboratory parameters in metachromatic leukodystrophy is given below.

Table Laboratory investigation of metachromatic leukodystrophy		
System	*Laboratory parameter*	*Notes*
Clinical biochemistry	Aspartate aminotransferase	Increased levels especially in initial stages
	Cerebrospinal fluid (CSF) protein	Levels may be normal or increased
	Urine sulphatide levels	Levels of the enzyme sulphatidase are deficient in MLD
Haematology	None specific	
Histology	Biopsy and microscopy: gallbladder, kidney, or peripheral nerve	Metachromatic granules may be seen; nerves stain yellow-brown with cresyl violet dye
Immunology	None specific	
Microbiology		
Other	Arylsulphatase A enzyme activity	Enzyme may be measured *in vitro* (leukocyte or skin fibroblast cultures); levels may also be low in arylsulphatase A pseudodeficiency (low enzyme levels in clinically normal individuals)

Organic disorders

227

Multiple sclerosis

Definition   A condition of unknown aetiology in which demyelination occurs in areas of the brain and spinal cord. The course is usually one of chronic relapse and remission.

Psychiatric symptoms   Depression (common), emotional lability, euphoria (rare), intellectual impairment, psychosis (rare), suicidality (associated wth degree of physical disability).

Clinical symptoms   Bladder disturbances (frequency, incontinence, urgency); visual (blurring, dimming, diplopia, loss of acuity, periocular pain especially on movement, reduced colour vision, vertigo); sensory symptoms (deafness, headache, impaired joint position/vibration sensation, L'Hermitte's sign (flexing the neck causes paraesthesiae in the legs and occasionally trunk and upper limbs), numbness, paraesthesiae).

Clinical signs   Cerebellar signs (abnormal eye movements, impaired balance, speech incoordination), impaired mobility, vomiting.

Laboratory investigation

The UK NICE has published guidelines for multiple sclerosis (MS) (http://guidance.nice.org.uk/CG8/guidance/English) and suggests that the diagnosis be made on clinical grounds, with laboratory investigation (e.g. of CSF) reserved for situations where there is clinical uncertainty or to rule out possible differentials. Specialist advice should therefore be sought prior to requesting laboratory investigations.

Possible alterations in laboratory parameters in multiple sclerosis are summarized below.

Table Laboratory parameters and multiple sclerosis

Medium	Laboratory parameter	Notes
Serum	Cholesterol	May be increased
	GGT	May be increased
CSF	Immunoglobulins	Protein electrophoresis may show discrete bands in gamma 4 and gamma 5 regions of immunoglobulin G (IgG) (oligoclonal bands) in 90% of cases. Note that these are not specific to MS and may also occur in conditions such as neurosyphilis and neurosarcoid. Neurosarcoid may present with extrapulmonary, non-specific CNS features such as personality change, delirium, dementia, seizures. CSF analysis is helpful (look for increased protein, lymphocytosis, decreased glucose, possibly oligoclonal bands) and serum angiotensin converting enzyme (ACE) levels may be raised. Magnetic resonance imaging (MRI) may be helpful
	Lymphocyte count	Usually normal but may be raised
	Total protein	Usually raised (<1 g/l), with increased IgG concentrations. Ratio of IgG/albumin may be greatly increased and will be abnormal in about 80% of cases of MS. Note that other conditions such as neurosyphilis and neurosarcoid will also show abnormally increased ratios

Organic disorders

229

Neuroacanthocytosis

Definition   Neuroacanthocytosis (also known as Levine–Critchley syndrome) is an extremely rare, progressive movement disorder due to degeneration of the basal ganglia.

Psychiatric symptoms   Anxiety, apathy, dementia (subcortical), depression, impulsivity, obsessive–compulsive disorder (OCD), paranoia/psychosis.

Clinical signs and symptoms   Diminished/absent deep muscle reflexes, movement disorders (chorea, dystonia, gait abnormalities, ororfacial dyskinesia, parkinsonism), muscle wasting, seizures, tics (motor and/or vocal); there may be weight loss secondary to eating dystonia.

Laboratory investigation

There are currently no NICE guidelines for neuroacanthocytosis. Specialist advice should be sought prior to requesting laboratory investigations.

Table Laboratory investigations in neuroacanthocytosis		
System	*Laboratory parameter*	*Notes*
Clinical biochemistry	Creatine phosphokinase	May be normal or elevated
	LFT	Serum transaminases may be elevated
Haematology	Blood smear for acanthocytes (irregularly contracted red cells, also known as 'spur' cells)	Normal level of acanthocytes in blood is <3%; in neuroacanthocytosis this may be raised up to 30%. Other conditions to be excluded include abetalipoproteinaemia, haemolytic anaemia, liver disease (especially advanced), splenectomy
Immunology	None specific	
Microbiology		

Phaeochromocytoma

Definition A rare tumour (incidence probably less than 1%) of the adrenal medulla which usually secretes norepinephrine, causing hypertension, and if untreated can lead to death from cardiovascular disease or cerebral haemorrhage.

Psychiatric symptoms Anxiety symptoms (may rarely mimic generalized anxiety disorder or panic disorder).

Clinical symptoms Abdominal discomfort, headache, nervousness.

Clinical signs Flushing, hypertension (may be greatly raised by exercise), pallor (rare), palpitations, paraesthesiae (rare), Raynaud's-type discolouration over extremities and joints, sweating.

Laboratory investigation

There are currently no NICE guidelines for phaeochromocytoma.

Organic disorders

Suggested laboratory investigations Urine 4-hydroxy-3-methoxyman-delic acid (HMMA) or vanillylmandelic acid (VMA); specialist advice needed.

Table Laboratory investigations and phaeochromocytoma		
System	**Laboratory parameter**	**Notes**
Endocrine	Plasma epinephrine	In most patients with phaeochromocytoma levels will be elevated at least two-fold (normal range <50 pg/ml)
	Urinary epinephrine (24-hour collection)	Usually raised (normal range <0.1 μmol/24 hours)
	Urinary hydroxymethoxymandelic acid (24-hour collection)	Usually raised (normal range <35 μmol/24 hours). Levels affected by diet (bananas, chocolate, coffee, tea, vanilla)
	Urinary norepinephrine (24-hour collection)	Usually raised (normal range <0.57 μmol/24 hours)
	Norepinephrine suppression tests	Pentolinium (ganglion-blocker) is usually used, although clonidine (alpha-blocker) may also be used; a normal response to an intravenous bolus of pentolinium 2.5 mg is a fall of plasma epinephrine and norepinephrine into the normal range or by 50% from baseline
Haematology	Erythrocytes	May be increased
	Haemoglobin	May be increased
Clinical biochemistry	Calcium	May be increased
	Free fatty acids	May be increased
	Glucose	Hyperglycaemia may be present as may glycosuria
	Phosphate	May be decreased
	Potassium	May be decreased
	Protein	May be increased

Organic disorders

Porphyria

Definition A group of inherited disorders of abnormal porphyrin metabolism. They may be classified into acute (acute intermittent, variegate; hereditary coproporphyria) and non-acute (congenital porphyria, erythropoietic proto-porphyria, porphyria cutanea tarda).

Psychiatric symptoms (found in 30–70% of patients with acute porphyrias) Agitation, anxiety (generalized), conversion disorder, delirium, dementia, depression, mania, psychosis (rare, usually occurring late; may mimic schizophrenia).

Clinical symptoms Abdominal pain, anorexia, neuropathy (usually starts peripherally).

Clincal signs Hypertension, nausea, tachycardia, vomiting.

Laboratory investigation (acute porphyrias)

There are currently no NICE guidelines for porphyria.

Suggested laboratory investigation Specialist advice required.

Organic disorders

Table Laboratory investigations and (acute) porphyria

System	Laboratory parameter	Notes
Endocrine	Catecholamines	Increased excretion may be present
	Glucose	Glucose tolerance test may be abnormal
	Thyroid function tests	May show elevated thyroxine levels in the absence of signs of hyperthyroidism
Haematology	Anaemia	Usually normocytic, normochromic
	Haemoglobin	May be decreased
	MCH	May be decreased
	MCV	May be decreased
	White blood cells	Leukocytosis may be present
Hepatic	Liver function tests	May be normal or show elevated alkaline phosphatase, bilirubin, and transaminases
Clinical biochemistry	Chloride	May be decreased
	Cholesterol	Hypercholesterolaemia may be present
	Coproporphyrin III	Levels may be measured in faeces and urine; high levels suggest hereditary coproporphyria; the enzyme coproporphyrinogen oxidase can be measured in leukocytes and skin fibroblasts to confirm the diagnosis
	Magnesium	Hypermagnesaemia may be present
	Porphobilinogen deaminase	Decreased activity (measured in red blood cells) can help to confirm diagnosis
	Potassium	May be decreased
	Sodium	May be decreased
	Urine chromatography	Quantitative measurement of aminolevulinic acid (ALA) and porphobilinogen (PBG) – increased in both plasma and urine
	Urinary porphyrin screening	Qualitative tests include the Watson–Schwartz and Hoesch tests which screen for porphobilinogens (ALA and PBG) during acute attacks
Renal	Proteinuria	May be present
	Urea and electrolytes	Hyponatraemia and/or hypokalaemia may be present (secondary to vomiting or syndrome of inappropriate antidiuretic hormone secretion (SIADH); urea may be increased

Systemic lupus erythematosus

Definition A multisystem, autoimmune disorder characterized by a chronic, relapsing and remitting course.

Psychiatric symptoms Cognitive dysfunction, delirium, depression, psychosis.

Clinical symptoms Arthralgia, arthritis, chest pain, migraine, shortness of breath, tendinitis.

Clincial signs Joints: 'Z' deformity of thumb may be seen; skin: bullous lesions, hair loss, oral ulceration, rash (characteristic facial 'butterfly' rash seen in about 40% of patients), Raynaud's phenomenon, urticaria.

Laboratory investigation

There are currently no NICE guidelines for systemic lupus erythematosus. Investigations should be guided by the clinical presentation.

Suggested laboratory investigations Immunology (antibodies): antinuclear antibodies (ANA), dsDNA, rheumatoid factor.

A summary of possible changes in laboratory parameters in SLE is given below.

Table Laboratory investigations and systemic lupus erythematosus

System	Laboratory parameter	Notes
Haematological	Anaemia	Haemolytic anaemia with reticulocytosis may be present; haptoglobin levels may be low and Coomb's test is positive
	Erythrocyte sedimentation rate	May correlate with disease activity
	Haemoglobin	May be decreased
	Leukocytes	May be decreased (neutropaenia may be present)
	Lymphocytes	May be decreased
	Partial thromboplastin time	May be increased
	Thrombocytopaenia	Usually $<100\,000/mm^3$

Table Laboratory investigations and systemic lupus erythematosus (Cont.)

System	Laboratory parameter	Notes
Hepatic function	C-reactive protein	Usually normal
	LFT	May be abnormal in patients with hepatic disease or who are taking non-steroidal anti-inflammatory drugs (NSAIDs). Persistent abnormalities may warrant biopsy
Immunology	ANA	May be a useful screening test as positive titres seen in about 95% of patients; if positive other autoantibodies may be measured
	Other autoantibodies: antiphospholipid, double-stranded DNA (dsDNA), La (SSB), ribonucleoprotein (RNP), Ro (SSA), Sm	May be useful in differentiating between 'spontaneous' and drug-induced forms of SLE; dsDNA, RNP, Sm rare in drug-induced forms. Antiphospholipid antibodies may be associated with thrombotic tendency
	Complement	Reduced in spontaneous SLE and normal in drug-induced forms
	Immune complexes	Elevated in spontaneous SLE and normal in drug-induced forms
	Venereal Disease Research Laboratory (VDRL)	False positive syphilis serology may be present prior to clinical manifestations becoming apparent
Renal	Proteinuria	Either >0.5 g/day if quantified or 3+ on urine dipstick (may reflect glomerulonephritis)
	Urea and electrolytes	May reflect renal involvement; nephritis occurs in at least 50% of patients; creatinine and urea may be increased
	Urinary analysis	Cellular casts may be present

Organic disorders

Uraemic encephalopathy (see also renal failure, Chapter 8)

Definition   A clinical syndrome in which there is severe azotaemia in association with renal failure.

Psychiatric symptoms (associated with degree of renal failure)   Early: apathy, drowsiness, irritability, poor concentration; late: confusion, hallucinations, stupor.

Clinical signs and symptoms   Asterixis, hypertension, myoclonic jerks, muscle twitching, myopathy, neuropathy, pruritus, seizures; in later stages, fasciculations, hiccups, stupor, coma.

Laboratory investigation

There are currently no NICE guidelines for uraemic encephalopathy.

Suggested investigations   As for chronic renal failure (see also Chapter 8).

Organic disorders

A summary of possible changes in laboratory parameters in uraemic encephalopathy is given below.

Table	Laboratory investigation and uraemic encephalopathy	
System	**Laboratory parameter**	**Notes**
Metabolic	Alkaline phosphatase	May be decreased in some patients
	Blood ammonia	Azotaemia may be present
	Calcium	Hypocalcaemia usually present
	Cholesterol	May be normal or slightly raised
	Glucose	May be normal or slightly raised
	Magnesium	May be raised (not normally clinically significant)
	pH	Metabolic acidosis may occur
	Phosphate	Hyperphosphataemia usually present with advanced disease
	Potassium	Usually raised, especially in advanced disease
	Triglycerides	Usually elevated
	Uric acid	Hyperuricaemia may be raised, especially in advanced disease (when GFR is at or below around 20% of normal)
Haematology	ESR	May be raised (these patients are more prone to infections)
	FBC	Anaemia with lowered haematocrits (15–20%) may be seen. Thrombocytopaenia may be present
Immunology	None specific	
Microbiology		

Water intoxication

Definition   Excess water intake due to a non-medical cause. Often associated with chronic schizophrenia.

Psychiatric symptoms   Anxiety, confusion, lethargy, psychosis.

Clinical symptoms   Seizures. Death may result in severe, untreated water intoxication.

Clinical signs   None specific – patients may present with an array of signs including arrhythmia, ataxia, dyspnoea, dysuria, movement disorders, tachycardia, tremor.

Differential diagnosis   Includes disorders associated with polydipsia, polyuria, or hyponatraemia:

- drugs: alcohol, lithium, some antibiotics (e.g. tetracycline)
- endocrine: Cushing's syndrome, diabetes insipidus (cranial, nephrogenic), diabetes mellitus; hyperaldosteronism, hyperparathyroidism
- iatrogenic diuretic therapy
- miscellaneous: sickle-cell anaemia
- renal: renal failure (chronic).

Laboratory investigation   Includes the following.

Table	Basic laboratory investigations and water intoxication	
Medium	*Parameter*	*Notes*
Blood	Calcium	May reveal underlying parathyroid disorder
	ESR	Raised in inflammatory disorders and malignancy
	FBC	Anaemia may be associated with renal failure or inflammatory disease
	Glucose	May reveal glucose intolerance/diabetes mellitus
	U&E	May reveal renal failure
Urine	Urine dipstick	Screen for underlying medical disorders
	Urine osmolality	Low in psychogenic polydipsia with low plasma osmolality; high plasma and low urine osmolality found in diabetes insipidus

Organic disorders

Additional laboratory investigations that may be useful in diagnosis of water intoxication are given below.

Table	Additional laboratory investigations and water intoxication	
Blood	Autoantibody screen	To rule out autoimmune illness such as SLE
	Hormone profile	To rule out suspected pituitary disease
	Serum electrophoresis	To rule out possible myeloma
Urine	24-hour collection	To determine possible proteinuria
	Urine electrophoresis	To rule out possible myeloma

There are currently no NICE guidelines for water intoxication/psychogenic polydipsia.

Wernicke–Korsakoff syndrome (see also thiamine, Chapter 8)

Definition   A clinical syndrome comprising Wernicke's syndrome (ataxia, delirium, nystagmus, and ophthalmoplegia) which progresses to include Korsakoff's syndrome, which is characterized by cognitive impairments, especially of recent and retrograde memory. It is due to thiamine deficiency and is associated especially with chronic alcohol use.

Psychiatric symptoms   Confabulation, hallucinations, memory loss, inability to form new memories.

Clinical symptoms   Gait ataxia, visual changes (double vision, nystagmus, ophthalmoplegia, ptosis).

Clinical signs   Abnormal reflexes, muscular atrophy, polyneuropathy, poor coordination; hypotension, hypothermia, and tachycardia may be present.

Differential diagnosis   Acquired immunodeficiency syndrome (AIDS), anorexia nervosa (including re-feeding), chronic haemodialysis, hyperemesis gravidarum, hypoglycaemia, hyponatraemia, malignancy (especially gastric), intestinal obstruction, malignancy, total parenteral nutrition, tuberculosis, uraemia.

Laboratory investigation

There are currently no NICE guidelines for Wernicke–Korsakoff syndrome.

Although the diagnosis is primarily clinical, a number of specific laboratory investigations may be helpful. Other investigations will be aimed at ruling out possible differential diagnoses, especially those secondary to dementia or chronic alcohol use (see also delirium, Chapter 2 and alcohol, Chapter 7).

Table Laboratory investigation of Wernicke–Korsakoff syndrome		
System	*Laboratory parameter*	*Notes*
Clinical biochemistry	Thiamine levels	May be normal or decreased
	Transketolase	Enzyme activity may be decreased (enzyme measurement provides a functional test for thiamine)
Haematology	Pyruvate	May be normal or elevated
Immunology	None specific	
Microbiology		

241

Wilson's disease (hepatolenticular degeneration)

Definition   An autosomal recessive disorder of copper metabolism in which excessive levels accumulate initially in the liver. If untreated the condition leads to cirrhosis and central nervous system damage.

Psychiatric symptoms   Anxiety, cognitive impairment/confusion, depression, lability of mood, mania, psychosis (rare).

Clinical symptoms   May initially present as chronic haemolytic anaemia or acute haemolysis, although in most patients it presents as a range of hepatic diseases (from non-specific, abnormal liver function tests to acute/chronic cirrhosis or even fulminant hepatic failure) with variable neurological symptoms (akinesia, chorea, drooling, dysarthria, dystonic spasms, fits (rarely), tremor) and psychiatric presentations (altered personality/behavioural change, conduct disorder, even frank psychosis).

Clinical signs   Keiser–Fleischer ring on slit-lamp examination; osteomalacia and rickets may result secondary to renal tubular loss of phosphate. Polyarthritis, hyperpigmented skin (especially blue-coloured nail lanulae), gynaecomastia, and menstrual disturbance may also occur.

Laboratory investigation

There are currently no NICE guidelines for Wilson's disease.

Suggested investigations   Copper (plasma, urine), FBC, glucose, LFT.

A summary of laboratory parameters in Wilson's disease is given below.

Table	Laboratory investigations and Wilson's disease	
System	**Laboratory parameter/condition**	**Notes**
Clinical biochemistry	Calcium	May be decreased
	Cholesterol	May be increased
	Glucose	Usually increased
	Hepatic copper (biopsy)	Raised in Wilson's: normal = 15–55 µg/g dry weight, Wilson's = 250–3000 µg/g dry weight
	LFT	May reflect hepatitis (chronic active) or hepatic failure; alanine aminotransferase, alkaline phosphatase, aspartate aminotransferase, bilirubin, and lactate dehydrogenase may all be increased
	Plasma caeruloplasmin	Low levels found in Wilson's: normal = 25–40 mg/dl, levels <25 characteristic of Wilson's
	Plasma copper	Decreased levels found in Wilson's disease: normal=11–24 µmol/l, Wilson's=3–10 µmol/l
	Urinary copper	24-hour collection increased in untreated disease (normal=<40 µg/24 h, Wilson's= 100–1000 µg/24 h)
Haematology	Haemolysis	Up to 15% of patients with Wilson's disease will have non-spherocytic, Coombs-negative intravascular haemolysis; severe haemolysis may be associated with fulminant hepatitis
	Haemoglobin	May be decreased
Renal	Renal tubular acidosis (RTA)	Aminoaciduria may occur, with variable urine pH and altered potassium levels depending on type of RTA (e.g. type 1: urine pH >6, low plasma K^+; type 2: urine pH <5.4, low plasma K^+; type 3: urine pH <5.4, high plasma K^+

Further reading

General

Axford J. (ed.) Medicine. Oxford: Blackwell Science, 1996.
Jacobs DS, DeMott WR, Grady HJ et al. Laboratory Test Handbook, 4th edn. Hudson, OH: Lexi-Comp, 1996.
Moore DP, Jefferson JW. Handbook of Medical Psychiatry, 2nd edn. Philadelphia: Elsevier Mosby, 2004.
Pomeroy C, Mitchell JE, Roerig J, Crow S. Medical Complications of Psychiatric Illness. Washington, DC: American Psychiatric Press, 2002.
Schiffer RB, Side RC, Klein RS. Medical Evaluation of Psychiatric Patients. London: Springer, 1988.
Young DS, Friedman RB. Effects of Disease on Laboratory Tests, 4th edn. Washington, DC: AACC Press, 2001.

Addison's syndrome

Anglin RE, Rosebush PI, Mazurek MF. The neuropsychiatric profile of Addison's disease: revisiting a forgotten phenomenon. J Neuropsychiatry Clin Neurosci 2006; 18: 450–9.
Nieman LK, Chanco Turner ML. Addison's disease. Clin Dermatol 2006; 24: 276–80.

Cushing's syndrome

Kelly WF. Psychiatric aspects of Cushing's syndrome. QJM 2006; 89: 543–51.
Newell-Price J, Grossman A. Biochemical and imaging evaluation of Cushing's syndrome. Minerva Endocrinol 2002; 27: 95–118.

Diabetes mellitus

Holt RJ. Diagnosis, epidemiology and pathogenesis of diabetes mellitus: an update for psychiatrists. Br J Psychiatry 2004; 47(Suppl): S55–63.
Llorente MD, Urrutia V. Diabetes, psychiatric disorders, and the metabolic effects of antipsychotic medications. Clin Diabetes 2006; 24: 18–24.

Hyperparathyroidism

Akerstrom G, Hellman P. Primary hyperparathyroidism. Curr Opin Oncol 2004; 16: 1–7.
Roman S, Sosa JA. Psychiatric and cognitive aspects of primary hyperparathyroidism. Curr Opin Oncol 2007; 19: 1–5.

Hyperthyroidism

McKeown NJ, Tews MC, Gossain VV, Shah SM. Hyperthyroidism. Emerg Med Clin North Am 2005; 23: 669–85.
Peiris AN, Oh E, Diaz S. Psychiatric manifestations of thyroid disease. South Med J 2007; 100: 773–4.

Hypoparathyroidism

Lynn J, Patel T. Blood testing diagnostic for parathyroid disease. Practitioner 2007; 251: 69–70, 72–3.
Yang SL, Wang CH, Feng YK. Neurologic and psychiatric manifestations in hypoparathyroidism. Clinical analysis of 71 cases. Chin Med J (Engl) 1984; 97: 267–72.

Hypopituitarism

Lynch S, Beshyah S, Merson S. Psychiatric aspects of hypopituitarism in adults. J R Soc Med 1995; 88: 603–4.
Rippere V. Psychiatric morbidity in adults with hypopituitarism. J R Soc Med 1995; 88: 721–2.
Soule SG, Jacobs HS. The evaluation and management of subclinical pituitary disease. Postgrad Med J 1996; 72: 258–62.

Hypothyroidism

Davis JD, Tremont G. Neuropsychiatric aspects of hypothyroidism and treatment reversibility. Minerva Endocrinol 2007; 32: 49–65.

Wong ET, Steffes MW. A fundamental approach to the diagnosis of diseases of the thyroid gland. Clin Lab Med 1984; 4: 655–70.

Iron-deficiency anaemia

Cook JD. Diagnosis and management of iron-deficiency anaemia. Best Pract Res Clin Haematol 2005; 18: 319–32.

Ghosh K. Non haematological effects of iron deficiency – a perspective. Indian J Med Sci 2006; 60: 30–7.

Metachromatic leukodystrophy

Baumann N, Masson M, Carreau V et al. Adult forms of metachromatic leukodystrophy: clinical and biochemical approach. Dev Neurosci 1991; 13: 211–15.

Multiple sclerosis

Feinstein A. The neuropsychiatry of multiple sclerosis. Can J Psychiatry 2004; 49: 157–63.

Lutterotti A, Berger T, Reindl M. Biological markers for multiple sclerosis. Curr Med Chem 2007; 14: 1956–65.

Neuroacanthocytosis

Danek A, Walker RH. Neuroacanthocytosis. Curr Opin Neurol 2005; 18: 386–92.

Phaeochromocytoma

Cameron OG. The differential diagnosis of anxiety. Psychiatric and medical disorders. Psychiatr Clin North Am 1985; 8: 3–23.

Zelinka T, Eisenhofer G, Pacak K. Pheochromocytoma as a catecholamine producing tumor: implications for clinical practice. Stress 2007; 10: 195–203.

Porphyria

Burgovne K, Swartz R, Anath J. Porphyria: reexamination of psychiatric implications. Psychother Psychosom 1995; 64: 121–30.

Dombeck TA, Satonik RC. The porphyrias. Emerg Med Clin North Am 2005; 23: 885–99.

Systemic lupus erythematosus

Benseler SM, Silverman ED. Systemic lupus erythematosus. Rheum Dis Clin North Am 2007; 33: 471–98.

Stojanovich L, Zandman-Goddard G, Pavlovich S, Sikanich N. Psychiatric manifestations in systemic lupus erythematosus. Autoimmun Rev 2007; 6: 421–6.

Water intoxication

Dundas B, Harris M, Narasimhan N. Psychogenic polydipsia review: etiology, differential, and treatment. Curr Psychiatry Rep 2007; 9: 236–41.

Illowsky BP, Kirch DG. Polydipsia and hyponatremia in psychiatric patients. Am J Psychiatry 1988; 145: 675–83.

Wernicke–Korsakoff syndrome

Sechi G, Serra A. Wernicke's encephalopathy: new clinical settings and recent advances in diagnosis and management. Lancet Neurol 2007; 6: 442–55.

Wilson's disease

Medici V, Rossaro L, Sturniolo GC. Wilson disease—a practical approach to diagnosis, treatment and follow-up. Dig Liver Dis 2007; 39: 601–9.

Organic disorders

chapter 7

Laboratory aspects of alcohol and drug use

General aspects

It is widely recognized that many substances, both illicit and prescribed, exert a wide range of effects on the brain that often translate into behaviour and presentations which may induce, mimic, worsen, or maintain signs of mental illness. It should be noted that effects may be related to both intoxication as well as withdrawal of the substance in question.

Although the laboratory can assist in making differential diagnoses, there are a number of important considerations when testing body fluids for the presence of drugs and their metabolites, and caution should be applied when interpreting all results. For example, it is recognized that sampling times, other treatments, ingestion of certain foodstuffs, and baseline physiological parameters as well as methodological limitations may influence findings. *Note*: quantitative analysis for drugs of abuse is not routinely performed.

Alcohol and drug use

It should be noted that the duration of detectability of agents varies widely, and this should be taken into account when considering routine drug analysis.

Table Duration of detectability of miscellaneous substances in urine	
Agent	*Approximate duration of detectability post-dose (hours)*
Alcohol	Up to 24
Amphetamine	48–72
Caffeine	Up to 12
Cannabis	72 hours (with heavy use, up to 10 days, more for chronic, heavy use)
Cocaine	6–8 (but up to 72 hours for the major metabolite benzoylecgonine)
Ecstasy	30–48
Gammahydroxybutyrate (GHB)	12–24
Ketamine	24–48
Khat	Up to 48
Nitrites	Unknown
Opioids	Codeine – approximately 24 hours; methadone – up to 9 days; propoxyphene – 6–48 hours
Phencyclidine	Up to 8 days
Steroids (anabolic)	Up to 3 weeks (oral), 3–6 months or more (injected)
Tobacco (nicotine)	Up to 12 hours

While the most common medium of analysis is urine, other tissues may be considered for analysis, depending on the substance under investigation; these include blood, breast-milk, breath, gastric contents, hair, saliva, sweat, and tears.

Table Body tissues and their utility in drug testing

Tissue	Detectable drugs	Notes
Blood	All	Second most commonly analysed body fluid after urine
Breast-milk	Amphetamine, cannabis, cocaine, methadone, morphine	Analysis of breast-milk not routinely performed
Breath	Alcohol, cannabis metabolites (tetrahydrocannabinol)	Only alcohol breath testing commonly undertaken
Gastric contents	All	Not routinely performed in clinical practice
Hair	Amphetamines, cannabis, cocaine, morphine	Analysis of hair, saliva, and sweat not routinely performed in clinical practice
Saliva	Amphetamine, cocaine, methadone, morphine, nicotine metabolites (cotinine)	
Sweat	Amphetamine, cocaine, methadone, morphine	
Tears	None	Currently under investigation; analysis of tears not routinely performed due to methodological limitations
Urine	All	Most widely studied body fluid in determination of illicit drug use

Alcohol and drug use

Of those illicit agents commonly utilized, a number of specific behavioural/ mental state effects have been identified, some specifically sought by the user and others experienced as adverse effects.

Table	Effects of illicit and selected other substances on mental state	
Agent	*Examples of specific effects sought*	*Examples of possible adverse psychiatric effects*
Alcohol	Impairment of judgement Increased risk-taking Reduction in inhibition	Aggression Delirium Lability of mood Slowing of mentation Specific syndromes: Korsakoff's, Wernicke's
Amphetamine	Decreased tiredness Increased alertness Increased self-confidence Increased garrulousness	Anxiety/agitation Confusion Delirium Depression Exhaustion/fatigue Hallucinations Insomnia Panic attacks Paranoia/psychosis Violent behaviour
Caffeine	Decreased fatigue Increased alertness Increased 'clear-headedness'	**Low levels of intake:** may be none or minor/mildly increased anxiety, insomnia **Higher levels of intake:** Anxiety (persistent) Auditory/visual disturbance Confusion Delirium Impaired concentration Insomnia Panic attacks Paranoia Psychomotor restlessness
Cannabis	Disinhibition Elation Increased sensory awareness Merriment Relaxation	**Acute effects:** may be none or minor/mildly increased: Anxiety Disorientation Dysphoria Hallucinations Psychosis **Effects of chronic use:** Anxiety Depression Flashbacks Sleep disturbance Social withdrawal

Table	Effects of illicit and selected other substances on mental state (Cont.)	
Agent	**Examples of specific effects sought**	**Examples of possible adverse psychiatric effects**
Cocaine	Alertness Elation Increased confidence	**Acute effects:** Anxiety Agitation Hallucinations Insomnia Panic attacks Psychosis Risk-taking/violent behaviour **Effects of chronic use:** Anxiety Depression Psychosis
Ecstasy	Enhancement of perceptions Euphoria Feeling of tranquillity	Anxiety Confusion Hallucinations/psychosis Panic attacks
GHB	Disinhibition Euphoria Relaxation	Agitation Confusion Delirium
Ketamine	Disorientation Out of body experiences Vivid dreams	Agitation/anxiety Flashbacks
Khat	Increased alertness Increased garrulousness Mild euphoria	Depression Lethargy Mania Psychosis
Nitrites	Decreased inhibition Feeling of being high ('rush')	None specific
Opioids	Euphoria Relaxation	Confusion Disinhibition Dysphoria Hallucinations Risk-taking behaviour
Phencyclidine	Delusions Euphoria Feeling of detachment from self/surroundings Hallucinations	**Acute effects:** Agitation Dysphoria Hallucinations Psychosis Risk-taking/violent behaviour **Effects of chronic use:** Anxiety Confusion Depression Flashbacks Personality change Psychosis

Alcohol and drug use

Table Effects of illicit and selected other substances on mental state (Cont.)

Agent	Examples of specific effects sought	Examples of possible adverse psychiatric effects
Steroids (anabolic)	Decreased fatigue Euphoria Increased aggression Increased confidence	Depression Paranoia Personality changes Psychosis Violent behaviour
Tobacco	Decreased anxiety Increased concentration Relaxation	**Effects of withdrawal:** Anxiety Emotional lability Insomnia Irritability Restlessness
Volatile solvents	Disinhibition Euphoria Hallucinations Increased sociability Perceptual disturbances	Aggression Confusion Depression Disorientation Insomnia Nightmares

The following substances will be considered in this chapter:

- alcohol
- amphetamine
- caffeine
- cannabis
- cocaine
- ecstasy
- gammahydroxybutyrate
- ketamine
- khat
- nitrites
- opioids
- phencyclidine
- steroids (anabolic)
- tobacco
- volatile solvents.

For each of these the following information will be provided:

- important facts
- clinical features of intoxication/complications
- features of withdrawal
- laboratory features
- blood/urine concentrations and qualitative testing.

Alcohol

Important facts

Many psychiatric patients consume alcohol on a regular basis, and the concept of 'dual diagnosis', referring to individuals with both serious mental health problems who also use drugs and/or alcohol, is now well established.

Current guidelines suggest that between 21 and 28 units/week for males and 14 and 21 units/week for females constitute the upper safety limit.

Clinical features of intoxication/complications

Alcohol affects all organ systems of the body, and chronic/excess use has a large number of medical and neuropsychiatric sequelae.

Table Possible sequelae of alcohol misuse

System	Condition	Notes	Laboratory investigations
Cardiovascular	Angina Arrhythmias (especially atrial fibrillation) Cardiomyopathy Heart failure Hypertension Ischaemic heart disease	Diagnosis and investigation are essentially clinical	Electrocardiogram (ECG) required; no specific laboratory investigations
Endocrine	Pseudo-Cushing's syndrome	Usually reversible on withdrawal of alcohol	24-hour cortisol excretion (<300 nmol/24 hours)
			Overnight dexamethasone suppression test (plasma cortisol <50 nmol/l at 09.00)
			Insulin hypoglycaemia test (plasma cortisol increased by at least 200 nmol/l in response to the hypoglycaemia)
	Hypogonadism	See Chapter 8	
Gastrointestinal	Alcoholic liver disease (see specific conditions below)	The Combined Clinical and Laboratory Index for Alcoholic Liver Disease looks at a number of clinical findings and laboratory parameters (albumin, alkaline phosphatase, AST, bilirubin, and prothrombin time) to assess the degree of illness severity. (see reference 1 for more details)	

		Note that an AST/ALT ratio >2 is suggestive of alcoholic liver disease, as is a GGT/ALP ratio >1.4 (>3.5 considered to be diagnostic)	
Alcoholic cirrhosis	Possible changes include anaemia, increased MCV, increased ALT, AST, bilirubin, CDT, and GGT; decreased albumin. Note that a discriminative scoring system has been devised to predict prognosis in patients with alcoholic cirrhosis; this looks at five laboratory parameters (AST, antithrombin III, factor V, total serum bilirubin, and transferrin) together with the presence of encephalopathy (see reference 2 for more details)	Carbohydrate-deficient transferrin levels (CDT), clotting screen, FBC, LFT	
Alcohol-induced fatty liver	Often hepatomegaly is the only clinical sign; abnormalities may be reversible on withdrawal of alcohol	FBC: increased MCV LFT: GGT and transaminases may be slightly elevated Carbohydrate-deficient transferrin levels may be raised	
Alcohol-induced liver fibrosis	As for alcoholic cirrhosis		
Alcoholic hepatitis	Possible leukocytosis and raised AST with normal or only slightly raised ALT; in severe cases, prolonged prothrombin time and renal failure may be evident; albumin may be low	Carbohydrate-deficient transferrin levels (CDT), clotting screen, FBC, LFT	

Alcohol and drug use

Table Possible sequelae of alcohol misuse (Cont.)

System	Condition	Notes	Laboratory investigations
	Gastritis	A clinical diagnosis aided by endoscopy	None specific
	Hepatic carcinoma	LFT may be abnormal but with non-specific changes; imaging required	Elevated serum α-fetoprotein may suggest primary liver cancer
	Mallory–Weiss syndrome	Vomiting-induced haematemesis due to a tear in the distal oesophagus or gastric fundus	None specific; diagnosis confirmed by endoscopy
	Oesophageal cancer	FBC may reveal anaemia, diagnosis confirmed by imaging and biopsy	None specific
	Oral squamous cell carcinoma	Diagnosis confirmed by biopsy	None specific
	Pancreatitis (acute)	Raised serum amylase (especially five times the upper limit of normal) suggests acute pancreatitis; laboratory tests may also show complications such as hypoalbuminuria, hypocalcaemia, disseminated intravascular coagulation (DIC), hypoglycaemia, or uraemia	Amylase, calcium, FBC, glucose, LFT, U&E
	Pancreatitis (chronic)	In chronic pancreatitis serum amylase may be normal; specialized pancreatic function tests may be needed	
	Pancreatic carcinoma	Possible increased ALP; diagnosis via imaging or biopsy	None specific

Haematological	Anaemia (macrocytic, iron deficiency, sideroblastic)	May be due to a variety of causes such as direct effects of alcohol on erythropoiesis, folate deficiency, gastrointestinal bleeding, or liver dysfunction	FBC
	Thrombocytopaenia	Due to direct effect of alcohol; usually reversible on withdrawal of alcohol	FBC
Infection	Tuberculosis	Alcohol excess is associated with suppression of macrophage function and is associated with infections such as tuberculosis (TB)	See Chapter 8
	Viral hepatitis	Hepatitis B, C, and D most commonly associated	Increased titres of hepatitis B surface antigen (HBsAg) together with parallel increases in ALT; HBsAg may be undetectable after 3 months but persisting levels after 6 months suggest a carrier state
Metabolic	Metabolic acidosis	Raised bicarbonate, PCO_2, pH; decreased hydrogen ion concentration	Arterial blood gases
	Haemochromatosis	Deposition of excess iron in various tissues especially liver, skin, pancreas, pituitary, heart, and joints	Serum ferritin (increased) Iron saturation >75% LFT (may be normal) Liver iron >180µg/g dry weight
	Hypertriglyceridaemia	Alcohol increases triglyceride synthesis	Lipid screen: increased high-density lipoprotein (HDL) common
	Hyperuricaemia	See Chapter 9	Uric acid

257

Table Possible sequelae of alcohol misuse (Cont.)

System	Condition	Notes	Laboratory investigations
	Hypocalcaemia	See Chapter 9	Serum calcium
	Hypoglycaemia	May occur secondary to alcohol-associated fasting; adrenocorticotropic hormone (ACTH) deficiency, malnutrition, or liver/pancreatic disease may contribute; alcohol increases release of insulin in response to glucose load	Blood glucose, glycolated haemoglobin (HbA1c)
	Hypokalaemia	See Chapter 9	U&E
	Hypomagnesaemia	See Chapter 8	Serum magnesium
	Hypophosphataemia	May occur secondary to malnutrition, malabsorption, or magnesium deficiency	FBC and blood film to screen for haemolysis. Electrolytes: calcium, magnesium, phosphate, potassium LFT (liver abnormalities may result secondary to hypophosphataemia)
	Ketoacidosis	A medical emergency – fluid replacement and correction of metabolic disturbances required; possible metabolic changes include glycosuria, hyperglycaemia, hyperkalaemia, ketonaemia, metabolic acidosis, uraemia	Blood gases, FBC, glucose, U&E, urinalysis

	Lactic acidosis	Alcohol intoxication usually causes a modest rise in lactate level; lactic acid may also result in association with protein malnutrition	Arterial blood gases Creatinine Electrolytes (to calculate the anion gap) Glucose Serum lactate Urea
Musculoskeletal	Avascular necrosis, especially of femoral head	May be asymptomatic, diagnosis confirmed radiologically	None specific
	Myopathy	Neurophysiological tests may be required	None specific; consider creatine kinase measurement (see Chapter 9)
	Rhabdomyolysis	May present with acidosis, hypoxaemia, hypothermia, and hypovolaemia, progress to renal failure. A number of enzyme levels may be raised	Enzymes: alanine transferase, amylase, aspartate transferase, creatine kinase, lactate dehydrogenase U&E/creatinine (rise in urea/creatinine may herald renal failure) Hyperkalaemia may be present Calcium (hypocalcaemia may be present)
Neurological	Alcoholic dementia Alcoholic seizures Cerebellar degeneration	Diagnoses based on clinical presentation and radiology	None specific
	Central pontine myelinolysis	Can result from rapid over-correction of low serum sodium	U&E
	Korsakov's syndrome	Related to thiamine deficiency, empirical treatment with thiamine can help some patients	None specific; thiamine levels and transketolase may be measured

Table Possible sequelae of alcohol misuse (Cont.)

System	Condition	Notes	Laboratory investigations
	Marchiafava–Bignami syndrome	Degeneration of the corpus callosum, may present with psychiatric disturbances or stupor/coma	None specific, in stupor/coma consider investigations for delirium including FBC, U&E, and possibly toxicology
	Peripheral neuropathy (sensorimotor polyneuropathy)	Neurophysiological tests may be required	None specific
	Toxic amblyopia Wernicke's syndrome	Linked to thiamine deficiency (see Chapter 8)	None specific
Nutritional	Folate deficiency	See Chapter 8	
	Nicotinic acid (niacin) deficiency (pellagra)	See Chapter 8	
	Vitamin B12 deficiency	See Chapter 8	
	Thiamine deficiency	See Chapter 8	
Psychiatric	Alcoholic hallucinosis	Can manifest with a range of hallucinations, but visual hallucinations are particularly associated with delirium tremens (see below)	None specific
	Behavioural abnormalities	Outbursts of anger, anxiety states, depressive disorders, paranoia	
	Cognitive impairment/ acute confusional state Deliberate self-harm and suicide	Variable presentations may be seen	
	Morbid jealousy	Also known as Othello's syndrome	
	Sexual dysfunction	Due to direct and indirect effects of alcohol	

Respiratory	Pneumonia (community-acquired, aspiration)	Findings will depend on organism and should be selected depending on clinical presentation; in all cases appropriate chest imaging is required	Culture (blood, sputum), ESR, FBC, LFT, U&E
	Pulmonary tuberculosis	Alcohol suppresses macrophage activity leading to immunosuppression and increased risk of TB	See Chapter 8
Skin	Seborrhoeic dermatitis	Clinical diagnosis, condition also associated with human immunodeficiency virus (HIV)	None specific
Other	Acute intoxication	Usually based on clinical presentation	None specific, blood glucose to distinguish between hyper- and hypoglycaemic states which may mimic acute intoxication
	Withdrawal syndrome	Delirium tremens (DT) is an acute alcohol withdrawal syndrome and is a *medical*, not psychiatric, emergency	DT is essentially a clinical diagnosis, hence laboratory investigations aimed at excluding medical comorbidity; see also Chapter 2 (delirium) and 'Features of withdrawal' below

Features of withdrawal

Alcohol withdrawal can result in a range of features which may mimic a range of conditions; judicious use of the laboratory may be helpful in diagnosis/ monitoring of these, although are not a substitute for good clinical observation and evaluation.

Withdrawal syndromes may be considered depending on the period of time elapsed from the last use of alcohol:

- short-term (within 24 hours of stopping use): a wide range of possible signs and symptoms, including convulsions (grand mal), depression, diaphoresis, hallucinosis (auditory, transient), hyperacusis, itching, muscle cramps, nausea, tinnitus, vomiting; can last for several days
- medium-term (within 1–3 days of stopping use): delirium tremens, including agitation, autonomic overactivity, confusion, delusions, hallucinations (visual), sleeplessness; delirium tremens constitutes a medical emergency and patients should be treated in a medical facility which has appropriate resuscitation facilities as mortality is approximately 10%
- longer-term (variable length of time after stopping use): Wernicke–Korsakoff syndrome (see Chapter 6); alcoholic hallucinosis, including auditory hallucinations in clear consciousness; usually resolves within a week but rarely may progress to amnesic, cognitive impairment or schizophreniform syndromes.

Laboratory features

Laboratory-related cautions with alcohol (conditions worsened by alcohol use) include:

- acute porphyria
- diabetes mellitus
- hepatic dysfunction.

Laboratory investigation
Selection of appropriate laboratory investigations in an alcoholic patient will depend on history and clinical findings, and whether the patient is a chronic alcoholic or may be acutely withdrawing from alcohol. At a minimum the following screening tests in alcoholism may be considered.

Table Baseline investigations in chronic alcoholic patients

Domain	Investigation	Notes
Clinical biochemistry	Carbohydrate-deficient transferrin (CDT)	CDT best used for monitoring rather than diagnosis. CDT levels are raised with heavy alcohol use, and can return to normal within 3 weeks of abstinence; may also be raised in primary biliary cirrhosis
	LFT	Raised bilirubin levels may indicate serious liver pathology GGT raised in about 70% of patients; ALT and AST are non-specific markers, relatively low sensitivity/specificity; AST may have longer-term prognostic utility. *Note*: a raised AST/ALT ratio (>1.5) is suggestive of liver disease, and a ratio above 3 is associated with acute myocardial infarction (see also Chapter 9)
	U&E	Magnesium, zinc, and potassium levels may be low in acute withdrawal; note that magnesium and zinc are not routinely measured
Haematology	FBC	Non-specific changes may occur as a direct or secondary consequence of alcohol use such as anaemia or neutrophilia
	MCV	MCV raised in approximately 30% of patients; it is a non-specific marker, also raised in folate deficiency and non-alcoholic liver disease (see Chapter 9)
Immunology Medical microbiology	None specific, investigations guided by clinical presentation	
Other	Alcohol breath levels Blood or urine level	See below

Alcohol and drug use

263

In acute alcohol intoxication the following parameters may be altered.

Table Altered laboratory parameters in acute alcohol intoxication

Domain	Test	Notes
Clinical biochemistry	11-Hydroxycorticosteroids	Plasma levels increased (remain unchanged in chronic alcoholics)
	Aldosterone	Plasma levels may be decreased
	Cortisol	Plasma levels may be increased
	Growth hormone	Serum levels may be increased
	Lactic acid	Increased blood levels may be seen, especially following binges
	Magnesium	Decreased serum levels may be seen
	Parathyroid hormone	Increased serum levels may be seen
	Phosphate	Decreased serum levels may be seen

A summary of possible altered laboratory parameters in alcoholism is given below.

Table Summary of altered laboratory parameters in alcoholism

Parameter	Decreased levels	Increased levels
25-OH vitamin D3	X	
Aldolase	X	
Alkaline phosphatase		X
ALT		X
Amylase	X	
Androgens	X	
Apolipoproteins		X
AST		X
Bilirubin		X
Cadmium		X
Cholesterol		X
Copper		X
Cortisol		X
Creatine kinase		X
Follicle stimulating hormone (FSH)		X
GGT		X
Glucose	X	
Glucose tolerance	X	
Growth hormone		X
HbA1c		X
Lactate dehydrogenase (LDH)		X
Lactic acid		X
Lipids		X
Luteinizing hormone (LH)		X
Magnesium	X	
MCV		X
Parathyroid hormone		X
Phosphate	X	
Platelets	X	
Potassium	X	
Testosterone		X
Urate		X

Alcohol and drug use

265

Blood, urine, and breath concentrations

Measurement of alcohol blood/urine concentrations
Utility

- diagnosis of alcohol intoxication
- screening/monitoring of treatment
- investigation of coma (to distinguish alcohol-related coma from, e.g. diabetic coma, drug overdose, or head trauma).

Practical information For blood sampling, use a gold top tube; grey (sodium fluoride) recommended for prolonged storage. For urine collection a sterile container is needed.

Reference ranges
Blood <80 mg/dl (<7.4 mmol/l); at 50–100 mg/dl (10.9–21.7 mmol/l) clinical signs of intoxication may be observed. Whole blood levels >300 mg/dl (>65.1 mmol/l) associated with severe toxicity (coma).

In the UK the legal blood alcohol limit for driving is 80 mg of alcohol per 100 ml of blood (7.4 mmol/l, 0.8% of blood alcohol concentration).

Note: blood alcohol level can be estimated from knowing the osmolar gap and applying the following equation:

Estimated blood alcohol level (in mmol/l)=osmolar gap (in mOsm/kg H_2O)×0.99 (To calculate osmolar gap (mOsm/kg H_2O)=(sodium in mmol/l× 2) +(glucose in mmol/l)+(urea in mmol/l).)

Note: the normal osmolar gap is <10.

Urine Negative (qualititative test); more advanced techniques (immunoassay, gas chromatography) are available for specific drug screening purposes. In the UK the legal urine alcohol limit for driving is 107 mg of alcohol per 100 ml of urine.

Cautions Other alcohols (ethylene glycol, isopropanol, methanol, *n*-propanol) in sufficiently high concentration may interfere with analysis.

Measurement of alcohol breath concentrations
A device such as the Lion Intoximeter 3000® is utilized; in the UK the legal breath alcohol limit for driving is 30 µg of alcohol per 100 ml of breath.

Cautions Diabetes mellitus (controversial), restrictive lung disease.

Amphetamine

Important facts

Amphetamine and its deritatives (such as methamphetamine and 3,4-methylenedioxyamphetamine) have a long hstory of abuse due to their stimulant properties; amphetamine is commonly administered via oral and parenteral (nasal inhalation and injection) routes.

In the past amphetamine has been used therapeutically for a number of neuropsychiatric conditions, but is currently classed as a class B drug under the Misuse of Drugs Act (1971).

The adverse effects of amphetamine, especially hyponatraemia, may be increased by concurrent use of SSRIs, notably fluoxetine, which has been reported to inhibit amphetamine metabolism.

Clinical features of intoxication/complications

Mental effects   Variable, but may include aggression, excitement, euphoria, irritability, lability of mood, paranoia, psychosis.

Physical effects   Abdominal discomfort, cardiac arrhythmia, chest pain, hyperpyrexia, hyperreflexia, hypertension, mydriasis, tachycardia.

Features of withdrawal

Anergia, depression/dysphoria, irritability, sleep disturbance, possible suicidal ideation (especially with methamphetamine use).

Laboratory features

Alterations in laboratory parameters are more likely with heavy and/or chronic use of amphetamine.

Table Possible laboratory sequelae of amphetamine use

System	Condition	Laboratory investigations	Notes
Gastrointestinal	Hepatotoxicity	LFT, clotting screen	A range of presentations has been described, ranging from mild hepatitis to fulminant liver failure
Metabolic	Hyponatraemia	U&E	Variable mechanisms may be responsible, may be mainly due to hyperpyrexia
Musculoskeletal	Rhabdomyolysis	Calcium, enzymes (see Notes), U&E, urinalysis for myoglobinuria	Raised enzymes: alanine transferase, amylase, aspartate transferase, creatine kinase, lactate dehydrogenase U&E/creatinine (rise in urea/creatinine may herald renal failure) Hyperkalaemia may be present Calcium (hypocalcaemia may be present)
Renal	Renal failure	U&E	May be a consequence of rhabdomyolysis or a result of hyperpyrexia

Blood/urine concentrations

Note: a number of sympathomimetic agents (phenethylamines) such as ephedrine, fenfluramine, tranylcypromine, and others may cause positive results on testing. Sodium chloride may cause a false negative on urine testing.

Blood
EDTA (ethylenediaminetetraacetic acid) sample required, therapeutic range approximately 20–30 ng/ml (148–222 nmol/l), toxic range >0.2 μg/ml (>1.48 μg/ml).

Urine
Random urine collection into sterile container, refrigerate after collection.

Note: alkalization of urine will decrease renal excretion of amphetamine whereas acidification will increase it. The half-life of amphetamine in urine is approximately 12 hours and amphetamine may be detectable in urine for up to 3 days post-administration.

Qualititative testing   Negative result.

Quantitative testing: Toxic concentration (method dependent) at approximately 25–250 μg/ml (180–1850 μmol/l).

Caffeine

Important facts

Caffeine is the most widely used stimulant but also has a number of therapeutic uses:

- use as bronchodilator in asthma (rare)
- use as a diagnostic tool (radiolabelled caffeine) to measure specific enzyme activity (xanthine oxidase, cytochrome P450, N-acetyltransferase) or to determine acetylator status
- pretreatment in electroconvulsive therapy (ECT) (rare)
- augmentation of warning symptoms of hypoglycaemia in diabetics
- treatment of neonatal apnoea
- treatment of mild orthostatic hypotension
- analgesic adjunct such as in treatment of migraine (coadministration with ergot)
- use as CNS stimulant.

The average cup of tea will contain approximately 60 mg of caffeine, a cup of brewed coffee may contain up to 120 mg caffeine, a cup of instant coffee may contain up to 70 mg of caffeine, and a can of caffeinated, carbonated drink may contain up to 50 mg of caffeine.

Note: caffeine has a number of important psychiatric associations and both toxicity and withdrawal are associated with mood and behavioural disturbances.

Caffeine consumption may be higher in patients with serious mental disorders.

Excess caffeine consumption in individuals with bipolar disorder may be associated with exacerbation of mania.

Caffeine may interefere with the metabolism of certain psychotropics such as clozapine (increased levels possible with caffeine) and lithium (decreased levels possible with caffeine).

Clinical features of intoxication

Mental effects   Agitation, anxiety, depression, excitement, nervousness, rambling speech (rambling thoughts).

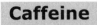

Alcohol and drug use

Physical effects Cardiac arrhythmia (often tachycardia), facial plethora, gastrointestinal disturbance, insomnia, muscle twitching, psychomotor agitation, restlessness, sleep disturbance, sweating.

Features of withdrawal

Features of withdrawal can begin as early as 3–6 hours post-cessation and last for several days.

Common Decreased concentration, drowsiness, fatigue, headaches, increased muscle tension, irritability, weakness.

Less common Anxiety, depression, nausea, tremor and vomiting.

Laboratory features/complications

Table	Possible laboratory sequelae of chronic caffeine use		
System	*Condition*	*Notes*	*Laboratory investigations*
Hepatic	Altered liver enzymes (raised ALT, lowered ALP and GGT)	Modest changes reported with unfiltered, 'boiled' coffee; not considered clinically significant	LFT
Metabolic	Altered lipid profiles (raised total cholesterol and low-density lipoprotein (LDL))	Effects especially associated with boiled coffee. Effect due to the presence of diterpenes (cafestol and kahweol). These ae not found in filtered coffee. Clinical significance unclear	Lipid screen
	Thiamine deficiency	Excessive consumption of tea required; tea contains an antithiamine factor, as does raw fish, which contains a microbial thiaminase	Blood thiamine levels, possible with determination of transketolase activity (a marker for thiamine deficiency)

Table	Possible laboratory sequelae of chronic caffeine use (Cont.)		
System	**Condition**	**Notes**	**Laboratory investigations**
	Hypoglycaemia	May occur in high doses secondary to catecholamine release. Hypokalaemia described in myositis (see below)	Blood glucose, HbA1c
	Hypokalaemia		U&E
	Lactic acidosis		Blood gases
	Musculoskeletal	Myositis	There is a single case report in the literature.[3] A 70-year-old male was admitted with a 1-week history of worsening muscle pain and weakness. The following laboratory abnormalities were found on extensive screening. **Increased**: creatinine (122 µmol/l), creatine kinase (5690 IU/l), lactate dehydrogenase (714 IU/l), alkaline phosphatase (146 IU/l), alanine transaminase (145 IU/l), total white cell count (11.6×10^9/l). **Decreased**: potassium (1.7 mmol/l, on two occasions), calcium (2.18 mmol/l) Other investigations were normal (autoantibodies, coagulation studies, serum hydroxocobalamin, folate, immunoglobulins, thyroid function, prostate-specific antigen, and ferritin), as were chest X-ray and abdominal ultrasound. ECG showed flat T waves and prominent U waves It soon transpired that this man had, over many years, consumed approximately 14 l of tea each day. He was successfully treated with steroids and potassium correction and advised to reduce his tea intake!

Blood/urine concentrations

Note: the half-life of caffeine is approximately 3.5 hours, and enzyme inducers such as barbiturates and phenytoin may *increase* the metabolism of caffeine. Agents such as erythromycin may *decrease* the metabolism of caffeine.

Blood   Serum sample, with time of last dose recorded.

No specific reference range, toxic range approximately >50 μg/ml (>155 μmol/l); fatal concentration reported to be >80 μg/ml (>410 μmol/l).

Urine   No specific reference range.

Cannabis

Important facts

Cannabis and its psychoactive metabolites (mainly Δ9-tetrahydrocannabinol, THC) are widely used for their psychoactive properties, but also as established therapies for a number of conditions, such as an appetite stimulant in patients with acquired immunodeficiency syndrome (AIDS) and for the control of nausea induced by chemotherapeutic agents. There is also some evidence for its use in the treatment of conditions as diverse as multiple sclerosis, glaucoma, and epilepsy.

Cannabis essentially consists of three main varieties, namely marijuana (heads and leaves of the plant, contains on average 5% THC), hashish (cannabis resin, contains up to 20% THC), and hash oil (contains up to 60% THC).

Clinical features of intoxication

Mental effects   Euphoria, increased perceptual awareness, relaxation.

Physical effects   Dry mouth, gynaecomastia, increased risk of conjunctival infection, respiratory tract infection, tachycardia.

Features of withdrawal

A withdrawal syndrome has been described for cannabis, but note that no specific laboratory measurements are indicated for this.

Table Possible features of the cannabis withdrawal syndrome	
Behavioural	Anxiety Insomnia Irritability Restlessness
Gastrointestinal	Anorexia Change in bowel habit
Nervous system	Headache
Miscellaneous	Sweating

Laboratory features

None specific.

Complicatons

Complications

Table	Possible sequelae of cannabis misuse		
System	*Condition*	*Notes*	*Laboratory investigations*
Behavioural	'Amotivational' syndrome	May be reported by chronic, heavy users	No specific investigations
	Anxiety and panic reactions	May be more pronounced in inexperienced users	
	Cognitive dysfunction	May include distortions of time and space with disturbed memory and impaired judgement; may be accompanied by motor incoordination	
	Elation Irritability Relaxation	Effects may vary depending on environment and individual factors	
Cardiovascular	Hypotension	Postural hypotension may be related to dilatation of peripheral veins; may lead to dizziness and fainting	
	Tachycardia	Commonly reported	
Gastrointestinal	Dry mouth Increased appetite Nausea and vomiting	Effects commonly associated with acute use	
Neurological	Coma	Reversible coma (with flumazenil) has been described in a single case in two children who ingested cannabis	
	Motor incoordination	Commonly associated with acute intoxication	
Psychiatric	Psychotic episodes	No clear link between cannabis and psychosis; effects may be more pronounced in inexperienced users, especially those using 'stronger' varities such as 'skunk'	
Miscellaneous	Hyperthermia	Uncommon effect	
	Visual disturbance	Cannabis causes dilatation of blood vessels in cornea	

Alcohol and drug use

Blood/urine concentrations

Measurement of urine concentrations
Utility

- evaluation of drug abuse
- assessment of toxicity.

Practical information   Urine collection in a sterile container. *Note*: deliberate dilution of urine will negate the result and cannabinoids can adhere to plastic. The half-life of cannabinoids ranges between 20 and 30 hours. Toxic ranges have not yet been defined and urinary metabolites of Δ9-tetracannabinol may be detectable for up to 3 weeks.

Blood
Blood collection is in a heparin or EDTA tube.

Reference ranges
Urine   <50 ng/ml.

Blood (tetrahydrocannabinol)   0.004–0.01 mg/l (0.01–0.03 µmol/l).

Cocaine

Important facts

Cocaine is obtained from the leaves of *Erythroxylum coca*, the coca plant, and has been used variously as a local anaesthetic as well as a psychoactive substance, famously by Sigmund Freud.

Various forms of cocaine exist, including cocaine hydrochloride and more recently 'crack' cocaine, a pure form of cocaine freebase. Cocaine may be taken orally, inhaled, injected, rubbed on the gums, or smoked.

Alcohol and drug use

275

Clinical features of intoxication/complications

Table Possible sequelae of cocaine misuse

System	Condition	Notes	Laboratory investigations
Cardiovascular	Arrhythmias	Supraventricular, sinus, and ventricular tachycardias; may result in sudden death especially in overdose. Note that many cardiovascular effects of cocaine are idiosyncratic, but patients with plasma cholinesterase deficiency are at particular risk of sudden death	ECG
	Cardiomyopathy	Especially dilated cardiomyopathy	ECG; some centres measure serum brain natriuretic peptide; levels >100ng/l suggest heart failure or cardiomyopathy
	Hypertension	May be severe, leading to aortic dissection or rupture, cerebrovascular accident (CVA), stroke	None specific
	Myocardial infarction/ischaemia	May manifest as ST elevation during cocaine withdrawal	Cardiac enzymes, troponins
	Myocarditis	ESR raised in at least half of patients, leukocytosis present in about 25%	ESR, FBC
	Peripheral ischaemia	May involve extremities, gut, kidney, spinal column, and spleen	None specific
Gastrointestinal	Anorexia	Often a longer-term effect	None specific except in the case of severe cases (see Chapters 2 and 8)
	Liver dysfunction	Non-specific effects reported	Clotting, LFT

Category	Condition	Description	Investigation
Haematological	DIC	Cocaine reported to stimulate platelet aggregation; thrombocytopaenia, prolonged prothrombin time (PT)/APTT and presence of D-dimers/fibrinogen degradation products suggestive	Clotting, FBC
	Thrombocytopaenia	Small number of case reports in the literature, may occur within 28 days following use	FBC
Metabolic	Hypokalaemia	May induce cardiac arrhythmias	U&E
	Plasma cholinesterase	Enzymes may be lower in patients with severe, life-threatening cocaine toxicity	Enzyme levels
Musculoskeletal	Rhabdomyolysis	May lead to renal failure	Enzymes: alanine transferase, amylase, aspartate transferase, creatine kinase, lactate dehydrogenase U&E/creatinine (rise in urea/creatinine may herald renal failure) Hyperkalaemia may be present Calcium (hypocalcaemia may be present)
Neurological	Dizziness Headache	Often associated with acute usage	None specific
	Myoclonic jerks/seizures	In overdose may lead to status epilepticus	
	Sweating Tremors	Associated with acute usage	
Psychiatric	Acute dysphoric syndrome Acute euphoric syndrome Psychotic syndrome	Associated with both acute and chronic use	

Table Possible sequelae of cocaine misuse (Cont.)

System	Condition	Notes	Laboratory investigations
Pulmonary	Bronchiolitis	Especially obliterative bronchiolitis	Blood gases may be helpful; imaging
	Exacerbation of asthma	May be life-threatening	Arterial blood gases; oxygen saturations
	Pneumomediastinum	May mimic cardiac pathology	Arterial blood gases, imaging
	Pneumonitis	Especially hypersensitivity pneumonitis	Analysis of bronchiolar lavage fluid helpful; in hypersensitivity pneumonitis, there may be eosinophilia, lymphocytosis, neutrophilia, and reduced CD4/CD8 ratio (<1)
	Pulmonary haemorrhage	Rare condition; can cause sudden death. May be associated with Goodpasture's syndrome (combination of glomerulonephritis and pulmonary haemorrhage)	Laboratory investigations for Goodpasture's: antiglomerular basement membrane antibodies (diagnostic), antineutrophilic cytoplasmic antibodies (found in about a third of patients), FBC, U&E, urinalysis
	Pulmonary oedema	May result from cardiac failure/cardiomyopathy	FBC, U&E
Renal	Renal failure/uraemia	Rare events, may be associated with rhabdomyolysis	U&E, urinalysis
Sexual	Infertility	Decreased sperm counts have been reported	See Chapter 8

Features of withdrawal

Anxiety, craving, dysphoria, fatigue, irritability, sleep disturbance.

Laboratory features

See above.

Blood/urine concentrations

Blood
Use serum or plasma sample (EDTA or heparin); sample should be stored on ice and assyed within 1 hour of collection. Note that the half-life of cocaine is approximately 1 hour.

Toxic range   >1000 ng/ml (<3300 nmol/l).

Urine
Use random urine collection into a sterile container, refrigerate sample immediately.

Reference ranges
Qualitative   Negative.

Quantitative   1–215 mg/l (2.69–578 µmol/l).

Ecstasy (MDMA, 3,4-methylenedioxymethamphetamine)

Important facts

Ecstasy, 3,4-methylenedioxymethamphetamine, is an amphetamine derivative which is commonly taken orally for its stimulant effects, although it was initially considered as an appetite suppressant.

It is associated with a state of tranquillity and is thought to suppress thoughts of violence and aggression.

Clinical features of intoxication

Mental effects   Anxiety, euphoria, increased perceptual awareness, paranoia, psychosis.

Physical effects   Anorexia, bruxism, diaphoresis, hyperthermia, tachycardia.

Alcohol and drug use

Features of withdrawal

Features may include anxiety, depression, fatigue, irritability, and restlessness.

Laboratory features

Table	Possible laboratory sequelae of Ecstasy use		
System	*Condition*	*Laboratory investigations*	*Notes*
Haematology	Disseminated intravascular coagulation	Clotting screen (prolonged APTT, thrombin, and prothrombin time; reduced fibrinogen level and raised D-dimers and fibrinogen degradation products); FBC (possible reduced platelet count)	Effects may be secondary to, or maintained by, hyperpyrexia
Hepatic	Acute hepatitis Hepatic fibrosis	LFT	
Metabolic	Hyponatraemia	U&E	
Musculoskeletal	Rhabdomyolysis	U&E, urinalysis for myoglobin	
Renal	Acute renal failure	U&E, creatinine	

Blood/urine concentrations

Note: the half-life of MDMA is approximately 10–30 hours.

Blood
As for amphetamine; EDTA sample required, therapeutic range approximately 20–30 ng/ml (148–222 nmol/l), toxic range >0.2 µg/ml (>1.48 µg/ml).

Urine
Random urine collection into sterile container, refrigerate after collection.

Qualitative   Negative result.

Quantitative   Cut-off range for screening 1000 ng/ml, for confirmation 500 ng/ml.

Gamma hydroxybutyrate

Important facts

Gamma hydroxybutyrate (GHB) is both a synthetic and a naturally occurring chemical which has been considered for a number of therapeutic uses, including as an anaesthetic, and as treatment for insomnia and narcolepsy. It has euphoric and relaxant properties and is often used by individuals attending nightclubs.

GHB is not currently classed under the Misuse of Drugs Act (1971).

Clinical features of intoxication

Mental effects Agitation, confusion, delirium, possible increased risk of violence.

Physical effects Bradycardia, dizziness, drowsiness, headache, hypotension, hypothermia, nausea, vomiting.

Features of withdrawal

A variety of symptoms have been reported (see below). Laboratory investigation is not normally required, except in complicated cases.

Symptoms include Agitation, anxiety, confusion, diarrhoea, hypertension, muscle cramps, nausea, tachycardia, tremors, vomiting.

Laboratory features

There are none specific, possibly U&E in cases of severe dehydration with diarrhoea/nausea/vomiting.

Blood/urine concentrations

No reference ranges are currently defined.

Ketamine

Important facts

Ketamine is used therapeutically as an anaesthetic, for relief of chronic pain, and in the treatment of severe cases of asthma that are unresponsive to other treatments. At lower doses it has stimulant properties and may be taken orally, inhaled, or injected.

Alcohol and drug use

Clinical features of intoxication

Mental effects Altered perceptions, especially of time and of one's body; anxiety, confusion, euphoria, flashbacks, hallucinations (often visual), vivid dreams reported.

Physical effects Chest pain, bronchodilatation, hyperpyrexia, hypertension, incoordination, nausea, tachycardia, visual disturbance, vomiting.

Features of withdrawal

There is no clear withdrawal syndrome described to date.

Laboratory features

No specific effects on laboratory parameters are identified to date; it may rarely be associated with abnormal LFT (raised AST and ALT) and rhabdomyolysis (measure U&E to check for increased potassium, urinalysis for myoglobin in urine; creatine kinase may be significantly raised).

Blood/urine concentrations

Note: the half-life of ketamine is between 2 and 4 hours.

Blood Plasma sample (EDTA), therapeutic reference range 0.5–6.5 µg/ml (2.1–27.4 µmol/l).

Urine No reference range currently defined.

Khat

Important facts

Khat is derived from the leaves of *Catha edulis*, a plant native to areas of Africa. Khat contains two active ingredients, cathine and cathinone, which have similar effects to amphetamines.

It is not classed as an illicit substance under the Misuse of Drugs Act (1971).

Clinical features of intoxication

Mental effects Increased alertness, increased sociability; less commonly euphoria and hallucinations.

Physical effects Anorexia, depression, hypertension, hyperthermia, lethargy, sleep disturbances; possible increased incidence of oral cancer and decreased male fertility (controversial).

Features of withdrawal

They are not commonly described, but may include depression, sleep disturbance, tremors.

Laboratory features

Table	Possible laboratory sequelae of khat use	
System	Condition	Notes
Musculoskeletal	Rhabdomyolysis	There is a single published case report.[4] A 46-year-old male with no previous medical history was admitted the day after ingesting 20 'Antidipositum X-112' tablets, each containing 25 mg of cathine hydrochloride, 8 mg of nikethamide, 10 mg of caffeine/sodium salicylate, and 19 other herbal substances. Regular medications included carbromal, diphenhydramine, and secobarbital The next morning, after vomiting and feeling drowsy, he was taken to hospital and noted to be confused, tachycardic, and sweating. He had also become oliguric and required haemofiltration and respiratory support Laboratory screening revealed increased levels of: creatine kinase (50 100 IU/l), uric acid (0.535 mmol/l), creatinine (initially 838 µmol/l then normalized over the next 4 weeks), serum myoglobin (18 600 µg/l, quoted normal range <70 µg/l), urine myoglobin (85 470 µg/l, quoted normal range <70 µg/l) and decreased levels of phosphate (0.59 mmol/l), calcium (1.98 mmol/l) Myoglobin and creatine kinase levels normalized within 3 weeks (details of management not described). The authors conclude that the cathine was causally implicated
Other	Oral cancer	Chonic khat consumption (25+ years) thought to be associated; no specific laboratory investigations

Blood/urine concentration

No reference ranges are currently defined.

Nitrites

Important facts

Three main types of nitrites, amyl, butyl, and isobuytyl nitrite, are commonly inhaled for their transient euphoriant effects. They are also referred to as 'poppers'.

Nitrates have also been used therapeutically for their vasodilatory effects.

Clinical features of intoxication

Mental effects Transient euphoria, dysinhibition; possible aphrodisiac effect.

Physical effects Dizziness, headache, nausea, tachycardia, 'warm' feeling.

Complications/laboratory features

Table Possible complications and laboratory sequelae of nitrite use

System	Condition	Notes	Laboratory investigations
Dermatological	Periocular, periorbital face rash	Erythematous rash, may involve cheeks and include symptoms of sinusitis	None specific
Haematological	Methaemoglobinaemia	Rare event, patients will usually present with cyanosis	FBC
Immunological	Possible weakening of non-specific defences	Controversial, mooted in the case of HIV but no clear evidence to date	None specific
Psychiatric	Psychosis	Rare event, may be more frequent in individuals with pre-existing mental illness	None specific

Features of withdrawal

There are none specific – see mental and physical effects above.

Blood/urine concentrations

No reference ranges are currently defined.

Opioids

Important facts

Opioids include a range of natural and synthetic compounds such as codeine, fentanyl, morphine, opium, papaverine, pethidine, and tramadol.

Opioids are also used therapeutically in anaesthesia and pain relief.

Clinical features of intoxication/complications

Mental effects   Anorexia, decreased activity, diminished libido, drowsiness, euphoria, personality change.

Physical effects   Bradycardia, constipation, meiosis, nausea, pruritus.

Features of withdrawal

Abdominal cramps, agitation, craving, diarrhoea, diaphoresis, mydriasis, piloerection, restlessness, tachycardia, yawning.

Laboratory features

System	Condition	Notes	Laboratory investigations
Table Possible laboratory features of opioid misuse			
Cardiac	Raised hydroxybutyric acid dehydrogenase	Cardiac-specific lactate dehydrogenase isoenzyme; peaks post-myocardial infarction at 2–3 days then declines over the following week; present in red cells, hence haemolysis interferes with measurement. May also rise in pulmonary embolism	Hydroxybutyric acid dehydrogenase
Endocrine	Hyperglycaemia	Rare events, may be exacerbated by chronic, heavy use	Random glucose; HbA1c
	Hyperprolactinaemia		Prolactin levels
	Thyroid dysfunction	T4 levels may be increased in heroin addiction	TFT
Gastrointestinal	Pancreatitis	Large doses especially associated	Amylase, lipase
	Altered liver function	ALT, AST may be raised	LFT
Haematological	Eosinophilia	May occur in about 25% of addicts	FBC
	Lymphocytosis	Common	FBC
	Thromobocytopaenia	Controversial effect, may be due to contaminants	FBC
Infectious	Hepatitis, HIV	Hepatitis C and HIV especially in injecting drug users	Hepatitis serology; HIV serology
	Venereal Disease Research Laboratory (VDRL)	False positives may be seen in about 20% of addicts	Syphilis serology

Table Possible laboratory features of opioid misuse (Cont.)

System	Condition	Notes	Laboratory investigations
Musculoskeletal	Rhabdomyolysis	Has been described in toxic doses sufficient to cause compression of skeletal muscle. May also present with acidosis, hypoxaemia, hypothermia, and hypovolaemia, progress to renal failure. A number of enzyme levels may be raised (see right-hand column)	Enzymes: alanine transferase, amylase, aspartate transferase, creatine kinase, lactate dehydrogenase U&E/creatinine (rise in urea/ creatinine may herald renal failure) Hyperkalaemia may be present Calcium (hypocalcaemia may be present)
Metabolic	Hypocholesterolaemia	Cholesterol levels may be decreased in chronic heroin addiction	Lipid profile
	Hypoxia	Larger doses cause respiratory depression	Blood gases, O_2 saturations
Renal	Myoglobinuria	Haematuria/ myoglobinuria may be early markers	U&E, urinalysis
Other	Anaphylaxis	Rare, especially after intravenous administration	None specific
	Diaphoresis, nausea, vomiting	May lead to dehydration and delirium	U&E

Alcohol and drug use

Blood/urine concentrations (morphine)

Note: the half-life of morphine is between 2 and 4 hours.

Blood
Use EDTA sample.

Reference ranges Therapeutic range 10–80 ng/ml (35–280 nmol/l), toxic range >200 ng/ml (>700 nmol/l).

Urine
Random sample collected into sterile container; refrigerate sample after collection.

Reference ranges Qualitative: negative; quantitative: confirmation 300 ng/ml; screening cut-off 300 ng/ml.

Note: false positives on urine testing may occur in individuals who have used medications containing opiates or who have eaten food containing poppy seeds (see, for example, reference 5).

Phencyclidine

Important facts

Phencyclidine has previously been used therapeutically as an anaesthetic agent and is abused for its dissociative and euphoric effects.

Clinical features of intoxication

Mental effects Behavioural changes, confusion, depersonalization, derealization, euphoria, hallucinations.

Physical effects Breathing disturbances including apnoea, convulsions, diaphoresis, hyperpyrexia, hypertension, nausea, nystagmus, tachycardia, vomiting.

Complications

With chronic use, anxiety, dependence, dysphoria, personality changes, psychosis.

Features of withdrawal

Variable effects, may include anergia, craving, depression.

Laboratory features

Table Possible laboratory sequelae of phencyclidine use

System	Condition	Notes	Laboratory investigations
Clinical biochemistry	Altered glucose metabolism	Hypoglycaemia possible	Plasma glucose, ketones may be noted on urine dipstick
	Abnormal LFT	No consistent patterns reported	LFT
Constitutional	Hyperpyrexia	May lead to dehydration or rhabdomyolysis	Raised enzymes: alanine transferase, amylase, aspartate transferase, creatine kinase, lactate dehydrogenase U&E/creatinine (rise in urea/creatinine may herald renal failure) Hyperkalaemia may be present Calcium (hypocalcaemia may be present)
Haematological	Leukocytosis	Common finding	FBC

Blood/urine concentrations

Note: the half-life of phencyclidine is 10–50 hours.

Blood
No reference range is currently defined.

Urine
Random urine sample collected into sterile container.

Reference ranges Cut-off for screening 25 ng/ml (100 nmol/l). Toxic range >30 ng/ml (120 nmol/l); coma possible at 30–100 ng/ml (120–400 nmol/l); death may occur at levels >500 ng/ml (>2000 nmol/l).

Steroids (anabolic)

Important facts

Anabolic steroids are used therapeutically in the treatment of some forms of hypogonadism and some forms of anaemia (aplastic, haemolytic, hypoplastic).

They are abused, often by athletes, for their stimulatory effects on muscle mass and for decreasing body fat.

Examples of agents include boldenone, dromostanolone, mesterolone, methandrostenolone, methenolone, methyltestosterone, nandrolone, oxandrolone, oxymetholone, and stanozolol.

Clinical features of intoxication

Mental effects (controversial)   Agitation, irritability, paranoia, personality changes, psychosis, sleep disturbance, violence.

Physical effects

- females: clitoral enlargement, decreased breast size, increased body/facial hair growth, increased libido, menstrual irregularities
- males: altered libido, decreased sperm production and quality, gynaecomastia, testicular atrophy.

Complications

Acne, dependence, growth retardation in children, hair loss, liver disease, musculoskeletal problems, psychiatric changes.

Features of withdrawal (especially in acute withdrawal)

Psychological   anxiety, apathy, depression, listlessness, mood swings, poor concentration, violent behaviour.

Other   Abdominal pain, anorexia, decreased libido, diarrhoea, fatigue, nausea, vomiting, weakness, weight loss.

Laboratory features

Table Possible laboratory sequelae of anabolic steroid use

System	Condition	Notes	Laboratory investigations
Endocrine	Feminization (males) Virilization (females)	Effects usually manifested clinically, laboratory analysis not usually required	Steroid hormone profiling
Gastrointestinal	Liver disease	Cholestatic hepatitis has been described; *note*: exercise can also cause abnormal LFT	Creatine kinase, GGT, LFT
Haematological	Thrombosis	Anabolic steroids may promote platelet aggregation and increase risk of atherosclerosis	Clotting screen, lipid screen
Metabolic	Hyperlipidaemia	Anabolic steroids may increase LDL and decrease HDL resulting in increased risk of atherosclerosis	Lipid screen
	Rhabdomyolysis	May result from sustained exercise	Enzymes: alanine transferase, amylase, aspartate transferase, creatine kinase, lactate dehydrogenase U&E/creatinine (rise in urea/creatinine may herald renal failure) Hyperkalaemia may be present Calcium (hypocalcaemia may be present)

Blood/urine concentrations

No reference ranges are defined; specific agents are usually detected on urinary analysis (contact receiving laboratory for details).

Tobacco

See also Chapter 4 (nicotine).

Important facts

Tobacco is derived from the leaves of *Nicotana tobaccum* and contains a large number of active compounds, in addition to nicotine, the main active ingredient.

Nicotine has stimulant properties and is an agonist on nicotinic acetylcholine receptors.

Clinical features of intoxication/complications

Mental effects Alleviates anxiety and promotes relaxation, decrease in appetite, and heightened concentration. Initially it provides the user with a mild 'high', an effect which dissipates with prolonged use.

Physical effects Hypertension, increased peristalsis, nausea (especially in early stages of use), tachycardia, vasoconstriction.

Complications

- bone disease (osteoporosis, fractures)
- cancers (especially bladder, kidney, larynx, lung, oesophagus, oral, pancreas, pharynx)
- eye disease (cataracts, macular degeneration)
- gastrointestinal disease (including peptic ulcer and ulcerative conditions such as Crohn's disease)
- heart disease (especially diseases related to atherosclerosis such as cerebrovascular disease, ischaemic heart disease, peripheral vascular disease)
- lung disease (chronic obstructive airway disease, exacerbation of asthma, pneumonia)
- reproductive disorders (birth defects, impotence, infertility).

Features of withdrawal

These usually begin within 24 hours of cessation and may include anxiety, craving, emotional lability, headaches, increased appetite, insomnia, irritability, weight gain.

Laboratory features

No specific effects on laboratory parameters are reported.

Blood/urine concentrations

Nicotine
Note: the half-life of nicotine is approximately 30 minutes.

Blood EDTA sample, reference range in smokers 0.01–0.05 mg/l (0.062–0.308 µmol/l); in non-smokers <0.006 mg/l (<0.037 µmol/l).

Urine Random sample, reference range in smokers 0.1–3.0 mg/l (0.616–18.48 µmol/l); in non-smokers <0.007 mg/l (<0.431 µmol/l).

Cotinine
Note: cotinine, a stable metabolite of nicotine, is a more useful marker of nicotine intake and has a plasma half life of 7–40 hours.

Blood Plasma sample, reference range in smokers 16–145 ng/ml (91–823 nmol/l); in non-smokers 1–8 ng/ml (6–45 nmol/l).

Urine Random urine sample, reference range in smokers 300–1300 ng/ml (1703–7378 nmol/l); in non-smokers 1–20 ng/ml (6–114 nmol/l).

Volatile solvents

Important facts

Volatile solvents tend to be used by younger individuals and include a range of inhalable substances including solvents (hexane, toluene), ketones (acetone), and chlorinated hydrocarbons found in various media such as dyes, glues, paints, and varnishes.

Effects tend to be rapid and in rare cases can lead to death.

Clinical features of intoxication/complications

Acute effects
Mental effects Feeling 'high': may be associated with disinhibition, feeling merry/euphoric, and increased sociability; may also include disorientation, hallucinations, and perceptual distortions.

Physical effects Coughing, headache, local irritation of eyes/mouth/throat, movement difficulties, tremor, weakness, wheezing.

Complications (especially with chronic use, may be reversible upon cessation of use)
Mental effects Cognitive impairment, depression, emotional instability, impairment of short-term memory, nightmares.

Physical effects Gait abnormalities, lethargy, nosebleed, sensory deficits, slurred speech, ulceration of nose and mouth, weight loss.

Alcohol and drug use

Note: Death may occur due to accidents, aspiration of vomit, cardiotoxicity, toxic effects on respiratory drive, or suffocation.

Features of withdrawal

There are not fully defined, but may occur after 48 hours and include non-specific features such as diaphoresis, delusions/psychosis, headaches, irritability, nausea, tachycardia, and tremor.

Laboratory features

Table	Possible laboratory sequelae of volatile solvent use	
Condition	**Laboratory investigation**	**Notes**
Haematological toxicity: Aplastic anaemia Bone marrow suppression Leukaemia	FBC	Associated with long-term use; bone marrow suppression may manifest with any or all of leukopaenia, anaemia, thrombocytopaenia, and haemolysis
Hepatotoxicity	LFT, clotting screen	Damage may be reversible upon abstinence; especially associated with methylene chloride and trichloroethylene
Hypoxia	Blood gases	Especially associated with dichloromethane due to its metabolism to carbon monoxide
Nephrotoxicity	U&E, urinalysis	Damage may include acid–base disturbance, acute renal failure, Fanconi's syndrome and renal tubular acidosis; toluene especially implicated

Blood/urine concentrations

No reference ranges are defined; specific agents are usually detected on urinary analysis (contact receiving laboratory for details).

Miscellaneous agents

A great many other agents have abuse potential, and a full consideration of these is beyond the remit of this text. However, it should be noted that use of the laboratory in cases of suspected overdose/poisoning should be guided by clinical presentation, and that many agents are amenable to toxicological analysis. In all cases expert advice should be sought, and basic laboratory investigations (such as FBC, U&E, LFT) should be performed in every patient, for both diagnostic and monitoring purposes. For other possible investigations in acute intoxication see also Chapter 2 (delirium).

References

1. Orrego H, Israel Y, Blake JE, Medline A. Assessment of prognostic factors in alcoholic liver disease: toward a global quantitative expression of severity. Hepatology 1983; 3: 896–905.
2. Ekindjian OU, Devanlay M, Duchassaing D et al. Multivariate analysis of clinical and biological data in cirrhotic patients: application to prognosis. Eur J Clin Invest 1981; 11: 213–40.
3. Trewby PN, Rutter MD, Earl UM, Sattar MA. Teapot myositis. Lancet 1998; 351: 1248.
4. Rumpt KW, Kaiser HF, Horstkotte H, Bahlmann J. Rhabdomyolysis after ingestion of an appetite suppressant. JAMA 1983; 250: 2112.
5. Narcessian EJ, Yoon HJ. False-positive urine drug screen: beware the poppy seed bagel. J Pain Symptom Manage 1997; 14: 261–3.

Further reading

General

Bjornaas MA, Hovda KE, Mikalsen H et al. Clinical vs. laboratory identification of drugs of abuse in patients admitted for acute poisoning. Clin Toxicol (Phila) 2006; 44: 127–34.

Gable RS. Acute toxic effects of club drugs. J Psychoactive Drugs 2004; 36: 303–13.

Jacobs DS, DeMott WR, Grady HJ et al. Laboratory Test Handbook, 4th edn. Hudson, OH: Lexi-Comp, 1996.

Taylor D, Paton C, Kerwin R. The Maudsley Prescribing Guidelines, 9th edn. London: Informa, 2007.

Wu AH, McKay C, Broussard LA et al. National Academy of Clinical Biochemistry Laboratory Medicine practice guidelines: recommendations for the use of laboratory tests to support poisoned patients who present to the emergency department. Clin Chem 2003; 49: 357–79.

Young DS. Effects of Drugs on Laboratory Tests, 5th edn. Washington, DC: AACC Press, 2001.

Young DS, Friedman RB. Effects of Disease on Laboratory Tests, 4th edn. Washington, DC: AACC Press, 2001.

Alcohol

Conigrave KM, Davies P, Haber P, Whitfield JB. Traditional markers of excessive alcohol use. Addiction 2003; 98 (Suppl 2): 31–43.

Sharpe PC. Biochemical detection and monitoring of alcohol abuse and abstinence. Ann Clin Biochem 2001; 38: 652–64.

Amphetamine

White SR. Amphetamine toxicity. Semin Respir Crit Care Med 2002; 23: 27–36.

Caffeine

Benowitz NL. Clinical pharmacology of caffeine. Ann Rev Med 1990; 41: 277–88.

Broderick P, Benjamin AB. Caffeine and psychiatric symptoms: a review. J Okla State Med Assoc 2004; 97: 538–42.

Cannabis

Ashton HC. Pharmacology and effects of cannabis: a brief review. Br J Psychiatry 2001; 178: 101–6.

Hall W, Solowij N. Adverse effects of cannabis. Lancet 1998; 352: 1611–15.

Maykut MO. Health consequences of acute and chronic marijuana use. Prog Neuropsychopharmacol Biol Psychiatry 1985; 9: 209–38.

Cocaine

Loper KA. Clinical toxicology of cocaine. Med Toxicol Adverse Drug Exp 1989; 4: 174–85.

Mueller PD, Benowitz NL, Olson KR. Cocaine. Emerg Med Clin North Am 1990; 8: 481–93.

Ecstasy

El-Mallakh RS, Abraham HD. MDMA (Ecstasy). Ann Clin Psychiatry 2007; 19: 45–52.

Hall AP, Henry JA. Acute toxic effects of 'Ecstasy' (MDMA) and related compounds: overview of pathophysiology and clinical management. Br J Anaesth 2006; 96: 678–85.

Gamma hydroxybutyrate

Ricaurte GA, McCann UD. Recognition and management of complications of new recreational drug use. Lancet 2005; 365: 2137–45.

Wong CG, Chan KF, Gibson KM, Snead OC. Gamma-hydroxybutyric acid: neurobiology and toxicology of a recreational drug. Toxicol Rev 2004; 23: 3–20.

Alcohol and drug use

Ketamine

Britt GC, McCance-Katz EF. A brief overview of the clinical pharmacology of 'club drugs'. Subst Use Misuse 2005; 40: 1189–201.
Pomarol-Clotet E, Honey GD, Murray GK et al. Psychological effects of ketamine in healthy volunteers: phenomenological study. Br J Psychiatry 2006; 189: 173–9.

Khat

Hassan NA, Gunaid AA, Murray-Lyon IM. Khat (Catha edulis): health aspects of khat chewing. East Mediterr Health J 2007; 13: 706–18.
Warfa N, Klein A, Bhui K et al. Khat use and mental illness: a critical review. Soc Sci Med 2007; 65: 309–18.

Nitrites

Brouette T, Anton R. Clinical review of inhalants. Am J Addict 2001; 10: 79–94.
Romanelli F, Smith KM, Thornton AC, Pomeroy C. Poppers: epidemiology and clinical management of inhaled nitrite abuse. Pharmacotherapy 2004; 24: 69–78.

Opioids

Foley KM. Opioids. Neurol Clin 1993; 11: 503–22.
Zollner C, Stein C. Opioids. Handb Exp Pharmacol 2007; 177: 31–63.

Phencyclidine

Baldridge EB, Bessen HA. Phencyclidine. Emerg Med Clin North Am 1990; 8: 541–50.
Dove HW. Phencyclidine: pharmacologic and clinical review. Psychiatr Med 1984; 2: 189–209.

Steroids (anabolic)

Brower KJ. Anabolic steroid abuse and dependence. Curr Psychiatry Rep 2002; 4: 377–87.
Talih F, Fattal O, Malone D Jr. Anabolic steroid abuse: psychiatric and physical costs. Cleve Clin J Med 2007; 74: 341–4, 346, 349–52.

Tobacco

Arabi Z. Metabolic and cardiovascular effects of smokeless tobacco. J Cardiometab Syndr 2006; 1: 345–50.
Benowitz NL. Clinical pharmacology of nicotine. Annu Rev Med 1986; 37: 21–32.
Glassman AH. Cigarette smoking: implications for psychiatric illness. Am J Psychiatry 1993; 150: 546–53.

Volatile solvents

Flanagan RJ, Ives RJ. Volatile substance abuse. Bull Narc 1994; 46: 49–78.
Flanagan RJ, Ruprah M, Meredith TJ, Ramsey JD. An introduction to the clinical toxicology of volatile substances. Drug Saf 1990; 5: 359–83.

Alcohol and drug use

chapter 8

Miscellaneous topics

Hepatic failure

The liver is a primary site of drug metabolism, and in addition produces a number of important substances, including plasma proteins and clotting factors.

Hepatic impairment may lead to a reduced ability to metabolize a wide range of substances (leading to possible metabolic encephalopathy and/or increased adverse effects of medications) and altered production of, e.g. albumin (leading to hypoalbuminuria) and clotting factors (leading to increased risk of bleeding), and increased drug toxicity due to altered protein binding.

There is no single entity known as hepatic impairment; rather, there are a number of related conditions with one or more of the following manifestations: hepatic encephalopathy, bleeding diathesis, ascites, and jaundice.

Psychiatric associations with hepatic failure include parasuicide (especially with paracetamol overdose), chronic alcoholism, certain types of recreational drug abuse, unusual forms of pica, and rarely related to psychotropic treatment.

Psychiatric symptoms in hepatic failure are usually related to hepatic encephalopathy and may include behavioural disturbance, confusion, and mental dulling.

Laboratory features of hepatic failure

Table Laboratory features of hepatic failure

Manifestation	Possible associated event	Laboratory test	Notes
Hepatic encephalopathy: stage 1: decreased attention, slowed thinking, irritability, altered sleep pattern; stage 2: drowsiness, agitation, abnormal behaviour, confusion, loss of sphincter control, disorientation; stage 3: stupor, incoherent speech, restlessness; stage 4: coma, variable response to painful stimuli)	Diarrhoea/vomiting	U&E	May lead to dehydration and electrolyte imbalance
	Anaemia	FBC	May be secondary to gastrointestinal (GI) haemorrhage
	Azotaemia	Blood ammonia	High levels may be neurotoxic (normal range 10–47 µmol/l); may cause encephalopathy or coma
	Hepatorenal syndrome	Urea, creatinine	Urea and creatinine measurements may not be reliable in hepatic failure due to decreased hepatic synthesis of urea and decreased tubular secretion of creatinine
	Hypoalbuminuria	Albumin	Secondary to decreased hepatic synthesis and increased plasma volume
Asterixis usually present in stages 2 and 3; electroencephalogram (EEG) changes present from stage 2	Hypoglycaemia	Blood glucose; glycolated haemoglobin (HbA1c)	Can worsen cerebral and hepatic function
	Hypoxia	Arterial blood gases	May be due to hepatopulmonary syndrome or pulmonary arteriovenous shunts in patients with cirrhosis
	Infection	C-reactive protein (CRP), culture	May induce dehydration, electrolyte disturbance, and increase protein catabolism

Bleeding diathesis	Impaired production of clotting factors	Prothrombin time FBC	Thrombocytopaenia may reflect hyposplenism; upper GI bleeding may result in anaemia; associated abnormalities of platelet structure and function may further accentuate bleeding
Ascites	Venous hypertension (cirrhosis, heart failure, hepatic outflow obstruction, Budd–Chiari syndrome, acute thrombosis causing blockage of portal vein)	Possible routine blood tests: U&E, LFT, FBC, TFT, amylase, CRP/ESR Analysis of ascites for protein, neutrophils, cytology, microbiology Specialized tests: ascitic adenine deaminase; ascitic neutrophil count (both raised in suspected tuberculous peritonitis) Ascitic amylase and ascitic neutrophil count (both raised in suspected pancreatic ascites) Serum alkaline phosphatase and raised ascitic protein in malignancy; raised serum α-fetoprotein may suggest hepatoma	Investigations should be chosen based on clinical suspicion and appropriate expert advice regarding choice of tests, and their interpretation should always be obtained
	Hypoalbuminuria (cirrhosis, nephritic syndrome, malnutrition, protein-losing enteropathy)		
	Malignancy (primary: lymphomas, leukaemias, mesotheliomas; secondary)		
	Infections (human immunodeficiency virus (HIV)), tuberculosis, fungal e.g. candida, cryptococcus; parasitic e.g. strongyloides, entamoeba		
	Miscellaneous: chylous, biliary, pancreatic, urinary, ovarian disease, myxoedema, eosinophilic gastroenteritis, Whipple's, sarcoidosis, SLE		

Miscellaneous

Summary of classification of liver failure

Psychiatrists may see patients at any stage of liver failure, or on occasion, post-transplant. End-stage liver disease necessitating transplant may be due to psychiatric disorders such as parasuicide (especially following paracetamol overdose) or chronic alcoholism resulting in alcoholic liver disease.

Table Summary of classification of liver failure

Condition	Main symptoms/signs	Laboratory tests	Notes
Acute liver failure	Jaundice	LFT	Elevated aminotransferases and prolonged prothrombin time common
Fulminant liver failure	Jaundice+ encephalopathy	LFT, prothrombin time (PT)	Syndrome occurs within 8 weeks of onset of liver disease; elevated aminotransferases and prolonged prothrombin time common
		Plasma factor V (proaccelerin)	Level less than 50% of normal occurring fewer than 2 weeks after onset of jaundice
Subfulminant hepatic failure	Jaundice+ encephalopathy	LFT/PT/plasma factor V	Plasma factor V level less than 50% of normal occurring 2 weeks to 3 months after onset of jaundice
Late-onset liver failure	Acute liver failure+ encephalopathy		Syndrome occurs 8–24 weeks after the onset of liver disease
Chronic liver failure	Chronic liver disease with at least one of the main manifestations of liver disease (hepatic encephalopathy, bleeding diathesis, ascites, and jaundice)		Chronic disease may include cirrhosis or hepatitis. Procollagen type III (serum reference range 2–12 μg/l) may be a useful marker of cirrhosis. A number of other tests of liver function have been described, which require expert advice prior to requesting. These include: bromosulphthalein and indocyanine green excretion tests, galactose tolerance test (to measure liver metabolism/excretion), 14C-aminopyrine demethylation and caffeine clearance tests (for microsomal enzyme activity), plasma glutathione S-transferase activity (to assess general liver damage)

Note: severity/prognosis of liver disease is facilitated using two different measures, the Child–Pugh Score and the Model for End-Stage Liver Disease (MELD), although MELD may be more applicable for liver transplants.

Child–Pugh Score (also known as the Child–Turcotte–Pugh Score) This utilizes five separate measures and assigns points depending on severity. A summation of these points provides a rough estimate of survival.

Table Child–Pugh Score

Parameter	1 Point	2 Points	3 Points
Albumin (g/dl)	>3.5	2.8–3.5	<2.8
Ascites	None	Controlled with medication	Unresponsive to medication
Bilirubin (μmol/l)	<34	34–50	>50
Hepatic encephalopathy	None	Grade I or II	Grade III or IV
INR	<1.7	1.71–2.2	>2.2

Table Child–Pugh Score and prognosis

Points	Category	Approximate 1-year survival (%)	Approximate 2-year survival (%)
5–6	A	100	85
7–9	B	81	57
10–15	C	45	35

Model for End-Stage Liver Disease (MELD)

$$MELD = 3.78[\text{Ln serum bilirubin (mg/dl)}] + 11.2[\text{Ln INR}] + 9.57[\text{Ln serum creatinine (mg/dl)}] + 6.43$$

The maximum score is 40.

Miscellaneous

Further Reading

General

Av SP. Hepatic encephalopathy: pathophysiology and advances in therapy. Trop Gastroenterol 2007; 28: 4–10.
Bauer M, Winning J, Kortgen A. Liver failure. Curr Opin Anaesthesiol 2005; 18: 111–16.
Crone CC, Gabriel GM, DiMartini A. An overview of psychiatric issues in liver disease for the consultation-liaison psychiatrist. Psychosomatics 2006; 47: 188–205.

Child–Pugh

Child CG, Turcotte JG. Surgery and portal hypertension. In: Child CG, ed. The Liver and Portal Hypertension. Philadelphia: Saunders, 1964: 50–64.
Pugh RN, Murray-Lyon IM, Dawson JL, Pietroni MC, Williams R. Transection of the oesophagus for bleeding oesophageal varices. Br J Surg 1973; 60: 646–9.

MELD

Kamath PS, Wiesner RH, Malinchoc M et al. A model to predict survival in patients with end-stage liver disease. Hepatology 2001; 33: 464–70.
Wiesner RH, McDiarmid SV, Kamath PS et al. MELD and PELD: application of survival models to liver allocation. Liver Transpl 2001; 7: 567–80.

Miscellaneous

Renal failure and dehydration

Renal failure is usually divided into acute and chronic forms, although there is some overlap. See also uraemic encephalopathy (Chapter 6), creatinine (Chapter 9), and glomerular filtration rate (Chapter 9). For information regarding dehydration see below.

Acute renal failure

Definition Presence of an abnormally low glomerular filtration rate (GFR) for less than 3 months; acute renal failure is usually reversible.

Normal GFR in a young adult is approximately 80–120 ml/minute, and it declines after age 25 by approximately 1 ml/minute/year.

Clinical presentation Initially with anuria or oliguria as well as a range of clinical features including anaemia, cardiac abnormalities (arrhythmias, hypertension), lethargy, malaise, myopathy, pulmonary oedema, nausea/vomiting, peripheral neuropathy, seizures, skin discolouration/rashes.

Causes

- psychiatric: a number of psychotropics are associated with renal failure – see Chapter 4 for details. Psychiatric disorders rarely result in acute renal failure, although may occur with severe, protracted vomiting in eating disorders (see, for example, Abe et al (1990) A case of anorexia nervosa with acute renal failure resulting from rhabdomyolysis. Acta Neurologica Scandinavica 81(1): 82–83). It may also rarely occur in alcohol/substance abuse disorders, as a sequela of rhabdomyolysis as may occur as a result of prolonged, complicated physical restraint or extreme exertion. It may also occur in association with decreased food/fluid intake as may occur in dementia, obsessive-compulsive disorder, some types of psychosis, or severe depression.
- other: autoimmune disorders (such as SLE), complications of pregnancy (such as eclampsia), diabetes mellitus, hepatorenal syndrome, HIV, hypertension, hypokalaemia, obstruction, primary glomerulonephritis, renal artery stenosis, urinary tract infections (such as acute pyelonephritis).

Laboratory features

Table	Basic laboratory investigations in acute renal failure	
Domain	Parameter	Notes
Clinical biochemistry	Arterial blood gases	May show acidosis
	Creatinine Phosphate Potassium Urea	All increased
	Glomerular filtration rate	Decreased
Haematology	FBC	Anaemia may manifest several days after onset
Immunology	Presence of autoantibodies	Antibody screen positive with autoimmune cause such as SLE
Medical microbiology	None specific (but consider urine/blood culture in suspected cases of infection)	

Chronic renal failure

Definition Presence of an abnormally low glomerular filtration rate (GFR) for more than 3 months; chronic renal failure is usually irreversible.

It may be divided into two stages:

- initial (low clearance stage): associated with worsening GFR and associated signs and symptoms (see below)
- established chronic renal failure ('end-stage'): in which dialysis or a renal transplant is required to maintain life.

Clinical presentation Anaemia, asterixis, bleeding disorders, cardiac abnormalities (cardiomyopathy, congestive cardiac failure, hypertension), drugs (such as some antibiotics, non-steroidal anti-inflammatory drugs (NSAIDs), hyperprolactinaemia, immunosuppression, infertility, intellectual impairment, lethargy, loss of libido, malaise, menstrual disorders, myopathy, nausea/vomiting, seizures, skin rash.

Causes

- psychiatric: as for acute renal failure
- others: as for acute renal failure.

Miscellaneous

Laboratory features

Table	Basic laboratory investigations in chronic renal failure	
Domain	**Parameter**	**Notes**
Clinical biochemistry	Arterial blood gases	May show acidosis
	Creatinine Glomerular filtration rate (see below and Chapter 9) Phosphate Potassium Urea	All increased
Haematology	Clotting time	May be increased
	FBC	Anaemia may manifest several days after onset
Immunology	Presence of autoantibodies	Antibody screen positive with autoimmune cause such as SLE
Medical microbiology	None specific (but consider urine/blood culture in suspected cases of infection)	

Glomerular filtration rate UK guidelines for chronic kidney disease in adults have been proposed (http://www.renal.org/CKDguide/full/CKDprint-edfullguide.pdf), and suggest that the estimated GFR be used as a major criterion in the classification of chronic kidney disease.

Miscellaneous

Table   Proposed classification of chronic kidney disease

Classification	GFR (ml/min/1.73m²)	Notes	Changes in other blood parameters
Normal	>90	Males normally have higher GFRs than women	None
Mild impairment	60–89	With other evidence of chronic kidney damage;* note: a GFR of 60–89 without other evidence of chronic kidney damage does not require further investigation and GFR should be corrected for gender (women may have lower GFRs) and ethnicity (African–Caribbeans may have higher GFRs)	Minimal elevation of parathyroid hormone may be present
Moderate impairment	30–59	Sequelae of chronic kidney damage will be present	More marked evelation of parathyroid hormone may be seen; altered lipoprotein metabolism may be seen; calcium absorption may be decreased, phosphate excretion may be reduced; anaemia may be present
Severe impairment	15–29		Hyperkalaemia and metabolic acidosis may be seen as well as the changes described above
Established renal failure	<15	'Established' renal failure suggested in place of 'end-stage' renal failure	Changes as above but more severe

*Evidence of chronic kidney damage may include persistent changes in laboratory parameters (haematuria, microalbuminaemia, proteinuria), radiological findings (structural abnormalities), or biopsy findings (such as glomerulonephritis).

Miscellaneous

Acute versus chronic renal failure

In general, acute renal failure is associated with:

- more severe symptoms
- often, more prominent fluid retention
- hyperkalaemia (more common)
- renal osteodystrophy, usually asymptomatic
- pruritus (less common).

Dehydration (see also Chapter 2 (delirium) and Chapter 9 (sodium))

Dehydration refers to fluid loss in the body and can be defined as:

- mild – 1–2% reduction in body weight due to fluid loss
- moderate – 3–5% reduction in body weight due to fluid loss
- severe – 5% or more reduction in body weight due to fluid loss.

There are two basic types of dehydration:

- **Hypo**natraemic – due to excessive water loss as a result of burns, diarrhoea, sepsis, surgery, trauma, vomiting.

  Psychiatric associations include alcohol and drug abuse, delirium, and vomiting secondary to medication treatment (especially antidepressants such as SSRIs and other agents associated with syndrome of inappropriate antidiuretic hormone secretion (SIADH)).

- **Hyper**natraemic – due to reduction in water intake.

  Psychiatric assocations include psychiatric syndromes (alcohol and drug abuse, delirium, eating disorders, some forms of obsessive–compulsive disorder, with severe depression, schizophrenia), or as sequelae to treatment (especially lithium, SSRIs).

Clinical signs and symptoms

Table Clinical signs and symptoms in dehydration

Symptom/sign	Mild	Moderate	Severe
Blood pressure	Normal	Normal or slightly raised	Reduced
Capillary refill	≤2 seconds	2–4 seconds	≥4 seconds
Eyes (intraocular pressure)	Normal	Sunken	Sunken
Glasgow Coma Scale	15/15	12–15	May be less than 12
Heart rate	Slight increase	Increased	Tachycardic
Mucous membranes	Normal	Dry	Extremely dry/cracked
Pulse	Normal	Thready/weak	May be impalpable
Respiratory rate	Normal	Increased	Increased
Skin turgor	Normal	Slow	Extremely slow
Tears	Normal	Decreased	Absent
Urine output	Decreased	Oliguria	Oliguria/anuria
Weight	Normal or decreased	Decreased	May be markedly decreased

Differential diagnosis
Water depletion

* non-psychiatric:

  renal – diabetes insipidus, diabetes mellitus, diuretic use, high protein diet, renal tubular disease

  extrarenal – diarrhoea (severe), dysphagia, hyperventilation, old age/infirmity, restriction of oral intake, sweating

* psychiatric:

  alcohol/drug abuse, dementias, eating disorders, obsessive–compulsive disorder (OCD) (rare), severe depression, severe psychosis.

Miscellaneous

Sodium depletion

- non-psychiatric:

  renal – acute tubular necrosis, diuretics, mineralocorticoid deficiency

  extrarenal – burns, cystic fibrosis, gastrointestinal disorders (vomiting, diarrhoea, fistulae, ileus), SIADH (see Chapter 3), sweating

- psychiatric:

  syndromes – cachexia (alcoholism, anorexia nervosa, depression; may be rarely associated with severe OCD); psychogenic polydipsia; Ecstasy use

  medications – benzodiazepines, carbamazepine, chlorpromazine, donepezil, duloxetine, haloperidol, lithium, memantine, mianserin, phenothiazines, reboxetine, rivastigmine, SSRIs, tricyclic antidepressants (amitriptyline).

Laboratory investigation

Table Laboratory investigation of dehydration			
Domain	*Parameter*	*Sodium depletion*	*Water depletion*
Clinical biochemistry	Albumin	Increased	Slightly increased
	Creatinine	Increased	Normal or increased
	Sodium	Normal or slightly decreased	Increased
	Urea	Increased	Normal or increased
	Urine concentration	Slightly increased	Markedly increased
	Urine volume	Decreased	Markedly decreased
Haematology	Haematocrit	Markedly raised (in absence of blood loss)	Normal or slightly increased

Further reading

Block CA, Schoolwerth AC. Acute renal failure: outcomes and risk of chronic kidney disease. Minerva Urol Nefrol 2007; 59: 327–35.
Meyer TW, Hostetter TH. Uremia. N Engl J Med 2007; 357: 1316–25.
http://www.renal.org/CKDguide/full/CKDprintedfullguide.pdf.

Miscellaneous

Physiological conditions specific to women

Menstrual disorders

Menstrual disorders may be defined as primary (a failure to start menstruation) or secondary (defined as the cessation of menstruation for >6 months in the absence of pregnancy). Secondary menstrual disorders include: amenorrhoea (complete absence of menstruation), dysmenorrhoea (painful periods), menorrhagia (excessive blood loss), and oligomenorrhoea (infrequent periods).

Patients on certain types of medications associated with blood dyscrasias (see Chapter 4), prolactin (see Chapter 9), and possibly severe liver disease (see Chapter 4) may have increased susceptibility to menstrual abnormalities. In addition, some psychiatric medications have been specifically associated with menstrual disturbances; these include the following.

Table Psychotropic medications specifically associated with menstrual abnormalities

Agent	Notes
Fluoxetine	Rarely associated with vaginal bleeding on withdrawal
Risperidone	Rarely associated with non-specific menstrual disturbances
Valproate	Rarely associated with amenorrhoea and oligomenorrhoea
Venlafaxine	Rarely associated with non-specific menstrual disturbances

Psychiatric syndromes and substances of abuse associated with menstrual disorders include the following.

Table Psychiatric syndromes and substances of abuse specifically associated with menstrual abnormalities

Condition	Notes
Alcohol dependence	May prolong/worsen dysmenorrhoea in women susceptible to this condition
Anabolic steroid use	Non-specific effects on menstruation, including possible amenorrhoea, dysmenorrhoea, menorrhagia, or oligomenorrhoea
Caffeine use	High caffeine intake has been reported to worsen dysmennorhoea
Cannabis use	May cause minor menstrual irregularities and has been suggested as a treatment for dysmenorrhoea
Eating disorders	Associated with a range of abnormalities, including amenorrhoea, dysmenorrhoea, and oligomenorrhoea (see also Chapter 2)
Smoking	Reported to aggravate dysmenorrhoea
Volatile solvent abuse	Possibly associated with increased risk of oligomenorrhoea

Miscellaneous

Table Possible laboratory tests and menstrual disorders

Condition	Laboratory tests	Notes
Amenorrhoea	Follicle stimulating hormone (FSH)	May be raised in premature menopause
	Luteinizing hormone (LH)	Raised in polycystic ovary syndrome (triad of obesity, acne, facial hirsutes, and infertility/menstrual disturbance); testosterone levels may also be raised
	Prolactin	High levels may suggest prolactinoma (see Chapter 9)
	TFT	Both hyper- and hypothyroidism may be associated
Dysmenorrhoea	Tests for possible pelvic pathology such as chronic sepsis (culture, ESR, urinalysis etc.)	May be primary (no organic pathology identified) or secondary
Menorrhagia	FBC	May be associated with a blood dyscrasia and/or may lead to iron-deficiency anaemia
	TFT	May be associated with hypothyroidism
Oligomenorrhoea	As for amenorrhoea, above	May be especially associated with polycystic ovary syndrome

Pregnancy

The laboratory diagnosis of pregnancy is usually via qualitative measurement of the hormone β-hCG (human chorionic gonadotropin). This can often be performed at the bedside via a qualitative urine test ('home pregnancy test'). A quantity of urine is added to a test strip which changes colour if positive. Note that false positives may occur, and a more precise laboratory test involving blood collection may be required.

Table Specialized quantitative laboratory tests used in the diagnosis of pregnancy

Test	Notes
Serum β-hCG	β-hCG may be seen within 2 weeks post-conception, with levels peaking by 12 weeks' gestation. May be required in complicated pregnancies, possibly with serial monitoring
Urine β-hCG	May be required to confirm serum level (e.g. if there is concern about a false negative result)
Serum progesterone	Performed after a positive β-hCG test if there is concern about possible ectopic pregnancy; low levels (<16.0 nmol/l) suggest a non-viable pregnancy

Pregnancy induces a large number of physiological changes, which affect a large number of laboratory parameters. Below is a summary of some of the possible alterations.

Table Alterations in laboratory parameters in pregnancy

Parameter (plasma)	Notes
Adrenocorticotropic hormone (ACTH)	Increased levels seen (despite increased cortisol secretion)
Albumin	Levels decrease during pregnancy
Aldosterone	Increased levels seen (secondary to rises in angiotensin, renin, and natriuretic effects of progesterone)
Alkaline phosphatase	May be increased up to twice normal levels
Calcium	Fall in ionized calcium seen despite a rise in plasma calcitonin
Cholesterol	Levels rise during pregnancy
Copper	May be increased up to twice normal levels
Cortisol	Increase in both total and free cortisol
Creatinine	May be decreased due to rise in glomerular filtration rate
Free fatty acids	Levels decline in early/mid-pregnancy and then rise towards term
Glucose (fasting)	Levels fall in first trimester, rise between weeks 16 and 32 and then fall towards term. Fasting levels usually maintained between 4.0 and 4.5 mmol/l. Some women develop gestational diabetes which usually resolves after delivery. Glycosuria is common

Miscellaneous

315

Table Alterations in laboratory parameters in pregnancy

Parameter (plasma)	Notes
Gonadotropins Growth hormone Haemoglobin concentration	Decreased levels seen
Human chorionic gonadotropin (hCG)	Produced by blastocysts in the placenta and can be used in the diagnosis of pregnancy. Plasma levels peak between weeks 10 and 12 of pregnancy and then decline towards term
Human placental lactogen	Hormone has multiple effects, including the antagonism of insulin, mobilization of free fatty acids, retention of potassium, nitrogen, and other substances
Insulin	Concentrations rise from first to third trimester but decline from 32 weeks to non-pregnant levels
Iron	Increased iron requirements may result in reduced levels/ anaemia
Melanocyte stimulating hormone	Increased levels seen
Neutrophils	Increased especially in third trimester
Oestrogen	Increases throughout pregnancy
Osmolality	Decreased post-conception but with no accompanying diuresis
Packed cell volume	Decreased levels seen
Platelet count	Decreased levels, especially in third trimester
Potassium	Normal or slightly increased levels seen
Progesterone	Increases throughout pregnancy
Prolactin	Increased levels seen
Red cell count	Decreased levels seen
Thyroxine Triiodothyronine	Increased production but normal blood levels seen due to increased production of thyroid-binding protein
Urea	May be decreased due to rise in glomerular filtration rate
White cell count	Increases especially in third trimester. Mainly due to increased neutrophil count (other white blood cell concentrations remain relatively stable)

Miscellaneous

316

Lactation

A number of laboratory parameters may be affected by lactation:

- decreases may be seen in serum albumin
- increases may be seen in serum caeruloplasmin and copper (temporary effects); prolactin (especially 10–40 days postpartum).

Further reading

Futterman LA, Rapkin AJ. Diagnosis of premenstrual disorders. J Reprod Med 2006; 51 (Suppl): 349–58.

Gronowski AM. Handbook of Clinical Laboratory Testing During Pregnancy. Humana Press, New Jersey: 2004.

Kouides PA. Menorrhagia from a haematologist's point of view. Part I: initial evaluation. Haemophilia 2002; 8: 330–8.

Young DS. Effects of Drugs on Laboratory Tests, 5th edn. AACC Press, Washington, DC: 2001.

Young DS, Friedman RB. Effects of Disease on Laboratory Tests, 4th edn. AACC Press, Washington, DC: 2001.

Miscellaneous

Laboratory aspects of sexual dysfunction

Psychiatric patients may complain of sexual dysfunction, which may be due to a wide range of aetiologies, not all of them readily identified. In a large number of cases problems may occur following treatment with psychotropics, especially neuroleptic agents due to their effects on prolactin, and antidepressants due to their effects on cholinergic/adrenergic receptors and other mechanisms. Symptoms, which range in severity and impact, may not be reported by patients, but when medication-related are usually reversible upon cessation of the offending agent.

In **females**, symptoms may include amenorrhoea, anorgasmia, breast enlargement, dysmenorrhoea, galactorrhoea, decreased or lack of libido.

In **males**, symptoms may include delay in orgasm/anorgasmia, decreased or lack of libido, ejaculatory disturbances, erectile dysfunction, galactorrhoea, gynaecomastia, priapism (rare, more commonly associated with alpha-blocking agents).

Careful assessment to rule out medical, psychological, social, and other possible non-medication-related factors should first be undertaken. Where there is a clear association with adverse medication effects, for example in patients receiving dopaminergic agents such as phenothiazines, measurement of serum prolactin can be a useful predictor of problematic side-effects (see Chapter 9 for further details).

In some cases, additional laboratory investigation may be required, which is rarely undertaken by psychiatrists. For completeness, the possible laboratory investigations in the assessment of infertility are described below.

Miscellaneous

In females

Table Laboratory investigations in the assessment of female infertility		
Domain	**Test**	**Notes**
Clinical biochemistry	FSH levels	Raised levels may suggest ovarian failure
	LH levels	Raised levels of LH (together with testosterone) may suggest polycystic ovary syndrome (triad of obesity, acne, facial hirsutes, and infertility/menstrual disturbance)
	LH surge	Looks for proof of ovulation as rise in progesterone on day 21 (luteal levels >30 nmol/l)
	LFT	Severe liver disease is associated with abnormal hormone levels
	Prolactin levels	Extremely raised levels with anovulation may suggest prolactinoma (see Chapter 9)
	Thyroid function tests	Both hyper- and hypothyroidism may be associated
	Testosterone levels	May be adrenal or neoplastic in origin
Haematology	None specific	
Immunology	Ovary, adrenal, and steroid-cell antibodies	Useful in identifying primary autoimmune ovarian failure, found in up to 50% of women with premature ovarian failure
Haematology	None specific	
Microbiology		

In males

Table Laboratory investigations in the assessment of male infertility

Domain	Test	Notes
Clinical biochemistry	FSH levels	May be raised in oligospermia
	LH levels Testosterone levels	Low levels may be seen in androgen deficiency
	Thyroid function tests	Both hyper- and hypothyroidism may be associated
Haematology	ESR	May be raised in genital tract infections and prostatitis
Immunology	Sperm antibodies	May be either immunoglobulin A (IgA) or IgG and found in cervical/seminal secretions or sperm
Microbiology	Semen culture, urethral swab	A wide range of organisms implicated including chlamydia, gonococci, and gram-negative enterococci

In addition to the above, analysis of sperm motility, morphology, and other characteristics may be considered.

Table Approximate normal values for sperm

Parameter	Notes
Liquefaction	Completion ≤15 minutes
Morphology	Normal forms ≥60%
Motility	Motile forms ≥75%
pH	7.2–8.0
Spermatocrit	Approximately 10%
Spermatocyte count	≥50 million/ml (age dependent)
Sperm (ejaculate) volume	Approximately 2.0–6.6 ml

Further Reading

Hafez B. Recent advances in clinical/molecular andrology. Arch Androl 1998; 40: 187–210.
Pauls RN, Kleeman SD, Karram MM. Female sexual dysfunction: principles of diagnosis and therapy. Obstet Gynecol Surv 2005; 60: 196–205.
Young DS. Effects of Drugs on Laboratory Tests, 5th edn. Washington, DC: AACC Press, 2001.
Young DS, Friedman RB. Effects of Disease on Laboratory Tests, 4th edn. Washington, DC: AACC Press, 2001.

Miscellaneous

Electroconvulsive therapy

Electroconvulsive therapy (ECT) involves the application of an electric current to the brain via the use of external electrodes in order to generate a seizure.

Although the precise mechanism of action is unclear, ECT has been shown to be effective in a number of presentations.

Table Indications for electroconvulsive therapy

Condition	Notes
Depression	Primary indication for ECT; usually considered in treatment-resistant cases, but may be used first-line in patients with severe depression (inanition, stupor, other high-risk states)
Mania	ECT has been reported to be as effective as lithium, and may be especially useful in treatment-resistant patients
Psychosis	ECT is not indicated for schizophrenia, but certain symptoms (depressive delusions, catatonia) may respond well to ECT treatment; ECT has also shown efficacy in the treatment of cycloid and atypical psychoses
Catatonia	ECT is reported to be especially effective in the treatment of lethal catatonia
Delirium	May help in certain types of idiopathic delirium; multiple treatments may be needed
Parkinson's disease	May decrease symptoms and maintenance ECT may reduce relapse
Other	ECT has been used (rarely) to good effect in patients with severe OCD, anorexia nervosa, and chronic pain syndrome, despite these not being commonly accepted indications for ECT

The pathology laboratory and ECT

All patients undergoing ECT require an appropriate history, physical examination, and investigations prior to initiation of treatment. These are mainly required due to the risks of anaesthesia.

Baseline laboratory investigations aim to rule out factors associated with anaesthetic risk, especially those which may contribute to cardiovascular side-effects.

Miscellaneous

Table Baseline laboratory investigations in patients referred for electroconvulsive therapy

Domain	Laboratory tests	Notes
Biochemistry	U&E, creatinine	Low potassium levels correlate with premature ventricular contractions; any dehydration should be corrected before ECT
Haematology	FBC	Anaemia may be associated with anaesthetic complications
Medical microbiology Immunology	None specific	

Other investigations may be required based on history and physical examination.

A number of laboratory-related events have been reported following ECT; these are usually benign and not of long-term clinical significance.

Table Important laboratory findings and electroconvulsive therapy

Parameter	Laboratory tests	Notes
Lithium treatment	Lithium levels	Lithium treatment has been found to prolong recovery time when given with barbiturates when lithium levels are above the therapeutic range, even when there are no signs of toxicity; lithium can also decrease the therapeutic response to ECT and is usually discontinued prior to ECT
Prolactin levels	Prolactin levels	10–50-fold increase in levels post-ictally; levels peak after 10–20 minutes and return to baseline within 120 minutes. No clear correlation between levels and clinical response
Eosinophils	FBC	Transient eosinopaenia has been noted
Cardiac enzymes (creatine kinase, lactate dehydrogense (LDH))	Enzyme levels	Levels rise significantly after ECT but significant rises in cardiac-specific isoenzymes have not been found up to 96 hours after ECT; glutamic oxalaminase transaminase levels do not rise
Thyroid stimulating hormone (TSH)	TFT	Acute release post-ECT has been reported. Correlation reported between prolactin responses to ECT and TSH

Table Important laboratory findings and electroconvulsive therapy (Cont.)

Parameter	Laboratory tests	Notes
Cortisol	Urinary cortisol	Levels rise post-ictally (dose-dependent) then fall with improvement of depressive symptoms; plasma levels of corticotropin acutely elevated after ECT with gradual return to baseline; equivocal results of dexamethasone depression test post-ECT
Growth hormone (GH)	GH (serum)	Levels usually unchanged or slightly decreased post-ECT
Oxytocin, vasopressin	Oxytocin (plasma); vasopressin (plasma)	Increased secretion post-ECT but no clear correlation with clinical effectiveness
β-Endorphin	β-Endorphin (plasma)	Transient increase post-ECT found in one study
Trace metals	Zinc, copper	Transient decline post-ECT in one study
	Manganese	Transient increase then decline noted in one study
Miscellaneous	Calcium Chloride Glucose Insulin secretion Lymphocytes Neutrophils Sodium Potassium	Transient increases post-ECT have been reported; not thought to be clinically significant; altered levels of sodium may reflect water retention related to ECT

Further reading

Abrams R. Electroconvulsive Therapy, 4th edn. New York: Oxford University Press, 2002.
Nuttall GA, Bowersox MR, Douglass SB et al. Morbidity and mortality in the use of electroconvulsive therapy. J ECT 2004; 20: 237–41.
Pandya M, Pozuelo L, Malone D. Electroconvulsive therapy: what the internist needs to know. Cleve Clin J Med 2007; 74: 679–85.
Zwil AS, Pelchat RJ. ECT in the treatment of patients with neurological and somatic disease. Int J Psychiatry Med 1994; 24: 1–29.

Miscellaneous

Analysis of cerebrospinal fluid

Examination of the cerebrospinal fluid (CSF) is a useful investigation of a number of pathological conditions with associated psychiatric sequelae which affect the central nervous system; these include infections (such as encephalitis, meningitis, tuberculosis, and syphilis), neurological conditions (such as Guillain–Barré syndrome, multiple sclerosis) and trauma (especially subarachnoid haemorrhage).

The need for a lumbar puncture to obtain CSF must always be discussed with a senior physician, and as a basic guide to interpretation of laboratory results, various characteristics of the CSF are included herein.

Macroscopic analysis of CSF

Table	Macroscopic analysis of cerebrospinal fluid	
Parameter	**Finding**	**Notes/associations**
Colour	**Normal**	**Clear, with a consistency like water**
	Brown	Suggestive of meningeal melanomatosis
	Green	Hyperbilirubinaemia Presence of pus
	Green/blue	Medications such as amitriptyline, doxorubicin, indometacin
	Orange	Excess ingestion of carotenoids (found in carrots, corn, squash)
	Pink	Blood breakdown products
	Yellow ('xanthochromia')	Acoustic neuroma Blood breakdown products Cerebral infarction (occasionally) Guillain–Barré syndrome Hyperbilirubinaemia High CSF protein levels ($\geq 150\,mg/dl$) Intracranial tumours (occasionally) Subarachnoid haemorrhage (xanthochromia may be detected within 12 hours of event and will be seen for up to roughly 3 weeks) 'Traumatic tap' (accidental injury to intrathecal vein) Xanthochromia may be part of Froin's syndrome, which is characterized by high CSF protein and xanthochromia. These findings suggest a blockage to the flow of CSF, commonly due to spinal meningitis or spinal tumour
Clot	Visible clot	Suggests fresh blood/fibrinogen and a 'web' may be seen in tuberculous meningitis; a clot may sometimes be seen in polyneuritis
Turbidity	Increased	Usually due to pus (e.g. as in acute meningitis) or subarachnoid haemorrhage

Laboratory analysis of CSF

Table Laboratory analysis of cerebrospinal fluid		
Parameter	**Finding**	**Notes/associations**
Chloride*	**Normal**	**Normal range is 115–125 mmol/l**
	Decreased	Low values found in purulent meningitis and tuberculous meningitis
	Increased	Will parallel any condition which increases serum chloride (such as dehydration)
Glucose*	**Normal**	**2.2–4.0 mmol/l** (or >70% of plasma glucose) CSF glucose is also normal in viral infections
	Decreased	Bacterial infections (including tuberculosis), especially meningitis
Lactate	**Normal**	**Normal range is 1.1–2.4 mmol/l**
	Increased	Usually increased in bacterial/fungal meningitis, normal in viral meningitis; increased lactate levels may also be seen in brain abscess, intracranial haemorrhage, multiple sclerosis, seizures, trauma, and other CNS insults
Lymphocytes	**Normal**	**Normal range is <4/mm^3**
	Increased	Increased in viral, fungal, and tuberculous meningitis
Polymorphs	**Normal**	**Normal range is 0/mm^3**
	Increased	Neutrophils seen in bacterial infections
Protein	**Normal**	**Normal range is <0.4 g/l**
	Increased: 0.5–0.9 g/l	Seen in viral infections
	Increased: >1 g/l	Seen with bacterial infections (including tuberculosis) causing meningitis Diabetes mellitus Hypothyroidism Multiple sclerosis
	Increased: >5 g/l	Acoustic neuroma Guillain–Barré syndrome

*Note that blood determinations for comparative purposes are needed for these parameters; blood for glucose should be taken 2 hours before performing the lumbar puncture.

CSF changes in various diseases

The following is a summary of the major changes in CSF in various conditions. Note that the following are not absolute, and variations often occur.

Table Common CSF changes in various diseases*

Condition	Main cell type	Protein	Glucose
Normal	**Lymphocytes**	**<0.4g/l**	**>2.2mmol/l (roughly 70% of plasma level)**
Brain abscess	Lymphocytes	↑	↔
Brain tumour	Lymphocytes	↑	↔
Cerebral haemorrhage	Erythrocytes	↑	↔
Cerebral thrombosis	Lymphocytes	↔ or ↑	↔
Guillain–Barré syndrome	Lymphocytes	↑	↔
Lead encephalopathy	Lymphocytes	↑	↔
Limbic encephalitis	Lymphocytes	↔ or ↑	↔
Meningitis: aseptic	Lymphocytes	↑	↑
Meningitis: pyogenic	Polymorphs	↑	↓
Meningitis: tuberculous	Lymphocytes	↑	↓
Neurosarcoid	Lymphocytes	↑	↓
Neurosyphilis	Lymphocytes	↑	↔
Tumour (spinal cord)	Lymphocytes	↔ or ↑	↔
Viral infections	Lymphocytes	↑	↔

↓=decreased; ↔=normal; ↑=raised.

Further reading

Reiber H, Peter JB. Cerebrospinal fluid analysis: disease-related data patterns and evaluation programs. J Neurol Sci 2001; 184: 101–22.
Smith SV, Forman DT. Laboratory analysis of cerebrospinal fluid. Clin Lab Sci 1994; 7: 32–8.
Swash M, Glynn M. Hutchinson's Clinical Methods, 22nd edn. London: WB Saunders, 2007.

Miscellaneous

Analysis of urine

When it is possible to obtain a urine sample from psychiatric patients, a great number of possible laboratory investigations may be performed. Although the most common are urinary drug screening and urine dipstick testing, macroscopic and other tests may be performed.

Macroscopic analysis of urine

Urine should be passed into a clean, sterile container using a sterile technique and refrigerated before analysis. To collect urine, the first morning sample is recommended, as is a mid-stream collection. For this, the patient is instructed to clean the vulva or glans penis with water (*not* antiseptic) then to void and discard the first 20–50 ml of urine. The next volume of urine is then passed into a clean, sterile container. The sample should be analysed immediately, or refrigerated at 4°C until analysis.

Table Macroscopic analysis of urine		
Parameter	*Finding*	*Notes/associations*
Colour	**Normal**	**Usually amber/yellow, but will depend on concentration of urochrome pigment**
	Dark (brown-black)	May occur with bile pigments, haemorrhage, medications (iron sorbitol, methyldopa, nitrofurantoin), poisoning (especially lead and mercury), rhabdomyolysis
	Green	Associated with bile pigments or asparagus consumption
	Green/blue	Methylene blue dye; some medications including amitriptyline, doxorubicin, indometacin
	Milky	Associated with fat globules or pus, especially with urinary tract infections (UTIs)
	Pale	Due to dilution as in diabetes insipidus
	Red	Excessive beetroot or rhubarb consumption, porphyrins; some medications including B vitamins, laxatives (senna), pyridium, rifampicin, warfarin

Table	Macroscopic analysis of urine (Cont.)	
Parameter	**Finding**	**Notes/associations**
Odour	**Normal**	**Aromatic**
	Acrid	Usually due to asparagus consumption
	Faecal	Suggests intestinal–urinary fistulae
	Fishy	Suggests cystitis
	Peppermint	Commonly due to menthol consumption
	Pungent/ammoniacal	Usually due to decomposition
	Spicy	May be due to ingestion of spices (e.g. saffron)
	Sweet	Associated especially with diabetes mellitus
Quantity	**Normal**	**1000–1500 ml/day depending on exercise, fluid/food consumption, habits, temperature, renal function, etc.**
	Decreased	Diarrhoea, eclampsia, fever, heart disease, low fluid intake, nephritis, vomiting
	Increased	Caffeine consumption, diabetes insipidus, diabetes mellitus, diuretics, nephritis (chronic)
	None	Mercury toxicity, nephritis (acute), uraemia, urinary retention
Transparency	**Normal**	**Clear**
	Cloudy	Not normally of pathological significance if it results upon standing
	Milky	Due to presence of fat (some hyperlipidaemias)
	Turbid	Non-pathological: due to precipitation of calcium phosphate Pathological: presence of pus (UTI), some hyperlipidaemias

Laboratory analysis of urine

Note that the following investigations are not first-line and must be discussed with the receiving laboratory prior to requesting. A fresh, mid-stream urine sample is required.

Miscellaneous

Table Laboratory analysis of urine

Parameter	Utility	Finding	Notes
Chloride	Investigation of electrolyte imbalance such as metabolic alkalosis	**Normal**	**Reference range (24-hour urine collection) 110–250 mmol/day, dependent on chloride intake**
		High	Suggests increased adrenocortical insufficiency, diuresis, potassium depletion, salt intake, tubulointerstitial disease
		Low	<10 mmol/day, associated with adrenocortical hyperfunction, diarrhoea, low salt intake, sweating, vomiting, water retention
Cortisol	Aid in diagnosis of Cushing's disease (special protocol required)	**Normal**	**Reference range 83–276 nmol/day (24-hour urine collection)**
		High	Increased values seen in infection, oral contraceptive use, pregnancy, pseudo-Cushing's, stress, trauma
		Low	A value of <28 nmol/day excludes Cushing's syndrome
Creatinine	Renal function test as part of creatinine clearance (special protocol required)	**Normal**	**Reference range (24-hour urine collection): males 8.8–17.7 mmol/day; females 7.1–15.9 mmol/day**
		High	Acromegaly, diabetes mellitus, exercise, hypothyroidism, infections, meat ingestion
		Low	Acute renal failure, advanced congestive cardiac failure, anaemia, hyperthyroidism, muscle disease, paralysis, poorly controlled diabetes mellitus, renal artery stenosis; may also suggest deliberate dilution in the case of urine drug screening

Miscellaneous

Table   Laboratory analysis of urine (Cont.)

Parameter	Utility	Finding	Notes
Osmolality	Evaluation of diabetes insipidus, renal disease, and SIADH	**Normal**	**Reference range 250–900 mOsm/kg of water**
		High	Increased urine/plasma ratio is seen in concentrated urine; carbamazepine may increase urine osmolality
		Low	Exercise, diabetes insipidus, primary polydipsia, starvation; lithium may decrease urine osmolality
Potassium	Evaluation of electrolyte imbalance (hypokalaemia)	**Normal**	**Reference range 26–123 mmol/ day – depends on diet and diurnal variation (greater levels at night)**
		High	>50 mmol/day suggests aldosteronism (primary or secondary), Cushing's syndrome, and renal tubular acidosis
		Low	<20 mmol/day excludes renal loss; low levels may be seen in Addison's disease and renal disease (glomerulonephritis, pyelonephritis)
Sodium	Evaluation of renal failure and hyponatraemia	**Normal**	**Reference range 27–287 mmol/ day – depends on diet and diurnal variation (levels lower at night)**
		High	>10 mmol/l suggests Addison's disease, diuretics, emesis, hypothyroidism, renal disease, or SIADH
		Low	<10 mmol/l suggests extrarenal sodium depletion (congestive cardiac failure, dehydration, liver disease, nephritic syndrome)

Table	Laboratory analysis of urine (Cont.)		
Parameter	**Utility**	**Finding**	**Notes**
Vanillylmandelic acid	Aids in diagnosis of phaeochromocytoma	**Normal**	**Reference range (24-hour urine): 35–45 mmol/day**
		High	Suggests phaeochromocytoma; disulfiram may increase levels
		Low	Low levels associated with MAOI treatment

Urine dipstick

The urine dipstick provides a quick, qualitative screening of urine and can provide a basis for requesting further laboratory tests. A fresh, mid-stream urine sample is required.

Table	Interpretation of urine dipstick findings	
Parameter	**Finding**	**Notes**
Bilirubin (normally non-detectable in urine)	Positive	Suggests bile duct obstruction/liver disease; note that false positives may occur with phenothiazine use and rifampicin is associated with false negatives
Glucose (<1.67 mmol/l may be excreted by the kidney – may occasionally result in false positive)	Positive	Suggests diabetes mellitus; false negative results may be found with high vitamin C intake, levodopa and salicylate use. *Note*: very high ketone levels (>4 mmol/l) may cause a false positive
Haemoglobin (normal range <100 μg/l)	Positive	Suggests haematuria, haemoglobinuria, or myoglobinuria; *note*: test may be positive in dehydration or menstruation. Bacteriuria and myoglobinuria may give false positives, and vitamin C use may result in false negative
Ketones (normally non-detectable in urine)	Positive	Suggests diabetic ketoacidosis, pregnancy; may be seen following starvation or rapid weight loss (e.g. as in anorexia nervosa); levodopa use may give false positive
Leukocytes (normally non-detectable in urine)	Positive	Suggests presence of white blood cells/pyuria; high levels of tetracycline or very high glucose levels (>160 mmol/l) may cause false negatives

Table Interpretation of urine dipstick findings (Cont.)

Parameter	Finding	Notes
Nitrites (normally non-detectable in urine)	Positive	Suggests bacteriuria
pH (normal range 4.5–8.0)	Acid	Suggests acidosis (metabolic and/or respiratory), diabetes mellitus, diarrhoea, emphysema, high meat intake, renal failure, sleep, starvation
	Alkaline	Suggests alkali therapy, alkalosis (metabolic and/or respiratory), ingestion of large quantities of citrus fruit, Fanconi's syndrome (proximal tubule dysfunction resulting in excess urinary excretion of glucose, bicarbonate, phosphates, uric acid, potassium, sodium, and certain amino acids), Milkman's syndrome (increased urinary loss of bicarbonate), urea-metabolizing bacteria such as *Proteus* spp., vegetable diet
Protein (normal range <150 mg/24 hours)	Positive	Suggests multiple myeloma or renal disease (glomerular renovascular or tubulointerstitial); may be positive in alkaline or dilute urine. Proteinuria may also be found in normal individuals as a result of upright posture. Not usually of significance with normal renal function. Microalbuminuria may be indicative of metabolic syndrome. Alkaline urine may give false positive
Specific gravity (normally 1.001–1.035)	Decreased	Suggests diabetes insipidus, diuresis, excessive intravenous fluid administration, excessive water consumption, hypothermia, renal disease (glomerulonephritis, pyelonephritis)
	Increased	Suggests antidiuretic hormone (ADH)-secreting tumours, adrenal insufficiency, congestive cardiac failure, dehydration, diabetes mellitus, diarrhoea, fever, proteinuria, SIADH, sweating, water restriction, vomiting. High quantities of protein in the urine may elevate the specific gravity.
Urobilinogen (normal range <16 μmol/l)	Positive	Positive results when urine urobilinogen is above about 33 μmol/l; suggests liver disease or increased breakdown of RBC

Miscellaneous

Qualitative urine drug screening

(See also 'General aspects' and individual agents in Chapter 7.)

It is recognized that many substances of abuse may induce changes in mental state, and qualitative urine drug screening can assist in diagnosis and monitoring. To perform a urine drug screen, collected urine is applied to test cells and the resulting colour change, or absence thereof, is noted. Note that in cases where there is doubt about the collected urine, urine dipstick analysis (see Chapter 8) may be indicated, as may determination of urine creatinine level, to rule out possible dilution or other interference. A urine creatinine of less than 4.0 mmol/l may suggest dilution and unreliability of the sample.

Most urine drug analysis kits currently in use look for the presence of the following substances or their metabolites:

- amphetamines
- benzodiazepines
- cocaine (metabolite)
- cannabinoid (50 µg/l cut-off)
- methadone metabolite (EDDP: 2-ethylidene-1, 5-dimethyl-3, 3-dipenylpyrrolidine)
- opiates.

In positive cases it may be necessary to perform quantitative analyses using advanced laboratory techniques (chromatography).

Note: a number of external confounding factors may influence urine drug screening, and it may be appropriate, for example, to observe the patient when providing the sample and/or have the patient pass urine into a sealed container.

Table Examples of possible confounders in point of care urine drug screening

Event	Possible effect on drug screen
Drinking water or clear tea (dilution effect) Using previously collected sample (whilst off drugs)	Negative
Using someone else's sample	Negative*
Use of chemicals/adulterants:	
alteration of urine pH (e.g. bicarbonate to make urine alkaline)	Negative (for amphetamine and other stong bases)
bleach commercial adulterants such as Clear Choice™ or Urine Luck™ liquid soap salt	Negative
Using previously collected sample (whilst on drugs)	Positive
Using prescribed drugs:	
codeine and derivatives	Positive for opiates
kaolin and morphine	Positive for morphine
methadone linctus	Positive for methadone
*Usually!	

Note: NICE has published guidelines (http://www.nice.org.uk/nicemedia/pdf/CG052fullversionprepublication.pdf) for opioid detoxification and recomends urine drug screening in addition to history and physical examination when there is concern re opioid dependence or tolerance.

Microbiological analysis of urine

For psychiatrists, the most common reason for requesting microbiological analysis of urine is for diagnosis of suspected urinary tract infection (UTI). Infection may affect the kidneys (pyelonephritis), bladder (cystitis), ureter, or urethra (urethritis).

Women are more prone to UTI (especially if pregnant), as are patients who are immobile, and/or immunosuppressed (especially with diabetes mellitus and HIV).

Signs of a UTI may include Altered urine characteristics (cloudy appearance, malodorous, presence of blood), fever (usually mild in uncomplicated UTI), increased frequency of micturition.

Symptoms of a UTI may include Abdominal pain, dysuria, hesitancy, malaise, urgency.

In severe UTI (pyelonephritis) there may also be severe abdominal pain, rigors, nausea, and vomiting.

Note:

• the above symptoms may also present in urinary tract obstruction
• some women may experience these symptoms in the absence of bacteri-uria; this condition has alternatively been termed urethral syndrome or abacterial cystitis.

To collect urine, the first morning sample is recommended, as is a mid-stream collection. For this, the patient is instructed to clean the vulva or glans penis with water (*not* antiseptic) then to void and discard the first 20–50 ml of urine. The next volume of urine is then passed into a clean, sterile container and the sample should be analysed immediately, or refrigerated at 4°C until analysis.

Common organisms implicated in UTI include the following: *Escherichia coli*, *Proteus*, *Pseudomonas*, *Staphylococcus* spp., *Streptococcus* spp.; if growth is found (i.e. >10^8 organisms/ml urine) then antibiotic sensitivity studies should be performed.

Note: some organisms causing UTI may be difficult to culture (e.g. atypical streptococci, *Mycobacterium tuberculosis*); in suspected cases of sterile pyu-ria, discussion with general medical colleagues and the receiving laboratory is recommended.

Further reading

Hammett-Stabler CA, Pesce AJ, Cannon DJ. Urine drug screening in the medical setting. Clin Chim Acta 2002; 315: 125–35.
Schwartz RH. Urine testing in the detection of drugs of abuse. Arch Intern Med 1998; 148: 2407–12.
Swash M, Glynn M. Hutchinson's Clinical Methods, 22nd edn. London: WB Saunders, 2007.
Toto RD. Microalbuminuria: definition, detection, and clinical significance. J Clin Hypertens (Greenwich) 2004; 6(11 Suppl 3): 2–7.

Miscellaneous

Laboratory aspects of clinical nutrition

Vitamins

Although patients with psychiatric disorders may present with features of vitamin deficiency, it is rarely necessary to determine blood vitamin levels and these assays are seldom performed, apart from determinations of vitamin B12 and folate. Where specific vitamin deficiency is suspected, it is advisable to seek expert advice prior to testing. Patients particularly susceptible to specific vitamin deficiencies include those with alcohol and substance abuse disorders, eating disorders, and possibly severe depression or psychosis.

The following vitamins will be discussed in this section:

- vitamin A
- biotin
- folate
- pantothenic acid
- vitamin B1 (thiamine)
- vitamin B2 (riboflavin)
- vitamin B3 (niacin)
- vitamin B6 (pyridoxine)
- vitamin B12
- vitamin C (ascorbic acid)
- vitamin D (cholecalciferol)
- vitamin E (α-tocopherol)
- vitamin K.

For each vitamin the following information will be provided:

- function
- dietary sources
- daily requirement
- reference range
- sampling
- possible associated changes in routine laboratory parameters with excess
- associations with raised levels
- associations with lowered levels.

Vitamin A

Function A fat-soluble vitamin, which plays important roles in maintenance of epithelial cell integrity as well as in the visual cycle.

Dietary sources Butter, cream, egg yolks, fish oils, liver; can also be converted in the intestine from green, leafy vegetables and yellow fruits.

Daily requirement 750–1000 μg daily; males may require more than females.

Reference range (serum) 30–95 μg/dl (1.05–3.32 μmol/l).

Sampling Plain tube (gold top); patients should be fasting and abstinent from alcohol for at least 24 hours prior to blood collection. Ideally the collection tube should be chilled. Haemolysed samples should be rejected and the sample should be protected from light. Samples are stable at 4°C for up to 1 month and up to 2 years at −20°C.

Possible associated changes in routine laboratory parameters with vitamin A excess include the following.

Table	Possible changes in laboratory parameters with vitamin A excess	
Parameter	*Decreased*	*Increased*
ALT		X*
ALP		X*
AST		X*
Bilirubin		X
Calcium		X*
Erythrocytes	X**	
ESR		X
Haematocrit	X	
Haemoglobin	X	
Leukocytes	X	
Prothrombin time		X

*Especially with acute intoxication.
**With chronic, high doses.

Associations with raised levels (*Note*: treatment with vitamin A analogues such as isotretinoin for acne may give rise to psychiatric symptoms)

- psychiatric: fatigue (non-specific), possibly visual hallucinations secondary to visual disorientation
- other: acute – fever, headache, nausea, skin changes (especially peeling skin), vertigo, visual disturbance, vomiting; chronic – alopecia, anorexia, dry skin, fatigue, hepatomegaly, increased intracranial pressure, joint pain, pruritus; increased levels may be associated with excessive intake (hypervitaminosis), chronic renal disease, diabetes mellitus, medications (steroids, oral contraceptives).

Associations with lowered levels

- psychiatric: chronic alcohol use
- other: eye signs and symptoms, including night blindness (main symptom), xerophthalmia, Bitot spots (conjunctival patches consisting of epithelia debris); late signs include corneal changes (ulceration, scarring) and retinal damage; reduced levels may be associated with carcinoid syndrome, hypothyroidism, gastrointestinal disease (bile duct obstruction, cirrhosis, coeliac disease, cystic fibrosis), malnutrition (kwashiorkor, marasmus, protein malnutrition, zinc deficiency), tuberculosis, and other chronic infections.

Biotin

Function Biotin is a water-soluble member of the B family of vitamins and plays important roles in a number of metabolic processes such as fatty acid biosynthesis. It also acts as a growth factor in cells.

Dietary sources Cereals (cooked), chocolate, egg yolks, pulses, nuts, vegetables (especially green and leafy vegetables).

Daily requirement Unclear, although an intake range of 10–70 μg/day has been suggested.

Reference range (whole blood) 200–500 pg/ml (0.82–2.05 nmol/l).

Sampling Sodium citrate tube (blue top); *note*: levels will be increased by chronic haemodialysis and decreased with certain medications (antibiotics, anticonvulsants). Excess consumption of egg whites will also decrease biotin levels.

Significant effects on routine laboratory parameters None reported.

Associations with raised levels

- psychiatric: none known
- other: none known.

Associations with lowered levels

- psychiatric: anorexia, depression, fatigue, irritability, poor sleep; treatment with antiepileptics (carbamazepine, phenytoin)
- other: alopecia, conjunctivitis, dermatitis (especially dry, scaly skin), hyperaesthesia, muscle pain, paraesthesia, smooth tongue; increased plasma lactic acid and fatty acid levels may be observed in biotin deficiency.

Folate (folic acid)

Function A water-soluble vitamin synthesized by intestinal bacteria and obtained from certain foods which plays important roles in cell division and protein synthesis.

Miscellaneous

Reference range (serum)   >2 ng/ml (>5 nmol/l).

Sampling   Plain tube (gold top); as levels are affected by diet, patients should fast overnight prior to sampling. Specimens should not be exposed to light and levels are unstable at room temperature (stable at 4°C for up to 24 hours, longer when frozen at −20°C). Haemolysed samples should be rejected.

Significant effects on routine laboratory parameters   None reported.

Associations with raised levels

- psychiatric: some eating disorders (malnutrition, strict vegan diet)
- other: gastrointestinal disorders (blind loop syndrome, distal small bowel disease); pernicious anaemia, vitamin B12 deficiency. *Note*: supplementation with high doses may be associated with a lymphocytosis.

Associations with lowered levels

- psychiatric: alcoholism, drugs (barbiturates, carbamazepine, valproate), eating disorders (especially malnutrition)
- other: achlorhydria, amyloidosis, B12 deficiency, Crohn's disease, coeliac disease, drugs (e.g. chloramphenicol, cycloserine, erythromycin, folate antagonists, isoniazid, metformin, oestrogens, oral contraceptives, penicillins, phenytoin, trimethoprim), exfoliative dermatitis (severe), haemodialysis (chronic), haemolytic anaemia, hyperalimentation/re-feeding, liver disease, old age, sideroblastic anaemia, ulcerative colitis, vitamin B6 deficiency, Whipple's disease.

Pantothenic acid
Function   A vitamin of the B class which is a precursor of a number of important coenzymes involved in a large number of metabolic pathways, including those of carbohydrate, lipid, protein, porphyrins, and haemoglobin.

Dietary sources   Meat, poultry, pulses, yogurt, avocado, mushrooms.

Daily requirement   Approximately 2–3 mg pantothenic acid/1000 kcal.

Reference range (serum)   0.2–1.8 μg/ml (0.9–8.2 μmol/l).

Sampling   Plain tube (gold top); ideally patients should be fasted prior to blood collection.

Significant effects on routine laboratory parameters   None reported.

Associations with raised levels

- psychiatric: none known, although there exists a pantothenic acid antagonist (known variously as pantoyl γ-aminobutyric acid, pantoyl-GABA,

homopantothenate, and hopantothenate) that is used in some parts of the world to treat cognitive impairment including Alzheimer's disease
- other: rarely diarrhoea with large quantities (diarrhoea has been reported with ingestion of very large quantities (10–20 g) of calcium pantothenate).

Associations with lowered levels

- psychiatric: chronic alcoholism is associated with increased excretion of pantothenic acid, although the clinical significance of this is unclear
- other: deficiency symptoms and signs include abdominal pain, cramps (typically described as 'burning'), 'nutritional erythromelalgia' (a condition of dilated blood vessels in the skin, especially in the foot, which results in severe pain), paraesthesia of extremities, poor wound healing; lowered levels have been reported in patients with cardiovascular disorders, peptic ulcer disease, chronic malnutrition, and rheumatism.

Vitamin B1 (thiamine)

Function A member of the B vitamin complex, which plays important roles in glycolytic pathways and the maintenance of cardiac muscle and peripheral nerves.

Dietary sources Brown rice, egg yolks, fish, grains, green vegetables, meat, nuts, pulses.

Daily requirement 1.0–1.5 mg/daily (there may be a higher requirement for women, especially those who are pregnant or nursing).

Reference range (whole blood) 275–675 ng/g Hb; *note*: transketolase activity may be a marker of thiamine deficiency and may be measured by some laboratories.

Sampling Heparin tube (green top); sample is stable for up to 2 months at –20°C.

Significant effects on routine laboratory parameters None reported.

Associations with raised levels

- psychiatric: none known
- other: levels have been reported to be raised in a variety of haemato-logical disorders including Hodgkin's disease, leukaemia, and polycythae-mia vera; *note*: supplementation with high doses may result in a lymphopaenia.

Associations with lowered levels

- psychiatric: alcoholism (especially chronic); specific associations include Wernicke's encephalopathy (presentation may include any of ataxic gait,

341

delirium (may include apathy, impaired attention, consciousness, and memory, and progress to stupor or coma), nystagmus, ophthalmoplegia (bilateral lateral rectus palsy, conjugate gaze palsy), polyneuropathy) and Korsakoff's psychosis (confabulation, impaired memory for recent events, retrograde amnesia, lack of global cognitive impairment, possible frontal lobe changes)

- other: chronic diarrhoea, decreased dietary intake, diabetes mellitus, excessive consumption of raw fish, excessive consumption of tea, febrile infections (chronic), increased lactate levels, increased metabolic requirements (such as rapid growth, pregnancy), neoplastic disease; the syndrome of beri-beri secondary to thiamine deficiency may be 'dry' (characterized by peripheral neuropathy with symmetrical sensory and motor impairment affecting distal limb segments more than peripheral) or 'wet' (characterized by peripheral neuropathy in association with cardiomegaly, cardiac failure, congestive heart failure, oedema).

Note: Pabrinex® is a parenteral form of thiamine used in the treatment of vitamin depletion/malabsorption as can occur especially in alcoholism. See Chapter 4 for further details.

Vitamin B2 (riboflavin)

Function Riboflavin is a water-soluble vitamin which plays an important role as a coenzyme in the flavoprotein system and hence many important metabolic processes.

Dietary sources Cheese, grains, leafy green vegetables, meat, milk, yogurt.

Daily requirement 1.2–1.7 mg/day.

Reference range (serum) 4–24 µg/dl (106–638 nmol/l); urine, >100 µg/day (>266 nmol/day).

Sampling Plain tube (gold top) for serum; patients should be fasted prior to blood collection and samples should be protected from light. Samples are stable for many weeks at –20°C; urine, 24-hour collection vessel.

Note: blood and urine samples are not especially sensitive indicators of riboflavin status, and measurement of the enzyme glutathione reductase in erythrocytes may be appropriate in some cases. Further increased enzyme levels may be seen in diabetes mellitus, in G6PD deficiency, during exercise, and after administration of nicotinic acid. Spurious values may be obtained in individuals receiving treatment with valproic acid.

Significant effects on routine laboratory parameters None reported.

Associations with raised levels

- psychiatric: none known
- other: none known (has been used as treatment of migraine in some individuals; no known toxic effects).

Causes of lowered levels

- psychiatric: acute agitation (theoretical possibility), alcoholism (especially chronic), eating disorders (especially anorexia nervosa)
- other: angular stomatitis, cheilosis, glossitis, hypothyroidism, liver disease, malabsorption states, photophobia, seborrhoeic dermatitis.

Vitamin B3 (niacin, nicotinic acid)

Function   Niacin is a water-soluble vitamin which plays important roles in a number of metabolic processes, specifically those involving mitochondrial electron transport.

Dietary sources   Liver, meat, nuts, and whole grains.

Daily requirement   Adult males approximately 14 mg/day; adult females approximately 16 mg/day; higher levels (up to 18 mg/day) may be required in pregnancy and lactation.

Sampling   24-hour urine collection for niacin metabolites.

Reference range (urine, male/non-pregant female)   2.4–6.4 mg/day (17.5–46.7 µmol/day).

Possible changes in laboratory parameters include the following.

Table   Possible changes in laboratory parameters with vitamin B3 excess

Parameter	Decreased	Increased
Albumin	X	
ALP		X
Bilirubin		X
Eosinophils	X	
Glucose tolerance		X*
Growth hormone (GH)		X
High-density lipoprotein (HDL)		X
Low-density lipoprotein (LDL)	X	

*Decreased glucose tolerance may be seen in diabetics.

Associations with raised levels

- psychiatric: none known
- other: toxicity may result in acanthosis nigricans (brownish hyperpigmentation on arms, groin, or neck) or flushing (secondary to histamine

Miscellaneous

release); occasionally hepatotoxicity may occur (usually as increased transaminases with jaundice, rarely fulminant liver failure or advanced hepatic encephalopathy) as may impaired glucose tolerance. Increased uric acid levels may also sometimes be seen.

Associations with lowered levels

- psychiatric: chronic alcoholism; cognitive changes, fatigue, and possibly psychosis secondary to pellagra (see below); may mimic chronic fatigue states in early stages (symptoms may include anxiety, apathy, depression, fatigue, irritability, sleep disturbance)
- other: carcinoid syndrome, Hartnup's disease (an autosomal recessive condition in which there is abnormal intestinal amino acid absorption; patients present with dermatitis, cerebellar ataxia, and aminoaciduria); nutritional deficiency (pellagra).

Pellagra is a clinical syndrome which occurs secondary to severe niacin deficiency. It presents with dermatitis (bilateral, with scaly skin on sun-exposed areas), dementia, gastrointestinal symptoms (constipation or diarrhoea, nausea). In some cases a characteristic skin sign ('Casal's necklace', a red, scaly band of affected skin around the neck and extending to the sternum) may be seen. Cognitive changes include apathy and delirium secondary to encephalopathy, resulting in agitation, arousal, dementia, hallucinations, and organic psychoses. There may also be extrapyramidal rigidity.

Vitamin B6 (pyridoxine)

Function A family of three related water-soluble compounds (pyridoxal, pyridoxamine, and pyridoxine) which act as cofactors in amino acid, carbohydrate, and lipid metabolism, and erythropoiesis.

Dietary sources Avocado, bananas, carrots, chicken, fish, wheat germ.

Daily requirement 1.4–2.0 mg/day (higher in pregnancy and lactation, approximately 2.0–2.6 mg/day).

Reference range (plasma) 5–30 ng/ml (20–121 nmol/l).

Sampling EDTA (ethylenediaminetetraacetic acid) tube (purple top); samples should not be exposed to light and should be analysed immediately due to lack of stabilty (50% of sample degrades at –20°C within 1 week).

Possible changes in laboratory parameters with B6 excess include the following.

Parameter	Decreased	Increased
Table Possible changes in laboratory parameters with vitamin B6 excess		
AST		X*
Lymphocytes	X**	
TSH	X	
*Especially in the elderly. *Especially with large doses.		

Possible changes in laboratory parameters with B6 deficiency include the following.

Parameter	Decreased	Increased
Table Possible changes in laboratory parameters with vitamin B6 deficiency		
ALT	X	
AST	X	

Associations with raised levels

- psychiatric: none known
- other: very high levels may result in peripheral neuropathy.

Associations with lowered levels

- psychiatric: chronic alcoholism, eating disorders (especially anorexia nervosa and those involving chronic malnutrition); medications – carbamazepine, disulfiram, phenelzine
- other: diabetes mellitus, dialysis, pre-eclampsia, gestational diabetes, hypochromic sideroblastic anaemia, lactation, malabsorptive states, malnutrition, niacin deficiency (pellagra), pregnancy, uraemia.

Medications associated with decreased B6 levels include: antituberculous agents (cycloserine, isoniazid, pyrazinoic acid; these may be associated with a sideroblastic anaemia), amiodarone, hydralazine, levodopa, oral contraceptives, penicillamine, theophylline.

Miscellaneous

345

Vitamin B6 deficiency may result in elevated serum homocysteine levels with an increased risk of thromboembolic events.

Vitamin B12

Function A group of related entities (cobalamins) which are not synthesized by humans and are vital for nucleic acid synthesis and other metabolic functions.

Reference range Ranges vary, but one accepted range is approximately 100–250 pg/ml (74–185 pmol/l); levels are generally higher in adult males as compared to females. Normal levels may not always be an accurate reflection of actual B12 status, and further tests (looking for elevated serum methylmalonic acid and elevated total homocysteine levels) may be required. *Note*: a raised MCV may be an early indicator of B12 deficiency.

Sampling Serum (gold top tube); a fasting specimen should be used, and specimens should be protected from light. Specimens are stable for up to 24 hours at 4°C and up to 2 months at –20°C.

Significant effects on laboratory parameters None reported, although a raised MCV may be an early indicator of B12 deficiency.

Associations with raised levels

- psychiatric: chronic alcoholism (in association with severe liver disease)
- other: carcinoma (especially those with liver metastases), chronic obstructive pulmonary disease, chronic renal failure, congestive heart failure, diabetes mellitus, drug-induced cholestasis, leukaemias (acute and chronic), leukocytosis, liver disease (cirrhosis, hepatic coma, hepatitis), obesity, polycythaemia vera; *note*: treatment may result in increased erythrocyte levels and a mild polycythaemia.

Associations with lowered levels (no clear causal link)

- psychiatric: affective, personality, psychotic, cognitive symptoms, and sometimes suicidal ideation may be associated with lowered levels (but no clear causal link); rarely associated with eating disorders (except in strict vegans)
- other: dietary deficiency (rare), malabsorption states (e.g. bowel resection, coeliac disease, pancreatic insufficiency, sprue), megaloblastic anaemia due to lack of intrinsic factor (gastrectomy, gastric atrophy, intrinsic factor antibody), may be associated with delirium; pernicious anaemia, pregnancy (especially in third trimester), rare congenital disorders (e.g. transcobalamin deficiency, Immerslung–Grösbeck syndrome), subacute combined degeneration of the pyramidal/dorsal column tracts of the spinal cord.

Vitamin C (ascorbic acid)

Function Vitamin C plays important roles in amino acid metabolism, the formation of collagen/connective tissue, iron absorption, wound healing, and many other metabolic processes.

Miscellaneous

Dietary sources Berries, broccoli, citrus fruits, spinach, tomatoes.

Daily requirement Adult males approximately 90 mg/day; adult females approximately 75 mg/day. Smokers require approximately an extra 35 mg/day.

Reference range (plasma) 0.6–2.0 mg/dl (34–114 µmol/l); levels are lower in males and heavy smokers.

Sampling Heparin tube (green top); ideally blood should be taken into a chilled tube and then kept on ice. Separated samples are stable for roughly 30 minutes at room temperature and 4 days at –20°C.

Significant effects on routine laboratory parameters None reported.

Associations with raised levels

• psychiatric: none known
• other: hypervitaminosis C-induced diarrhoea; induction of oxaluria with resultant kidney calculi has been reported but is rare.

Associations with lowered levels

• psychiatric: affective changes including depression, chronic alcoholism, eating disorders (especially anorexia nervosa), fatigue (may theoretically mimic chronic fatigue syndromes); medications – barbiturates
• other: cancer, hyperthyroidism, malabsorption, pregnancy, renal failure, rheumatoid disease, smoking (associated with lower blood levels).

Medications associated with decreased plasma vitamin C levels include aspirin, oral contraceptives, paraldehyde.

Primary vitamin C deficiency results in scurvy, a clinical syndrome character-ized by arthralgia, bleeding disorders (bleeding gums, ecchymoses, petechiae), hyperkeratosis, leg pain, lethargy, neuropathy (especially of proximal lower limbs), respiratory distress, and generalized weakness.

Vitamin D (cholecalciferol)
Function A fat-soluble group of related chemicals, which act as a prohormone and play a major role in calcium absorption and normal bone formation.

Dietary sources Milk, fish (salmon, tuna), fortified cereals.

Daily requirement Requirement increases proportional to age: 5 µg/day up to age 50, 10 µg/day between the ages of 51 and 70, and 15 µg/day after age 70.

Reference range (serum) 25-Hydroxy vitamin D3 10–60 ng/ml (25–150 nmol/l); *note*: a number of environmental factors will affect the reference range, including clothing, diet, ethnicity (Asian females, especially

Miscellaneous

347

elderly, more likely to be deficient), geography/season (degree of exposure to ultraviolet light), and medical comorbidity (vitamin D is influenced by endocrine disorders such as diabetes mellitus and thyroid disease, amongst others).

Sampling   Plain tube (gold top); patients should be fasted prior to sampling and samples are stable for up to 3 days at room temperature (refrigeration preferred) with spun samples stable for many months at −20°C. Note that many authorities advocate measuring parathyroid hormone together with vitamin D due to the complex control of calcium metabolism.

Possble changes in laboratory parameters include the following.

Table   Possible changes in laboratory parameters with vitamin D excess

Parameter	Decreased	Increased
ALP		X
Calcium		X
Cholesterol		X
Creatinine		X
Phosphate		X
Urea		X

Associations with raised levels

- psychiatric: excess intake especially in association with some eating disorders (some 'fad' diets, pica)
- other: exposure to sunlight can raise levels (but does not cause toxicity), hypercalcaemia (iatrogenic, idiopathic, secondary to excess intake), hyperparathyroidism (primary), lactation, lymphoma (occasionally), neoplasms ('oncogenic osteomalacia'), pregnancy, sarcoidosis, tuberculosis.

Associations with lowered levels

- psychiatric: anorexia nervosa (rare); chronic alcoholism (rare); lack of exposure to sunlight, theoretically possible in severe agoraphobia
- other: hyperalimentation/re-feeding, hypoparathyroidism, lead toxicity, osteoporosis (postmenopausal), pseudohypoparathyroidism, psoriasis, renal disease (chronic azotemic renal failure, renal osteodystrophy), rickets.

Rickets refers to a number of disorders secondary to vitamin D deficiency which are characterized by non-specific symptoms including bone pain, proximal myopathy, and possibly fractures of the rib and long bones.

Vitamin E (α-tocopherol)

Function   A lipid-soluble vitamin, which exists in eight different forms and acts as an antioxidant in addition to having roles in immune function and DNA repair.

Dietary sources   Fortified cereals, green leafy vegetables, nuts.

Daily requirement   15 mg/day (22.5 IU/day); pregnant and lactating women may require higher levels (19 mg/day, 28.5 IU/day).

Reference range (serum)   0.8–1.5 mg/dl (19–35 μmol/l).

Sampling   Plain tube (gold top); samples should be protected from light. Samples are stable for 4 weeks at 4°C or up to 1 year at −20°C.

Significant effects on routine laboratory parameters   None reported.

Associations with raised levels

- psychiatric: none known
- other: hyperlipidaemia secondary to obstructive liver disease; note that supplementation may result in a lymphocytosis.

Causes of lowered levels

- psychiatric: none known
- other: abetalipoproteinaemia, ceroid (a wax-like material found as crystals in certain pathological states) deposition in bowel muscle, malabsorption states.

Vitamin K (see also prothrombin time)

Function   Vitamin K is a fat-soluble vitamin which exists in two forms: K1 (phylloquinone) and K2 (menaquinone). There is also a synthetic form, K3 or menadione, which is metabolized to K2. The vitamin is involved in the maintenance of clotting factors including factors II, VII, IX, X and proteins C and S.

Dietary sources   Cereals, leafy green vegetables, soybeans; K2 is also synthesized by intestinal bacteria.

Daily requirement   Approximately 1 μg/kg body weight.

Reference range (serum)   0.13–1.19 ng/ml (0.29–2.64 nmol/l); *note*: levels correlate with triglyceride and vitamin E concentrations. The determination of prothrombin time provides a measure of vitamin K status.

Sampling   Plain tube (gold top); patients should be fasting. Samples are stable for 2–3 months at −20°C and should not be exposed to ultraviolet light.

Possible changes in laboratory parameters include the following.

Table	Possible changes in laboratory parameters with vitamin K excess	
Parameter	**Decreased**	**Increased**
Bilirubin		X*
Erythrocytes	X*	
Haematocrit	X*	
Haemoglobin	X*	
Leukocytes	X	
Platelets	X	
Prothrombin time	X	
*Especially in G6PD.		

Associations with raised levels

• psychiatric: none known
• other: none known.

Note: hypervitaminosis K is rarely associated with excess ingestion of supplements (toxicity is associated more with menadione than with the other forms); symptoms are non-specific and are more likely in babies and young children. Symptoms include flushing, sweating; in some cases haemolytic anaemia, hyperbilirubinaemia, and jaundice may develop.

Associations with lowered levels

• psychiatric: carbamazepine, phenobarbital, phenytoin, and valproate may reduce vitamin K levels (secondary to enzyme induction), especially in pregnancy. Dietary deficiency, as could occur in alcoholism or eating disorders, is reported to be rare
• other: cystic fibrosis, fat malabsortion states, hypoprothrombinaemia, increased bleeding/bruising tendency (cerebral haemorrhage, nosebleeds, bleeding peptic ulcer, urinary tract bleeding), obstructive jaundice, pancreatic disease.

Further reading

General

Bourre JM. Effects of nutrients (in food) on the structure and function of the nervous system: update on dietary requirements for brain. Part 1: micronutrients. J Nutr Health Aging 2006; 10: 377–85.

Bourre JM. Effects of nutrients (in food) on the structure and function of the nervous system: update on dietary requirements for brain. Part 2: macronutrients. J Nutr Health Aging 2006; 10: 386–99.

Moore DP, Jefferson JW. Handbook of Medical Psychiatry, 2nd edn. Philadelphia: Elsevier Mosby, 2004.

Petrie WM, Bann TA. Vitamins in psychiatry. Do they have a role? Drugs 1985; 30: 58–65.

Young DS. Effects of Drugs on Laboratory Tests, 5th edn. Washington, DC: AACC Press, 2001.

Young DS, Friedman RB. Effects of Disease on Laboratory Tests, 4th edn. Washington, DC: AACC Press, 2001.

Biotin

Fernandez-Majia C Pharmacological effects of biotin. J Nutr Biochem 2005; 16: 424–7.

Folate

Bottiglieri T. Folate, vitamin B12, and neuropsychiatric disorders. Nutr Rev 1996; 54: 382–90.

Hutto BR. Folate and cobalamin in psychiatric illness. Compr Psychiatry 1997; 38: 305–14.

Pantothenic acid

Tahiliani AG, Beinlich CJ. Pantothenic acid in health and disease. Vitam Horm 1991; 46: 165–228.

Vitamin A

Penniston KL, Tanumihardjo SA. The acute and chronic toxic effects of vitamin A. Am J Clin Nutr 2006; 83: 191–201.

Strahan JE, Raimer S. Isotretinoin and the controversy of psychiatric adverse effects. Int J Dermatol 2006; 45: 789–99.

Vitamin B1 (thiamine)

Davis E, Icke GC. Clinical chemistry of thiamin. Adv Clin Chem 1983; 23: 93–140.

Martin PR, Singleton CK, Hiller-Sturmhofel S. The role of thiamine deficiency in alcoholic brain disease. Alcohol Res Health 2003; 27: 134–42.

Thomson AD. Mechanisms of vitamin deficiency in chronic alcohol misusers and the development of the Wernicke-Korsakoff syndrome. Alcohol Alcohol Suppl 2000; 35: 2–7.

Vitamin B2 (riboflavin)

Powers HJ. Riboflavin (vitamin B-2) and health. Am J Clin Nutr 2003; 77: 1352–60.

Vitamin B3 (niacin)

Guyton JR, Bays HE. Safety considerations with niacin therapy. Am J Cardiol 2007; 99(6A): 22C–31C.

Vitamin B6 (pyridoxine)

Spinneker A, Sola R, Lemmen V et al. Vitamin B6 status, deficiency and its consequences—an overview. Nutr Hosp 2007; 22: 7–24.

Wilson RG, Davis RE. Clinical chemistry of vitamin B6. Adv Clin Chem 1983; 23: 1–68.

Vitamin B12

Bottiglieri T. Folate, vitamin B12, and neuropsychiatric disorders. Nutr Rev 1996; 54: 382–90.

Miscellaneous

Davis RE. Clinical chemistry of vitamin B12. Adv Clin Chem 1985; 24: 163–216.
Dommisse J. Subtle vitamin-B12 deficiency and psychiatry: a largely unnoticed but devastating relationship? Med Hypotheses 1991; 34: 131–40.

Vitamin C (ascorbic acid)

DeSantis J. Scurvy and psychiatric symptoms. Perspect Psychiatr Care 1993; 29: 18–22.

Vitamin D (cholecalciferol)

Schneider B, Weber B, Frensch A, Stein J, Fritz J. Vitamin D in schizophrenia, major depression and alcoholism. J Neural Transm 2000; 107: 839–42.
Stumpf WE, Privette TH. Light, vitamin D and psychiatry. Role of 1,25 dihydroxyvitamin D3 (soltriol) in etiology and therapy of seasonal affective disorder and other mental processes. Psychopharmacology (Berl) 1989; 97: 285–94.

Vitamin E (α-tocopherol)

Mustacich DJ, Bruno RS, Traber MG. Vitamin E. Vitam Horm 2007; 76: 1–21.
Rodrigo R, Guichard C, Charles R. Clinical pharmacology and therapeutic use of antioxidant vitamins. Fundam Clin Pharmacol 2007; 21: 111–27.

Vitamin K

Cranenburg EC, Schurgers LJ, Vermeer C. Vitamin K: the coagulation vitamin that became omnipotent. Thromb Haemost 2007; 98: 120–5.

Miscellaneous

Malnutrition

Malnutrition is encountered amongst psychiatric patients for various reasons, with multiple metabolic effects that may be reflected in routine laboratory assessment. Malnutrition may be of two types, primary (inadequate, inappropriate, or occasionally excessive intake) or secondary to endogenous factors such as abnormalities with digestion, absorption, transport, storage, metabolism, or excretion of nutrients.

Starvation (see also 'Eating disorders', Chapter 2)

This may also be primary (due to privation) or secondary to a range of physiological and other factors. In addition, dehydration may be coexistent with starvation and may not be apparent on routine laboratory analysis.

Table	Laboratory effects of starvation	
Laboratory parameter	**Laboratory tests**	**Notes**
Albumin	LFT	May be normal or slightly reduced; often a late change
Anaemia	Hb, MCV, serum iron/ transferritin/ferritin; LFT/B12 (may reveal a cause for macrocytic anaemia)	May be due to bleeding or folic acid deficiency. Iron-deficiency anaemia may show a reduced MCV. Macrocytic anaemia may suggest folic acid deficiency, which can be confirmed by a serum or red cell folate assay. Associated dehydration with subsequent rehydration may lead to decreased Hb levels
Glucagon	Plasma glucagons	May be high
Insulin	Fasting blood insulin (serum)	May be low
Total amino acids	Random, morning urine required for qualitative urine amino acid screen	Plasma levels elevated with some variation: alanine falls progressively; glycine rises usually after a delay; valine rises slowly over 10 days or so and then falls
Total fatty acids	Lipid panel	May be elevated
Urea	U&E	May be decreased in prolonged protein deficiency

Miscellaneous

Protein–calorie malnutrition

Two main types have been described, marasmus, which is due mainly to caloric deprivation, and kwashiorkor, in which protein deficiency is predominant. There is not always a clear delineation, and both states may coexist.

Table Altered laboratory parameters in malnutrition

Laboratory parameter	Laboratory tests	Notes
Acidosis (metabolic)	Arterial blood gases	Decreased [H+], increased pH, PCO_2, [HCO_3]
Albumin	LFT	Slight lowering may be present in moderate to severe cases, especially in kwashiorkor
Amino acids	Random, morning urine required for qualitative urine amino acid screen	Plasma levels of essential amino acids (especially 'branched chain') low; an 'overflow' aminoaciduria may be present, especially in kwashiorkor
Amylase	Serum amylase	May especially be associated with kwashiorkor
Anaemia	FBC, haematinics	Usually iron-deficiency anaemia
β-Lipoprotein	Fasting plasma lipoprotein	Low plasma levels, especially in kwashiorkor
Calcium	Calcium	Decreased in protein malnutrition
Cholesterol	Lipid profile	Decreased in protein malnutrition and kwashiorkor
Copper	Serum copper and caeruloplasmin	Especially in kwashiorkor
Cortisol	Patients with depression (up to 50% reported) may have abnormal findings on overnight dexamethasone suppression test (normal <3 µg/dl (<0.08 µmol/l), Cushing's >10 µg/dl (>276 nmol/l), depression >5 µg/dl (<138 nmol/l))	High plasma levels, especially in kwashiorkor
Creatinine	U&E	Decreases usually seen

Miscellaneous

Table Altered laboratory parameters in malnutrition (Cont.)

Laboratory parameter	Laboratory tests	Notes
Electrolytes	K, Mg	Electrolytes may be depleted
ESR	ESR	Decreased in cachexia
Folate	Serum folate	May be decreased
Glucose	Fasting blood glucose	Low plasma levels, especially in kwashiorkor
Growth hormone	Serum growth hormone levels (patients should be rested and not stressed prior to sampling)	Increased levels, especially in kwashiorkor
Haematocrit	FBC	Decreased levels seen
Haemoglobin	FBC	Decreased levels seen
Insulin	Fasting blood insulin (serum)	Increased levels, especially in kwashiorkor
Leukocytes	FBC	Decreases seen
Lipase	Serum lipase	Decreased levels seen, especially in kwashiorkor
Lymphocytes	FBC	Decreases seen
Magnesium	Serum magnesium	Decreases seen
3-Methylhistidine	Urinary determination	Increased urine levels indicate muscle breakdown
Potassium	U&E	Characteristic of kwashiorkor
Thyroxine	TFT	May be decreased with a normal TSH
Transferrin	Plasma transferrin	Reduced level especially in kwashiorkor
Urate	Plasma urate	May be increased
Urea	Plasma urea	Reduced levels
Vitamin A	Blood vitamin levels	Usually decreased
Vitamin B12	Blood vitamin levels	May be increased, especially in kwashiorkor
Zinc	Plasma zinc	May be decreased

Obesity

Obesity may be loosely defined as body weight above 120% of the average for age, sex, and height.

It is further defined using the Quetelet's body mass index (BMI):

$$BMI = (\text{weight in kilogrammes}) \div (\text{height in metres})^2$$

Hence, an individual weighing 70 kg and 1.80 m tall will have the following BMI:

$$BMI = (\text{weight in kilogrammes}) \div (\text{height in metres})^2$$
$$BMI = (70)/([1.80] \times [1.80])$$
$$BMI = (70)/(3.24)$$
$$BMI = 21.60$$

The UK NICE has published guidance relating to obesity (http://guidance.nice.org.uk/CG43/guidance) and suggests the following parameters for the BMI.

Classification	BMI (kg/m²)
Healthy weight	18.5–24.9
Overweight	25–29.9
Obesity I	30–34.9
Obesity II	35–39.9
Obesity III	40 or more

Note that the BMI is not an absolute measure of obesity, and NICE therefore suggests that BMI and waist circumference be considered together.

BMI classification	Waist circumference		
	Low	High	Very high
Overweight	No increased risk	Increased risk	High risk
Obesity I	Increased risk	High risk	Very high risk

For men, waist circumference of less than 94 cm is low, 94–102 cm is high, and more than 102 cm is very high.
For women, waist circumference of less than 80 cm is low, 80–88 cm is high, and more than 88 cm is very high.

Note further: NICE does *not* consider bioimpedance as a suitable measure of obesity.

Psychiatric conditions associated with weight gain/loss

A number of psychiatric conditions are associated with weight gain and loss, which should be evident following appropriate screening. A number of medical conditions are associated with obesity (see below), and other risk factors

356

include treatment with medications associated with weight gain (see below), a past history of obesity, poor housing/income, lack of exercise, and others. The psychiatric syndromes especially associated with weight changes are summarized below.

Table	Psychiatric conditions associated with weight gain/loss	
Condition	*Associated weight changes*	*Notes*
Anxiety disorders	Often weight loss but gain possible	Weight changes may be related to medication, lifestyle factors, or inability to obtain appropriate food or partake of physical activity
Bipolar disorder	Weight gain or loss may occur	Weight gain may be related to medication or manic episodes. Weight loss may sometimes occur in depressive or manic phases
Dementia	Obesity recently reported to increase risk of dementia in later life	Recent research suggests that risk factors for heart disease are also risk factors for developing dementia
Depression	Often weight loss but gain possible	Atypical depression especially associated with weight gain; obesity is especially associated with depression in females. Obesity often lowers self-esteem and can worsen depression
Eating disorders	Weight loss common	Anorexia nervosa especially associated
Obsessive–compulsive disorder	Weight loss possible (rare)	Weight loss may be apparent in those with severe OCD such as with fears concerning contamination
Schizophrenia	Usually weight gain	May be related to antipsychotic treatment, lifestyle factors, and many others; risk factors for weight gain appear to include male gender, previous history of weight gain, age (fourth decade and above), and others

Medical conditions associated with obesity
Obesity has a number of aetiologies, including genetic, environmental, and medical disorders; of these, a number of medical conditions may be amenable to laboratory investigation.

Miscellaneous

357

Table Examples of medical conditions associated with obesity

Condition	Laboratory investigation	Notes
Cushing's syndrome	See Chapter 6	
Growth hormone deficiency	Serum growth hormone levels (patients should be rested and not stressed prior to sampling)	May manifest with non-specific symptoms in adulthood and be associated with hypercholesterolaemia and hypoglycaemia
Hyperthyroidism	See Chapter 6	
Hypogonadism	See Chapter 8	
Hypothalamic disease	U&E, fasting glucose, FBC, lipid panel; ACTH, dexamethasone suppression tests, FSH/LH, GH, 17β oestradiol (women), prolactin, testosterone (males), TFT	May be secondary to radiation, trauma, surgery, or tumours Tests selected depending on clinical presentation following consultation with expert authorities
Hypothyroidism	See Chapter 6	
Insulinoma	Blood glucose, serum C-peptide, serum insulin	Raised levels of C-peptide and serum insulin seen with low glucose
Nesidioblastosis		Raised levels of C-peptide and serum insulin seen with recurrent hypoglycaemia. The condition is due to islet cell abnormalities
Polycystic ovary syndrome	LH levels	Raised levels of LH (together with testosterone) may suggest polycystic ovary syndrome (triad of obesity, acne, facial hirsutes, and infertility/menstrual disturbance)
Pseudoparathyroidism	Parathyroid hormone levels (fasting, morning serum sample), calcium, phosphate	Condition due to defect in adenyl cyclase and the resulting lack of response to parathyroid hormone; high parathyroid hormone levels noted together with hyperphosphataemia and hypocalcaemia

Medical complications of obesity

In addition to the medical conditions associated with obesity in terms of aetiology, obesity also has a number of recognized medical complications.

Table	Medical complications of obesity (incomplete list)	
System	**Condition**	**Notes**
Cardiovascular	Atherosclerotic heart disease Cerebrovascular disease Congestive cardiac failure Hypertension Oedema Venous stasis	Leading cause of morbidity and mortality in Western world
Gastrointestinal	Gallbladder disease Gastrointestinal reflux disease	Gallbladder disease less common in males
Metabolic	Diabetes mellitus Dyslipoproteinaemia Hypercholesterolaemia Metabolic syndrome	Effects contribute to other pathologies, especially cardiovascular
Renal	Urinary incontinence	Related to increased abdominal pressure (stress incontinence)
Reproductive	Menstrual irregularity Ovulatory failure	May manifest as polycystic ovary syndrome
Respiratory	Restrictive lung disease Sleep apnoea	Disturbed sleep can significantly impact on quality of life
Rheumatological	Degenerative arthritis Gout Osteoarthritis	May decrease mobility and independence
Skin	Adiposis dolorosa	Also called Dercum's disease, this condition consists of: (a) painful and multiple lipomas; (b) generalized obesity, usually in menopausal women; (c) psychiatric symptoms such as confusion, depression, and lability of mood; (d) weakness and fatigue

Table	Medical complications of obesity (incomplete list) (Cont.)	
System	**Condition**	**Notes**
Other	Increased risk of cancer	Males: colon, prostrate, rectum; females: breast, cervix, endometrium, gallbladder, ovary
	Pregnancy risks	Increased risk of diabetes and toxaemia
	Pseudotumour cerebri	Pseudotumour cerebri is defined clinically by the following criteria: (a) elevated intracranial pressure on lumbar puncture; (b) normal cerebral anatomy on imaging; (c) normal cerebrospinal fluid composition; (d) signs and symptoms of increased intracranial pressure, usually including papilloedema
	Anaesthetic and surgical risks	Increased risk of anaesthetic complications, pneumonia, poor wound healing, thromboembolism

Psychotropics associated with weight loss

Rarely, psychotropics may be associated with weight loss, although data remain incomplete in most cases.

Table	Psychotropics associated with weight loss
Agent	**Notes**
Bupropion	Clinically insignificant weight loss noted usually with longer-term treatment
Duloxetine	Weight loss has been reported
Fluoxetine	Weight loss especially associated with high doses
Fluvoxamine	Weight loss usually not clinically significant
Tranylcypromine	One study suggests that weight loss is more likely than gain
Venlafaxine	Often associated with weight loss

Psychotropics associated with weight gain

Patients with psychiatric disorders may be more prone to obesity due to a number of inter-related factors, such as sedentary lifestyle, lack of access to appropriate food, lack of appropriate education and guidance regarding diet, medical comorbidity, and use of medications, especially antipsychotics.

Table Psychotropics associated with weight gain

Class	Example	Risk of weight gain	Notes
Antidepressants	Citalopram Fluvoxamine Lofepramine Paroxetine Sertraline	Low	Risk of weight gain especially in the elderly; other SSRIs thought to be weight neutral in the short-term
	Mirtazepine Phenelzine Tricyclics	Moderate	Of the MAOIs, phenelzine is most commonly implicated, tranylcypromine rarely, and moclobemide intermediate to these
	Mianserin Reboxetine Trazodone	Insufficient data	
Antipsychotics	Chlorpromazine Clozapine Perphenazine Olanzapine Thioridazine Zotepine	High	Effects appear worse during first year of treatment with clozapine Increased risk of metabolic effects (including metabolic syndrome) in obese individuals at start of treatment
	Quetiapine Risperidone	Moderate	
	Amisulpride Aripiprazole Fluphenazine Haloperidol Loxapine Sulpiride Trifluoperazine Ziprasidone	Low	A number of complex effects may interact to cause weight gain; these include alterations in neurotransmitters, increased sedation, anticholinergic effects, effects on insulin, and possible changes in leptin levels (leptin is a polypeptide produced by fat cells which acts to reduce appetite)
	Benperidol Flupentixol Levomepromazine Promazine Pericyazine Pimozide Pipotiazine Zuclopentixol	Insufficient data	
Benzodiazepines	Alprazolam Clobazam	Low	Few data available
Mood stabilizers	Gabapentin Lamotrigine	Low	Effects variable
	Carbamazepine	Moderate	Lithium is associated with both increased thirst and insulin release which results in adipogenesis
	Lithium	High	
	Valproate		Risk increased when valproate is prescribed with clozapine

Baseline blood tests in obese patients

Laboratory investigations for obese individuals will be determined by clinical presentation and history together with the physical and mental state examinations. Obese patients receiving antipsychotics should also be considered for screening for metabolic side-effects associated with the specific medication or medications that they are being treated with. Note that NICE only recommends fasting glucose and fasting lipid panel.

For non-complicated/non-medicated patients an extended basic scheme is suggested below.

Table Suggested baseline laboratory investigations for obese patients

Domain	Laboratory investigation	Notes
Clinical biochemistry	Calcium	Obesity predisposes to cardiac arrhythmias
	Fasting glucose	Increased risk of glucose intolerance/ diabetes mellitus
	Fasting lipid panel	Increased risk of hypercholesterolaemia and dyslipoproteinaemias
	LFT	Increased risk of liver (gallbladder) disease and possibly also of alcohol use; note that ALT and AST may be higher in obese subjects in the absence of any significant hepatic disease
	TFT	Hyperthyroidism (rarely) and more often hypothyroidism are associated with obesity
	U&E	Obesity predisposes to cardiac arrhythmias
	Uric acid/urate	To support any clinical suggestion of gout
	Urinalysis	Increased risk of proteinuria, renal cancers, and UTI in obese individuals
Haematology	FBC	Polycythaemia and increased Hb may be seen in some patients with sleep apnoea (secondary to chronic hypoxia)
Immunology	No specific tests required	
Microbiology	No specific tests required – possible mid-stream urine sample if UTI suspected	

Miscellaneous

NICE guidelines The UK NICE has published guidance relating to obesity (http://guidance.nice.org.uk/CG43/guidance) and suggests that the medical assessment of obese individuals may include fasting glucose and a fasting lipid profile.

Changes in laboratory parameters associated with obesity Serum – β-endorphins, cholesterol, free fatty acids, glucagon, growth hormone, insulin, triglycerides; urine – 17-hydroxycorticosteroids.

Hyperalimentation and re-feeding

Definition Hyperalimentation, also known as total parenteral nutrition (TPN), is the administration of nutrients and vitamins given to a person in liquid form via parenteral routes. In psychiatry the most common indication is in the treatment of severe eating disorders and occasionally in severe depressive episodes, severe OCD, and severe, chronic alcoholism. Note that the UK NICE has published guidelines relating to TPN (http://guidance.nice.org.uk/CG32). Related to hyperalimentation is the re-feeding syndrome, which accompanies the electrolyte and fluid shifts that occur during hyperalimentation in cases of malnutrition. Note that the UK NICE (http://guidance.nice.org.uk/CG32) has published guidelines relating to total parenteral nutrition and includes specific advice regarding laboratory monitoring (see table below).

Related to hyperalimentation is the re-feeding syndrome, which accompanies the electrolyte and fluid shifts that occur during hyperalimentation in cases of malnutrition.

Clinically, a number of problems may occur, including neurological/psychiatric (delirium, epilepsy, movement disorders, muscle problems including fasciculations, paraesthesia and weakness, Wernicke's), cardiovascular (cardiac arrhythmia, heart failure), electrolyte disturbances (see Table below), gastrointestinal upset (abdominal pain, change in bowel habit). *Note*: the re-feeding syndrome may mimic rhabdomyolysis/neuroleptic malignant syndrome (see Chapter 3).

Table Possible metabolic associations with hyperalimentation

Laboratory tests	Notes
Albumin	May be decreased
Bicarbonate	Metabolic acidosis may occur (decreased: [H+], increased pH, PCO_2, $[HCO_3]$)
Blood glucose	Hyper- or hypoglycaemia may be seen
Calcium	May be decreased or increased
Chloride	Hyperchloraemia may be seen
Copper	May be decreased
Creatine phosphokinase	May be raised
Erythrocytes	Haemolysis may occur as a result of severe hypophosphataemia
Folate	Deficiency may be seen (see Chapter 8) and may result in anaemia
INR	May be altered
Iron	Deficiency may be seen (may result in anaemia)
Liver function tests	Non-specific derangements may be seen; in chronic hyperalimentation the AST/ALT ratio may be <1, especially in the disorder known as non-alcoholic steatohepatitis. This disorder may progress to cirrhosis
Linoleic acid	Deficiency may be seen; linoleic acid is an essential fatty acid, deficiency of which is associated with poor wound healing, hair loss, and (controversially) mood disorders and cardiac arrhythmias
Magnesium	May be decreased
Phosphate	Hypophosphataemia frequently occurs and may be severe, leading to rhabdomyolysis and cardiomyopathy
Potassium	Hypokalaemia may be seen
Selenium	May be decreased
Sodium	Hyponatraemia (usually mild) may occur; hypernatraemia is rare
Urea	Raised after high protein meal and in hyperalimentation
Vitamin D (25-OH)	Levels may be decreased
Zinc	May be decreased

Miscellaneous

NICE guidelines suggest the following system of laboratory monitoring (blood).

Parameter	Suggested frequency of monitoring
Albumin	At baseline, then weekly
Calcium	
Copper	At baseline, then every 2–4 weeks depending on results
C reactive protein	At baseline, then 2–3 times/week until stable
Creatinine	At baseline, then daily until stable, then 1–2 times/week
Ferritin	At baseline, then every 3–6 months
Folate	At baseline, then every 2–4 weeks
Full blood count	At baseline, then 1–2 times/week until stable, then weekly
Glucose	At baseline, then 1–2 times/day until stable, then weekly
Iron	At baseline, then every 3–6 months
Liver function tests (including INR)	At baseline, then twice weekly until stable then weekly
Magnesium	At baseline, then daily if at risk of re-feeding syndrome, then 3 times/day until stable, then weekly
Manganese	Every 3–6 months (if on home parenteral nutrition)
Mass cell volume	At baseline, then 1–2 times/week until stable, then weekly
25-OH vitamin D	Every 6 months (if on long-term support)
Phosphate	At baseline, then daily if at risk of re-feeding syndrome, then 3 times/day until stable, then weekly
Potassium	At baseline, then daily until stable, then 1–2 times/week
Selenium	At baseline if at risk of depletion; further testing dependent on baseline
Sodium	At baseline, then daily until stable, then 1–2 times/week
Urea	
Vitamin B12	At baseline, then every 2–4 weeks
Zinc	At baseline, then every 2–4 weeks depending on results

Further reading

Hyperalimentation and re-feeding syndrome

Catani M, Howells R. Risks and pitfalls for the management of refeeding syndrome in psychiatric patients. Psychiatr Bull 2007; 31: 209–11.
Ukleja A, Romano MM. Complications of parenteral nutrition. Gastroenterol Clin North Am 2007; 36: 23–46.

Malnutrition

Akuyam SA. A review of some metabolic changes in protein-energy malnutrition. Niger Postgrad Med J 2007; 14: 155–62.

Obesity

Bray GA. The Metabolic Syndrome and Obesity. New Jersey: Humana Press, 2007.
McIntyre RS, Konarski JZ. Obesity and psychiatric disorders: frequently encountered clinical questions. Focus 2005; 3: 511–19.
Ogden CL, Yanovski SZ, Carroll MD, Flegal KM. The epidemiology of obesity. Gastroenterology 2007; 132: 2087–102.
Sacks FM. Metabolic syndrome: epidemiology and consequences. J Clin Psychiatry 2004; 65 (Suppl 18): 3–12.

Psychotropics and weight gain/loss

Newcomer JW. Antipsychotic medications: metabolic and cardiovascular risk. J Clin Psychiatry 2007; 68 (Suppl 4): 8–13.
Schwartz TL, Nihalani N, Jindal S, Virk S, Jones N. Psychiatric medication-induced obesity: a review. Obes Rev 2004; 5: 115–21.
Tschoner A, Engl J, Laimer M et al. Metabolic side effects of antipsychotic medication. Int J Clin Pract 2007; 61: 1356–70.
Vanina Y, Podolskaya A, Sedky K et al. Body weight changes associated with psychopharmacology. Psychiatr Serv 2002; 53: 842–7.

Miscellaneous

Vegetarian/vegan diets
Definitions

- veganism: the voluntary practice of not eating meat (including poultry, fish, and seafood), eggs, dairy products, or by-products of these
- vegetarianism: the voluntary practice of not eating fish, meat, poultry, or seafood or by-products of these
- Ovo-lacto vegetarian: a vegetarian who also eats eggs, milk, and by-products of these.

Metabolic risks associated with chronic, strict vegetarian diets include the following.

Table Possible metabolic risks associated with vegetarian diets		
Condition	**Laboratory tests**	**Notes**
Anaemia	FBC, haematinics	Especially present in female ovo-lacto vegetarians (possibly up to 3%)
Carnitine deficiency	Carnitine levels	Carnitine is an amino acid derivative which plays an important role in mitochondrial processes; deficiency is rare, with primary deficiency usually found in infants and children and secondary deficiency which may present at any age with encephalopathy accompanied by hypoketotic hypoglycaemic episodes. It is associated with use of phenobarbital and valproic acid. Increased blood levels of carnitine may be found with alcohol use and severe renal disease
Protein deficiency	Total protein, U&E	Urea is decreased in low protein/high carbohydrate diets
Trace element deficiency (e.g. calcium, zinc)	Calcium levels; zinc levels	See Chapters 8 (zinc) and 9 (calcium)
Vitamin deficiency (B2, B3, B12)	Vitamin levels	See Chapter 8: increased serum folate and decreased serum vitamin B12 have been noted

Note: vegans/vegetarians who do not eat fish often have decreased levels of essential fatty acids.

Other changes in laboratory parameters have been described increased – serum folate, decreased – serum vitamin B12, urine creatinine.

Miscellaneous

Further reading

Bernstein AM, Treyzon L, Li Z. Are high-protein, vegetable-based diets safe for kidney function? A review of the literature. J Am Diet Assoc 2007; 107: 644–50.

Hunt JR. Bioavailability of iron, zinc, and other trace minerals from vegetarian diets. Am J Clin Nutr 2003; 78(Suppl): 633S–9S.

Obeid R, Geisel J, Schorr H, Hubner U, Herrmann W. The impact of vegetarianism on some haematological parameters. Eur J Haematol 2002; 69: 275–9.

Rajaram S. The effect of vegetarian diet, plant foods, and phytochemicals on hemostasis and thrombosis. Am J Clin Nutr 2003; 78(Suppl): 552S–8S.

Young DS. Effects of Drugs on Laboratory Tests, 5th edn. Washington, DC: AACC Press, 2001.

Young DS, Friedman RB. Effects of Disease on Laboratory Tests, 4th edn. Washington, DC: AACC Press, 2001.

Miscellaneous

Special populations

The following changes may be noted in some individuals as normal variants, but in all cases clinical presentation should always be taken into account when interpreting laboratory findings.

Age

Although the remit of general adult psychiatry is for patients between the ages of 18 and 65 years, on occasion patients ouside these ranges may be seen, usually at the upper end of the age spectrum and who are not deemed suitable for old-age services.

A number of laboratory parameters may show age-related changes in elderly patients (aged over 65 years).

Table	Possible age-related changes in laboratory parameters
Parameter (plasma)	**Usual age-dependent effect**
Albumin	Decreased
Alkaline phosphatase	Increased
Calcium	Decreased
Cholesterol	Increased
Creatine kinase	Decreased
Creatinine	Decreased
CRP	Increased
Erythrocyte sedimentation rate	Increased
Glomerular filtration rate	Decreased
Glucose	Increased
Haemoglobin	Increased
Mean cell volume	Increased
Protein (total)	Decreased
Urate	Increased

Miscellaneous

Ethnicity

Note: these effects are not universal and are not usually clinically significant.

Afro-Caribbeans versus Caucasians

Decreased

- cholesterol levels (controversial): especially after age 40
- haemoglobin levels: lower levels in black persons as compared to Caucasians (approximately 4–10 g/l lower)
- leukocyte counts (associated with benign ethnic neutropaenia)
- neutrophil counts (benign ethnic neutropaenia): lower WCC with neutrophil count between 1 and 2.5; may be detected prior to commencement of medications such as clozapine, carbamazepine, or mirtazepine and is not usually clinically significant
- red cell counts (may affect ESR)
- triglyceride levels observed (0.11–0.23 mmol/l lower)
- vitamin B12: in European women versus African women.

Increased

- cotinine levels
- creatine kinase levels observed in healthy subjects compared to Caucasians, with Afro-Caribbean females generally showing slightly higher levels than in males; caution is therefore advised in interpretation of creatine kinase levels in individuals from these populations
- estimated glomerular filtration rate.

South Asians versus Caucasians Increased rates of diabetes mellitus and metabolic syndrome (insulin resistance, low HDL cholesterol, high plasma lipids, central adiposity); decreased vitamin D levels especially in Asian women who do not receive adequate exposure to the sun.

Gender

Some laboratory parameters may have different reference ranges depending on gender, although this can vary and these should always be considered in relation to clinical presentation.

Lower levels in females (non-pregnant, non-lactating) compared to males:

- alanine transferase (minimal difference)
- alkaline phosphatase (slightly higher in men up to/including 5th decade)
- aspartate transaminase (slightly higher in men up to/including 5th decade)
- bilirubin (minimal difference)
- calcium (ionized) (minimal difference)
- creatine kinase (20–25% lower)*
- creatinine (difference depends on muscle mass, may be up to 20% lower)
- ferritin (minimal difference)
- gamma glutamyl transferase (may be up to 25% lower)
- glomerular filtration rate

- glucose (compared to males less than age 60)
- haematocrit (up to 10% lower)
- haemoglobin (up to 20% lower)
- red cell count (up to 10% lower)
- serum iron (up to 10% lower)
- urate (up to 25% lower)
- urea (minimal difference except compared to males age 70+).

*Levels may be higher in Afro-Caribbean females compared to Afro-Caribbean males.

Higher levels in females (non-pregnant, non-lactating) compared to males:

- amylase (approximately 16% higher)
- CD4 count (in healthy subjects – note that CD4 counts may fluctuate with the menstrual cycle)
- copper (plasma) (up to 20% higher)
- erythrocyte sedimentation rate (minimal difference)
- immunoglobulins (especially IgM) (minimal difference)
- transferrin (minimal difference)
- prolactin (minimal difference).

Females (non-pregnant, non-lactating) may have **greater** requirements for the following vitamins: B1 (thiamine), B3 (niacin), B12, C (ascorbic acid); **males** may have **greater** requirements for vitamin A.

Further reading

Bain BJ. Ethnic and sex differences in the total and differential white cell count and platelet count. J Clin Pathol 1996; 49: 664–6.
Gorman LS. Aging: laboratory testing and theories. Clin Lab Sci 1995; 8: 24–30.
Young DS. Effects of Drugs on Laboratory Tests, 5th edn. Washington, DC: AACC Press, 2001.
Young DS, Friedman RB. Effects of Disease on Laboratory Tests, 4th edn. Washington, DC: AACC Press, 2001.

Miscellaneous

Miscellaneous behavioural states

Hyperventilation
Effects seen are secondary to respiratory alkalosis:

- decreased – serum ionized calcium, serum phosphate
- increased – blood pH.

Hyperthermia
The following effects may be seen especially in prolonged exposure to heat such as in heat stroke:

- decreased – calcium, glucose, platelet count, potassium, protein
- increased – alanine transaminase, albumin, bilirubin, bleeding time, chloride, creatinine, haemoglobin, ketones, leukocytes, lymphocytes, monocytes, phosphate, prothrombin time.

Note: increased exposure to heat may result in increased water loss and thence dehydration (see Chapter 8).

Hypothermia
Effects may be secondary to acid–base disturbances, hypotension, or hypoxia:

- decreased – bicarbonate, pH, PO_2
- increased – aspartate transaminase, creatine kinase, free fatty acids, hydroxybutyrate dehydrogenase, PCO_2.

Note: prolonged ice-eating may be associated with decreased haemoglobin levels.

Psychomotor agitation
The following effects may be more prominent in non-athletic individuals and are usually benign:

- decreased – bicarbonate, iron, thyroxine (with strenuous/prolonged activity)
- increased – albumin, ammonia, calcium, caeruloplasmin, chloride, creatine kinase, haematocrit, ketones, lactate, leukocytes, phosphate, platelets, protein, prothrombin time, transferrin.

Psychomotor retardation
The following effects may be more prominent following prolonged inactivity:

- decreased – glucose
- increased – ionized calcium, phosphate.

Further reading

General

Young DS. Effects of Drugs on Laboratory Tests, 5th edn. Washington, DC: AACC Press, 2001.
Young DS, Friedman RB. Effects of Disease on Laboratory Tests, 4th edn. Washington, DC: AACC Press, 2001.

Hyperthermia

LoVecchio F, Pizon AF, Berrett C, Balls A. Outcomes after environmental hyperthermia. Am J Emerg Med 2007; 25: 442–4.

Hyperventilation

Bass C, Gardner WN, Chambers J. Hyperventilation syndromes in medicine and psychiatry. J R Soc Med 1987; 80: 722–3.
Lum LC. Hyperventilation syndromes in medicine and psychiatry: a review. J R Soc Med 1987; 80: 229–31.
Moe OW, Fuster D. Clinical acid-base pathophysiology: disorders of plasma anion gap. Best Pract Res Clin Endocrinol Metab 2003; 17: 559–74.

Hypothermia

Tisherman SA. Hypothermia and injury. Curr Opin Crit Care 2004; 10: 512–19.

Psychomotor agitation

Schillerstrom TL, Schillerstrom JE, Taylor SE. Laboratory findings in emergently medicated psychiatry patients. Gen Hosp Psychiatry 2004; 26: 411–14.

Psychomotor retardation

Adamu B, Sani MU, Abdu A. Physical exercise and health: a review. Niger J Med 2006; 15: 190–6.

Miscellaneous

Trace metals and psychiatry

The trace elements/metals discussed below are those in which psychiatric complications have been reported. Other metals may have rarely reported effects on mental state (e.g. barium, boron, cadmium, platinum, silicon, tellurium) but are not included herein. *Note*: trace metal toxicity is usually associated with a number of changes in routine laboratory parameters which may confound diagnosis.

Although patients with psychiatric disorders may present with features of trace metal deficiency, it is rarely necessary to determine blood levels of trace metals and these assays are rarely performed in routine practice. Where specific deficiency is suspected, it is advisable to seek expert advice prior to testing. Psychiatric patients particularly susceptible to specific deficiencies include those with alcohol and substance abuse disorders, eating disorders, and occasionally severe depression or psychosis. A thorough history, including occupational history, is recommended in all patients.

Note: some laboratories offer a heavy metal screen to check for suspected toxicity. As special collection techniques may be required for most heavy metals, it is advisable to contact the receiving laboratory prior to sample collection.

The following trace metals will be discussed:

- aluminium
- arsenic
- bismuth
- chromium
- cobalt
- copper
- gold
- iron
- lead
- magnesium
- manganese
- mercury
- nickel
- selenium
- thallium
- tin
- vanadium
- zinc.

For each metal the following information will be provided:

- routes of exposure
- normal range
- associated changes in laboratory parameters
- associations with excess
- associations with deficiency.

Aluminium

Routes of exposure Antacid ingestion, dialysis, foods, industrial exposure, parenteral nutrition.

Normal range (serum) 0–0.22 μmol/l (<54 μg/l). *Note*: levels are highest in the morning (09.00) and lowest in the evening (18.00).

The desferoxamine infusion test has been used to diagnose aluminium toxicity.

Associated changes in routine laboratory parameters (aluminium excess) Microcytic anaemia (hypochromic, normochromic); blood smear may show a number of changes including anisocytosis, basophilic stippling, chromophilic cells, and poikilocytosis.

Hypercalcaemia may be seen in some cases.

Associations with excess

- psychiatric: possible association with Alzheimer's dementia (controversial) and a dementia secondary to dialysis has been reported. This is in patients on intermittent, long-term dialysis, which presents initially as a speech disorder and then progresses to convulsions, myoclonus, and dementia. An association with amyotrophic lateral sclerosis and a form of parkinsonism/dementia in certain individuals from the Island of Guam has also been reported. Occupational exposure has been associated with encephalopathy, with cognitive changes, stuttering, disturbed gait, seizures, coma, and dementia
- Other: aluminium bone disease (a rare condition in patients undergoing dialysis against water with high aluminium content or when aluminium-containing phosphate binders are used. It is a type of renal osteodystrophy characterized by pathological fractures, bone pain, skeletal deformity and possibly dementia and anaemia); cystic fibrosis, Hodgkin's disease, renal failure, antacids containing aluminium. Additional symptoms related to aluminium toxicity include proximal myopathy, cardiac disturbances (secondary to myocardial dysfunction), microcytic anaemia. There may also be an increased risk of infection.

Associations with deficiency

- psychiatric: none known
- other: none known.

Arsenic

Routes of exposure Exposure to insecticides/rodenticides, industrial exposure.

Normal range (whole blood) <23 μg/l (<0.31 μmol/l); blood levels useful only for acute poisoning (due to short half-life of arsenic in blood); for chronic poisoning, hair, nail, or urine analysis is required.

Possible changes in routine laboratory parameters *Note*: effects include cirrhosis and renal failure, and hence laboratory testing in suspected arsenic toxicity should include FBC, LFT, and U&E.

Table Summary of possible changes in laboratory parameters with arsenic		
Parameter	*Decreased*	*Increased*
ALP		X
ALT		X
AST		X
Bilirubin		X
Cholesterol		X
Creatinine		X
Eosinophils		X
Erythrocytes	X	
ESR		X
Glucose	X	
Haematocrit	X	
Haemoglobin	X	
Leukocytes	X	
Reticulocytes		X
Urea		X

Associations with excess

- psychiatric: non-specific anorexia/fatigue (may present as depression), cognitive impairment, psychosis (rare)
- other: symptoms of acute intoxication include abdominal pain, cardiovascular collapse, diarrhoea and vomiting; symptoms of chronic intoxication include skin changes (hair loss, hyperkeratosis of palms and soles, 'Mees' lines' (transverse, white lines on fingernails), pigmentation, scaling). Haematological changes (anaemia, basophilic stippling, leukopaenia, thrombocytopaenia) may occur. Production of arsene gas may result in haematuria, haemoglobinuria, haemolysis, and acute renal failure.

Associations with deficiency

- psychiatric: none known
- other: none known.

Bismuth

Route of exposure Cosmetics, iatrogenic (treatment of gastrointestinal disorders).

Normal range (plasma) 0.1–3.5 µg/l (0.5–16.7 nmol/l).

Associated changes in routine laboratory parameters None specific, although patients with renal impairment may be at higher risk of toxicity. It is therefore suggested that tests of renal function (U&E, eGFR) be included in cases of bismuth toxicity.

Associations with excess

- psychiatric: non-specific anxiety, delusions (rare), depression, insomnia, irritability; hallucinations in any modality may occur, as can cognitive impairment, dementia, and delirium
- other: encephalopathy (secondary to bismuth-containing medications and reversible upon cessation of treatment), fetor, fever, generalized rheumatic pain, gum discolouration, motor problems (ataxia, myoclonus, tremor), renal failure; intoxication may occur following ingestion of bismuth-containing medications.

Associations with deficiency

- psychiatric: none known
- other: none known.

Chromium

Route of exposure Industrial exposure.

Normal range (serum) 0.05–0.5 µg/l (1–10 nmol/l).

Associated changes in routine laboratory parameters None specific, although anaemia, hepatotoxicity, and renal failure have been reported. It is therefore suggested that FBC, LFT, and U&E be measured in cases of chromium toxicity.

Associations with excess

- psychiatric: somatoform disorders (controversial association with industrial exposure)
- other: dermatitis, lung disease (asthma, bronchitis, carcinoma); acute intoxication may result in acute hepatitis, acute tubular necrosis, convulsions, and proteinuria.

Associations with deficiency

- psychiatric: depression (controversial)
- other: association with glucose intolerance and elevated plasma fatty acids in patients on long-term parenteral nutrition. It has been reported that

chromium supplementation may improve glucose tolerance in some patients, but this remains controversial. Levels have been reported to be lower in pregnant women compared to non-pregnant women.

Cobalt

Route of exposure Industrial exposure.

Normal range (serum) 0.11–0.45 µg/l (1.9–7.6 nmol/l).

Associated changes in routine laboratory parameters None specific, although chronic toxicity may be associated with hypothyroidism and renal dysfunction; it is thus recommended that TFT and U&E be obtained in suspected cobalt toxicity.

Associations with excess

- psychiatric: Alzheimer's dementia (controversial)
- other: allergic dermatitis, cardiomyopathy, goitre (chronic toxicity), hypertension, interstitial fibrosis, nausea, nerve damage (deafness, giddiness, tinnitus), polycythaemia, vomiting.

Associations with deficiency (as per vitamin B12 deficiency – cobalt plays a structural role in vitamin B12: see Chapter 8)

- psychiatric: fatigue (controversial)
- other: pernicious anaemia.

Copper (see also Wilson's disease in Chapter 6)

Route of exposure Essential element found in nature (found in many metalloenzymes).

Normal range (plasma) Males 56–111 µg/l (8.8–17.5 µmol/l), females 69–169 µg/l (10.7–26.6 µmol/l).

Associated changes in routine laboratory parameters None specific.

Associations with excess

- psychiatric: alcoholism, psychosis (controversial); Menkes' disease (Menkes' kinky hair syndrome) – a rare, inborn error of copper metabolism manifested by failure to thrive, neurological impairment, and severe mental retardation. Most affected individuals die before the age of 3 years. Low concentrations of copper are found in brain and liver with high concentrations elsewhere. Note that carbamazepine and other agents (oestrogens, oral contraceptives, phenobarbital, phenytoin) may increase serum levels of copper
- other: anaemia (microcytic or normocytic, occasionally haemolytic, thalassaemias), abdominal pain, coma, diarrhoea, gastrointestinal irritation (may cause bleeding), glomerulonephritis, haemochromatosis, headache,

hyperalimentation/re-feeding, hyperparathyroidism, hypotension, Indian childhood cirrhosis, infections (bacterial pneumonia, pulmonary tuberculosis (TB), rheumatic fever, septicaemia, typhoid, viral hepatitis), jaundice (secondary to hepatocellular necrosis), melaena, multiple sclerosis, nausea, neoplasms, ovarian hyperfunction, pregnancy, renal tubular necrosis, rheumatological disorders (dermatomyositis, Sjögren's, SLE, systemic sclerosis, rheumatoid arthritis), thyroid disorders, vomiting. Brain infarction will cause rises in CSF levels, and increased copper may also be found in the synovial fluid of individuals with rheumatoid arthritis.

Associations with deficiency

• psychiatric: Wilson's disease (see Chapter 6)
• other: anaemia (non-responsive to iron), bone disease (may resemble scurvy), chronic ischaemic heart disease, coeliac sprue, decreased skin pigmentation, growth failure, male infertility, nephritic syndrome, neutropaenia, osteoporosis, ovarian hypofunction, protein malnutrition.

Gold

Route of exposure As treatment of rheumatoid arthritis, industrial exposure (gold-plating).

Normal range (serum) 0–0.1µg/ml (0–0.5µmol/l); therapeutic range 1.0–3.0µg/mL (5.1–15.2µmol/l).

Associated changes in routine laboratory parameters None specific.

Associations with excess

• psychiatric: delirium, depression, hallucinations
• other: albuminuria, anaemia, dermatitis, eosinophilia, leukopaenia, nephrosis, proteinuria, pruritus, stomatitis, thrombocytopaenia; severe toxicity may induce cholestasis, gastrointestinal inflammation (small and large bowel), haematuria, peripheral neuropathy, pulmonary infiltrates.

Associations with deficiency

• psychiatric: none known.
• other: none known.

Iron (see also Chapter 6)

Route of exposure Essential element found in nature and certain foods (enzymatic cofactor, role in oxygen transport and in metabolic pathways such as the electron transport chain), genetic, iatrogenic (dialysis, blood transfusion, treatment of iron-deficiency anaemia), overdose.

Normal range (serum) Males 50–160µg/dl (9.0–28.8µmol/l), females up to 10% lower. *Note*: levels are highest in the morning and subjects should be fasted prior to specimen collection.

Miscellaneous

Associated changes in routine laboratory parameters None specific; there may be abnormal LFT or glucose.

Associations with excess

- psychiatric: lethargy (may mimic chronic fatigue syndrome)
- other: acute intoxication – abdominal pain, black stools, cyanosis, gastrointestinal bleeding, haematemesis, hyperglycaemia, hypotension, leukocytosis, liver damage, metabolic acidosis, renal failure, shock, vomiting; chronic intoxication – abnormal liver function, diabetes mellitus; haemochromatosis is an inherited disorder of increased intestinal iron absorption and deposition in various organs. Middle-aged males are more commonly affected and haematinics may show increased serum ferritin, increased serum iron, decreased total iron binding capacity.

Associations with deficiency (anaemia)

- psychiatric: tiredness, lassitude, depression, pica (rare); may contribute to symptoms of chronic fatigue, somatization, other functional disorders, or personality disorders (e.g. those involving deliberate self-harm)
- other: angular stomatitis, dysphagia (may be secondary to Plummer–Kelly syndrome – association of dysphagia with oesophageal web, especially in middle-aged women), glossitis, and nail signs (brittle, flattened nails; rarely koilonychia); hyperalimentation/re-feeding.

Lead

Route of exposure Cosmetics, exposure to lead paint or lead petrol, industrial exposure.

Normal range (whole blood) $<10\,\mu g/dl$ ($<0.5\,\mu mol/l$).

Note: the predominant effects of lead toxicity are neurological, and lead may affect renal function, especially the renal tubules. Thus U&E, phosphate, and glucose should be measured in suspected lead toxicity.

Associated changes in routine laboratory parameters Are given below.

Table	Summary of toxic effects of lead on laboratory parameters	
Parameter	*Decreased*	*Increased*
Aldolase		X
Aminolevulinic acid		X
Basophilic stippling		X
Bilirubin		X
Eosinophils		X
Erythrocytes	X	
ESR		X
Haematocrit	X	
Haemoglobin	X	
Iron		X
Lead		X
Leukocytes	X	
MCH	X	
MCHC	X	
MCV	X	
Red cell osmotic fragility	X	
Platelet count	X	
Reticulocytes		X
Urate		X
Urea		X

Associations with excess ('plumbism')

- psychiatric: altered mood, cognitive changes, delirium, hallucinosis, irritability, lethargy, mania, mental handicap (may be irreversible); has been reported in some cases of chronic fatigue syndrome (controversial)
- other: acute intoxication – abdominal discomfort, aminoaciduria, anaemia (microcytic or normocytic hypochromic anaemia), basophilic stippling, constipation, encephalopathy, glycosuria, gum discolouration, increased urinary zinc protoporphyrin, interstitial fibrosis, lethargy, peripheral phosphaturia, neuropathy, vomiting.

Miscellaneous

Associations with deficiency

- psychiatric: none known
- other: none known.

Other blood tests are described in lead poisoning.

Table Additional blood tests described in lead poisoning	
Test	*Notes*
Free erythrocyte protoporphyrin	May be raised in chronic lead poisoning and iron-deficiency anaemia
Red blood cell zinc protoporphyrin	May be raised in chronic lead poisoning
Serum aminolevulinate dehydratase	May be decreased in lead poisoning
Urine aminolevulinic acid Urinary coproporphyrin	Levels may be raised in lead poisoning (and porphyria)

Magnesium

Route of exposure Essential element (roles in energy production, enzymes, and muscle function); certain foods (cereals, meat, nuts, seafood), iatrogenic (antacids, cathartics, treatment of acute nephritis and eclampsia), industrial exposure, water.

Normal range (serum) 1.5–2.3 mg/dl (0.60–0.95 mmol/l).

Associated changes in routine laboratory parameters Deficiency may be associated with hypocalcaemia and hypoparathyroidism; toxicity may be associated with dehydration secondary to osmotic diarrhoea, and hence measurement of U&E may be helpful in cases of magnesium toxicity.

Associations with excess

- psychiatric: none known
- other: cardiac arrhythmia (cardiac arrest with severe hypermagnesaemia), loss of deep tendon reflexes, renal impairment, respiratory embarrassment; industrial exposure – conjunctivitis or production of discoloured sputum may be present.

Associations with deficiency

- psychiatric: chronic alcoholism, chronic sleep deprivation, eating disorders (especially those involving starvation), possibly secondary to treatment with medications causing SIADH (implicated agents include all antidepressants, carbamazepine, clozapine, haloperidol, olanzapine, phenothiazines, pimozide, quetiapine, risperidone)

- other: cardiac arrhythmias, convulsions, delirium, hyperalimentation/re-feeding, hypocalcaemia, hypokalaemia, irritability, kidney stones, tetany, tremor, weakness.

Manganese

Route of exposure Essential element found in nature (enzyme cofactor), foods (grains, nuts, tea, vegetables), iatrogenic (parenteral nutrition), industrial exposure (mining, manufacture of chlorine gas and lead-free petrol).

Normal range (serum) 0.43–0.76 ng/ml (7.8–13.8 nmol/l).

Associated changes in routine laboratory parameters None specific in deficiency or excess, although there may be non-specific changes in liver function in manganese toxicity.

Associations with excess

- psychiatric: anxiety, ataxia, cognitive changes, fatigue, hallucinosis, mania, insomnia, psychotic state resembling schizophrenia; with severe, chronic toxicity ('manganism') there may be compulsive behaviour manifested by dementia, increased physical activity, irritability, parkinsonian syndrome, and personality changes
- other: headache, liver failure, nausea, vomiting, respiratory disease (with industrial exposure).

Associations with deficiency

- psychiatric: none known
- other: possible association with epilepsy and bone abnormalities in Perthes' disease (avascular necrosis of the femoral head in children).

Mercury

Route of exposure contaminated foods (fish, pork), cosmetics, industrial exposure; *note*: there is no definitive evidence for toxicity resulting from dental amalgam.

Normal range (whole blood) <0.06 µg/ml (<0.3 nmol/l).

Note: renal dysfunction and non-specific changes in liver function tests may be apparent, and hence LFT, U&E, and urine dipstick analysis are suggested in cases of mercury toxicity.

Possible associated changes in laboratory parameters Increased blood leukocytes, blood pyruvate, urinary albumin, urine erythrocytes, urine protein, decreased serum bicarbonate, serum sodium.

Associations with excess (metallic mercury)

- psychiatric: apathy, cognitive changes, depression, emotional lability, fatigue, hallucinosis, insomnia, irritability, social withdrawal; there is a

383

specific syndrome ('erythism') associated with mercury intoxication, which includes nervousness, personality changes, social withdrawal and possible loss of self-control

- other: acute intoxication – anaemia, chest pain, colitis, cough, gastroenteritis, headache, nausea, peripheral neuropathy, pneumonitis (following inhalation), renal failure, stomatitis; acute/chronic intoxication – two syndromes have been identified: acrodynia ('pink disease', also known as Selter's disease, or Swift–Feer disease) is a syndrome of peeling of hands and feet, associated with erythema and pain as well as weight loss, personality change, lability of blood pressure, excess salivation, and hyperhydrosis; Minamata disease is a neurological syndrome secondary to mercury poisoning which initially includes ataxia, muscle weakness, and visual disturbance, and which may progress to behavioural disturbance, intellectual decline, paralysis, coma, and death; chronic intoxication – abnormal sweating, gingivitis, headache, hypersalivation, lassitude, renal failure, tremor.

Associations with deficiency

- psychiatric: none known
- other: none known.

Nickel

Route of exposure Environmental and industrial exposure; exposure to nickel-containing jewellery.

Normal range (serum) $0.14–1.0\,\mu g/l$ $(2.4–17.0\,nmol/l)$.

Associated changes in routine laboratory parameters *Note*: leukocytosis may occur in nickel deficiency but there are no specific alterations of blood parameters in toxicity.

Associations with excess

- psychiatric: cognitive changes (non-specific), delirium
- other: contact dermatitis (common); acute aerosol exposure – abnormal liver function tests, chest pain, drowsiness, dyspnoea, fever, headache, nausea, vomiting
- severe intoxication: convulsions, cyanosis, respiratory distress, and possibly death.

Associations with deficiency

- psychiatric: none known
- other: none known.

Selenium

Route of exposure Essential element (roles in thyroid hormone synthesis and antioxidant production), industrial exposure (paints, dyes, pigments, fungicides, maufacture of semiconductors and electronic equipment).

Normal range (serum) 95–165 ng/ml; levels >500 ng/ml are especially associated with toxicity.

Associated changes in routine laboratory parameters None specific.

Associations with excess

- psychiatric: none known
- other: glucocorticoid therapy; hair loss, nail changes (brittle nail, possibly with appearance of white lines); other signs/symptoms may include fatigue, fetor, irritability, nausea, and vomiting.

Associations with deficiency

- psychiatric: alcoholism, cognitive decline (possible association with Alzheimer's), depression; possible association between low selenium levels and schizophrenic patients treated with clozapine
- other: Balkan nephropathy (chronic interstitial nephropathy thought to be of viral origin and found in Bulgaria, Romania, and former Yugoslavia), HIV infection, hyperalimentation/re-feeding, hypothyroidism, inflammatory bowel disease, Kashin–Bek disease (a form of generalized osteoarthritis endemic in parts of Siberia, Korea, China, and Tibet), Keshan disease (a form of dilated cardiomyopathy endemic in some parts of China), kwashiorkor, liver disease (cirrhosis, hepatitis), low protein diet, myxoedematous endemic cretinism, peripartum cardiomyopathy (in sub-Saharan Africa), pregnancy, renal failure, total parenteral nutrition.

Thallium

Route of exposure Industrial exposure, may be found in certain dyes, as well as jewellery and optical lenses.

Normal range (serum) <10 ng/dl (<49 nmol/l); urine <10 µg/24 hours. Urine testing is considered more reliable than serum. There may be a delay of some weeks before clinical effects are manifest.

Associated changes in routine laboratory parameters None specific; there may be disturbances of renal function and electrolytes, and potassium specifically should be monitored in thallium overdose.

Associations with excess

- psychiatric: cognitive changes, delirium, dementia, depression, hallucinosis, psychosis
- other: acute toxicity ⁻ abdominal pain, ataxia, diarrhoea, fever, haematemesis, headache, hyperhydrosis, insomnia, lethargy, myalgia, nausea, vomiting; chronic toxicity – alopecia (primarily of the head), cardiac arrhythmia, hepatic necrosis, myoclonus, peripheral neuropathy, renal tubular necrosis, visual disturbances (including blindness).

Miscellaneous

Associations with deficiency

- psychiatric: none known
- other: none known.

Tin

Route of exposure Industrial exposure, exposure in cidal agents.

Normal range (serum) 0.40–0.64 µg/l (3.4–5.4 nmol/l).

Associated changes in routine laboratory parameters Reported changes, especially with chronic exposure to organic tin, include anaemia, hepatic damage (alterations in ALP, ALT, AST reported) and renal dysfunction (decreased potassium and increased creatinine, eGFR, and urea). Organic tin compounds may be associated with hyperglycaemia.

Associations with excess (organic tin compounds)

- psychiatric: cognitive changes, delirium, fatigue, personality change
- other: ataxia, fits, headache, hearing loss, nystagmus, paresis, paraesthesia, vertigo, visual impairment; aerosol exposure may cause pneumoconiosis ('stannosis').

Associations with deficiency

- psychiatric: none known
- other: none known.

Vanadium

Route of exposure Fat-containing foods, industrial exposure.

Normal range (serum) 0.014–0.230 µg/l (0.27–4.51 nmol/l).

Associated changes in routine laboratory parameters None specific.

Associations with excess

- psychiatric: depression (rare)
- other: abdominal pain, anorexia, blackened tongue, bronchitis/bronchopneumonia, nausea, palpitations, renal damage, tremor, visual disturbance, vomiting.

Associations with deficiency

- psychiatric: none known
- other: none known.

Zinc

Route of exposure Essential element present in nature, iatrogenic (dialysis).

Normal range (serum) 66–110 µg/dl (10.0–16.8 µmol/l).

Patients undergoing dialysis may be at increased risk of toxicity.

Associated changes in laboratory parameters

- decreased: blood copper, blood iron (may be associated with sideroblastic or hypochromic microcytic anaemia) leukocytes, neutrophils
- increased: alkaline phosphatase, calcium, serum cholesterol.

Associations with excess

- psychiatric: cognitive changes, delirium, fatigue/lethargy
- other: gastrointestinal dysfunction, possibly including diarrhoea, nausea, and vomiting.

Associations with deficiency

- psychiatric: anorexia nervosa (controversial); emotional lability (controversial)
- other: abdominal pain, acrodermatitis enteropathica (in babies), acquired immunodeficiency syndrome (AIDS), anaemia, burns patients, cerebellar ataxia, decreased ability to taste and smell, dermatitis, diarrhoea, folate treatment in pregnancy, geophagia (deficiency secondary to chelation), growth retardation, hepatosplenomegaly, histidine treatment, hyperalimentation/re-feeding, immunodeficiency (lymphopaenia may occur in severe cases), malabsorption states, poor wound healing, rash, tremor; zinc deficiency is also associated with vitamin A deficiency.

Miscellaneous

Further reading

General

Baldwin DR, Marshall W. Heavy metal poisoning and its laboratory investigation. Ann Clin Biochem 1999; 36: 267–300.
Ibrahim D. Heavy metal poisoning: clinical presentations and pathophysiology. Clin Lab Med 2006; 26: 67–97.
Yung CY. A synopsis on metals in medicine and psychiatry. Pharmacol Biochem Behav 1984; 21 (Suppl 1): 41–7.

Aluminium

Becaria A, Campbell A, Bondy SC. Aluminum as a toxicant. Toxicol Ind Health 2002; 18: 309–20.
D'Haese PC, Couttenye MM, Goodman WG et al. Use of the low-dose desferrioxamine test to diagnose and differentiate between patients with aluminium-related bone disease, increased risk for aluminium toxicity, or aluminium overload. Nephrol Dial Transplant 1995; 10: 1874–84.

Arsenic

Graeme KA, Pollack CV Jr. Heavy metal toxicity, Part I: arsenic and mercury. J Emerg Med 1998; 16: 45–56.
Kapaj S, Peterson H, Liber K, Bhattacharaya P. Human health effects from chronic arsenic poisoning–a review. J Environ Sci Health A Tox Hazard Subst Environ Eng 2006; 41: 2399–428.

Bismuth

Bradley B, Singleton M, Lin Wan Po A. Bismuth toxicity—a reassessment. J Clin Pharm Ther 1989; 14: 423–41.

Chromium

Barceloux DG. Chromium. J Toxicol Clin Toxicol 1999; 37: 173–94.
Costa M, Klein CB. Toxicity and carcinogenicity of chromium compounds in humans. Crit Rev Toxicol 2006; 36: 155–63.
http://www.food.gov.uk/multimedia/pdfs/evm_chromium.pdf.

Cobalt

Barceloux DG. Cobalt. J Toxicol Clin Toxicol 1999; 37: 201–6.
http://www.atsdr.cdc.gov/toxprofiles/tp33-p.pdf.
http://www.food.gov.uk/multimedia/pdfs/evm_cobalt.pdf.

Copper

Barceloux DG. Copper. J Toxicol Clin Toxicol 1999; 37: 217–30.
http://www.food.gov.uk/multimedia/pdfs/evm_copper.pdf.

Gold

Tozman EC, Gottlieb NL. Adverse reactions with oral and parenteral gold preparations. Med Toxicol 1987; 2: 177–89.

Iron

Mills KC, Curry SC. Acute iron poisoning. Emerg Med Clin North Am 1994; 12: 397–413.
Palatnick W, Tenenbein M. Leukocytosis, hyperglycemia, vomiting, and positive X-rays are not indicators of severity of iron overdose in adults. Am J Emerg Med 1996; 14: 454–5.

Miscellaneous

388

Lead

Brodkin E, Copes R, Mattman A et al. Lead and mercury exposures: interpretation and action. CMAJ 2007; 176: 59–63.
Kosnett MJ, Wedeen RP, Rothenberg SJ et al. Recommendations for medical management of adult lead exposure. Environ Health Perspect 2007; 115: 463–71.

Magnesium

Topf JM, Murray PT. Hypomagnesemia and hypermagnesemia. Rev Endocr Metab Disord 2003; 4: 195–206.
Touyz RM. Magnesium in clinical medicine. Front Biosci 2004; 9: 1278–93.
http://www.food.gov.uk/multimedia/pdfs/evm_magnesium.pdf.

Manganese

Crossgrove J, Zheng W. Manganese toxicity upon overexposure. NMR Biomed 2004; 17: 544–53.
http://www.food.gov.uk/multimedia/pdfs/evm_manganese.pdf.

Mercury

Ekino S, Susa M, Ninomiya T, Imamura K, Kitamura T. Minamata disease revisited: an update on the acute and chronic manifestations of methyl mercury poisoning. J Neurol Sci 2007; 262: 131–44.
Magos L, Clarkson TW. Overview of the clinical toxicity of mercury. Ann Clin Biochem 2006; 43: 257–68.
http://www.atsdr.cdc.gov/toxprofiles/tp46.pdf.

Nickel

Barceloux DG. Nickel. J Toxicol Clin Toxicol 1999; 37: 239–58.
Sunderman FW Jr. A review of the metabolism and toxicity of nickel. Ann Clin Lab Sci 1977; 7: 377–98.
http://www.food.gov.uk/multimedia/pdfs/evm_nickel.pdf.

Selenium

Barceloux DG. Selenium. Clin Toxicol 1999; 37: 145–72.

Thallium

Galvan-Arzate S, Santamaria A. Thallium toxicity. Toxicol Lett 1998; 99: 1–13.
Mulkey JP, Oehme FW. A review of thallium toxicity. Vet Hum Toxicol 1993; 35: 445–53.

Tin

Winship KA. Toxicity of tin and its compounds. Adverse Drug React Acute Poisoning Rev 1988; 7: 19–38.

Vanadium

Barceloux DG. Vanadium. J Toxicol Clin Toxicol 1999; 37: 265–78.

Zinc

Barceloux DG. Zinc. J Toxicol Clin Toxicol 1999; 37: 279–92.
Fosmire GJ. Zinc toxicity. Am J Clin Nutr 1990; 51: 225–7.

Miscellaneous

The microbiology laboratory and psychiatry

Infective agents can cause, as well as exacerbate, psychiatric presentations, with manifestations ranging from specific brain infections (such as encephalitis) to systemic infections such as herpes, HIV, and syphilis. Additionally, these infections may be primary or secondary to lifestyle (such as tuberculosis in the homeless mentally ill, or hepatitis in substance-abusing populations) or even occur following hospital admission (such as MRSA (methicillin resistant *Staphylococcus aureus*) or infective gastroenteritis).

While a complete discussion of microbiology and psychiatry is beyond the scope of this book, some general principles will be presented, together with selected specific examples of infectious agents especially associated with psychiatric sequelae.

General principles

Patients with psychiatric disorders may present with a range of infections or infestations which may be pre-existing (e.g. urinary tract infection), associated with specific syndromes (e.g. HIV or hepatitis secondary to intravenous drug use, tuberculosis in chronic alcoholism complicated by homelessness), nosocomial/acquired *de novo* whilst in hospital (e.g. gastroenteritis, MRSA, respiratory tract infections), or as a consequence of treatment (e.g. increased risk of infection secondary to clozapine-induced agranulocytosis or neutropaenia).

Hence the clinician should be aware of the general manifestations of infections and so utilize the microbiology laboratory appropriately. Clnical manifestations of acute infections may include features of local or systemic inflammation which may start insidiously and include non-specific, constitutional signs and symptoms such as malaise, weakness, listlessness, possibly with anorexia, arthralgia, headache, myalgia, and, commonly, fever, tachycardia, and tachypnoea.

Changes in a number of routine laboratory investigations may suggest infection.

Table General laboratory findings and infections		
Domain	*Laboratory investigations*	*Notes*
Clinical biochemistry	Albumin	May be decreased in bacterial sepsis (albumin is a negative-acute phase protein)
	CRP	May be raised especially in acute infections; may be a useful marker of disease progression
	LFT	Altered LFT may result from haemolysis (e.g. as with malaria) or hepatocellular damage (e.g. hepatitis, infectious mononucleosis)
	U&E	Pre-renal azoturia may occur which can lead to increased blood urea (but usually with normal creatinine) Shock may result in hypotension and rises in serum creatinine
	Urinalysis	May reveal haematuria/proteinuria or transient glyosuria
Haematology	Clotting screen	Gram-negative septicaemia may be associated with disseminated intravascular coagulation (with prolonged bleeding time and thrombocytopaenia)
	ESR	May be raised in acute and chronic infections; may be a useful marker of disease progression
	FBC	Anaemia may be present (due to bleeding or haemolysis/red cell destruction); chronic infections may present with an anaemia characterized by decreased plasma iron/TIBC/transferrin Basophilia is not usually associated with infections Eosinophilia may suggest a parasitic infection (especially helminthic) Lymphocytosis may be found in many viral infections Monocytosis may present with some infections such as tuberculosis or syphilis Neutrophilia is common in many bacterial infections but severe infections may result in a neutropaenia due to depleted neutrophil stores and decreased productive capacity of bone marrow

Miscellaneous

391

Where the clinical presentation suggests a link between infection and symptoms (physical and/or psychiatric), appropriate investigations should always be performed after consultation with the microbiology laboratory.

Serology

The psychiatrist is most likely to encounter the need for serological investigation in specific patient groups, namely patients with substance abuse disorders (especially with injected agents), those with putative chronic fatigue syndrome (see Chapter 2 for further details), and physically unwell patients presenting with signs and symptoms suggestive of specific dignoses.

Commonly, the following tests will be requested:

* investigation of chronic fatigue syndrome
* herpes simplex
* HIV*
* syphilis
* viral hepatitis*.

* Note: the patient must provide informed consent.

Prior to requesting serology, advice should be sought from the serology laboratory.

In almost all cases, the specimen material will be clotted blood (brown top tube).

In some cases further confirmation tests may be required.

Table Serology: basic diagnostic and confirmatory tests

Condition	Diagnosic tests	Confirmatory tests
Cytomegalovirus	IgG, IgM	—
Epstein–Barr virus	IgG, IgM	IgM
Hepatitis A	IgG, IgM	—
Hepatitis B	Surface antigen	Surface antigen by neutralization
	Core antibody Core IgM e antigen Surface antibody	—
Hepatitis C	Virus antibody	—
HIV	Antibody	Antibody 1p24 antigen
Syphilis	IgM Treponemal total antibody Rapid plasma reagin	—

Note: for suspected acute hepatitis based on clinical and laboratory presentation including jaundice and abnormal LFT, the following serology screen may be performed:

• hepatitis A: IgM
• hepatitis B: surface antigen
• hepatitis C: antibody.

In addition, the following optional tests may also be requested:

• cytomegalovirus IgM
• Epstein–Barr virus: IgM, viral core antigen.

For patients with a previous history of hepatitis, the following tests may be requested:

• hepatitis A: IgG
• hepatitis B: core total antigen
• hepatitis C: antibody.

For occupational health purposes, hepatitis B titres may be measured to provide an indication of immunity. An adequate level is >100 mIU/ml. Between 10 and 100 mIU/ml suggests a poor response and a booster may be required. Levels below 10 mIU/ml may require a repeat course.

Miscellaneous

Notifiable diseases in the UK

The following conditions are notifiable diseases in the UK (under the Public Health (Infectious Diseases) Regulations, 1988; UK Health Protection Agency, 2006):

- acute encephalitis
- acute poliomyelitis
- anthrax
- cholera
- Creutzfeldt–Jakob disease
- diphtheria
- dysentery
- food poisoning
- leprosy
- leptospirosis
- malaria
- measles
- meningitis

  - meningococcal
  - pneumococcal
  - *Haemophilus influenzae*
  - viral
  - other specified
  - unspecified

- meningococcal septicaemia (without meningitis)
- mumps
- ophthalmia neonatorum
- paratyphoid fever
- plague
- rabies
- relapsing fever
- rubella
- scarlet fever
- smallpox
- tetanus
- tuberculosis
- typhoid fever
- typhus fever
- viral haemorrhagic fever
- viral hepatitis

  - hepatitis A
  - hepatitis B
  - hepatitis C
  - other

- whooping cough
- yellow fever.

Specific infections

The following infectious syndromes will be considered in this chapter:

- brucellosis
- Creutzfeldt–Jakob disease
- herpes simplex
- HIV
- infectious mononucleosis
- Lyme disease
- malaria (cerebral)
- meningitis
- neurosyphilis
- tuberculosis.

For each condition the following information will be provided:

- definition
- transmission
- incubation period
- psychiatric symptoms
- clinical symptoms
- clinical signs
- complications
- differential diagnosis
- laboratory investigation.

Brucellosis

Definition *Brucella* species are gram-negative, aerobic coccobacilli with three species (*B. abortus, B. melitensis, and B. suis*) known to be pathogenic in man.

Transmission Brucellosis is primarily a disease of agricultural workers, veterinary staff, and abattoir workers, with exposure via contact with infected cattle (genital secretions or fetal material), by drinking unpasteurized milk or eating cheese (sheep, goats), or occasionally in laboratory workers. All ages may be affected, but adults are most commonly affected.

Incubation period Acute brucellosis (usually *B. melitensis*) – approximately 1–3 weeks; chronic brucellosis (usually *B. abortus*) – in untreated patients approximately 1 month to 1 year.

Psychiatric symptoms (usually with chronic infection) Anxiety, depression, fatigue, lassitude; may rarely lead to suicide.

Clinical symptoms Acute – anorexia, fatigue, fever (may be undulant), headache, joint pains, lassitude, weakness; chronic – recurrent episodes of backache, flu-like illnesses, headaches, lassitude, and psychiatric symptoms (anxiety, depression).

Clinical signs Acute – hepatosplenomegaly and/or lymphadenopathy (occasionally), profuse sweating, rash (erythematous, papular, found on extremities); chronic – swollen, painful joints; weight loss.

Complications Arthritis, encephalitis, endocarditis, hepatitis, meningoencephalitis, orchitis, radiculitis, thrombophlebitis.

Differential diagnosis Non-infective disease (collagen disorders such as sarcoidosis, lymphoma); other infections (bacterial endocarditis, enteric fever, Q fever, tuberculosis).

Laboratory investigation

Table Laboratory investigations and brucellosis		
Domain	*Investigation*	*Notes*
Clinical biochemistry	None specific	CRP may provide an indication of severity of acute infection. Liver enzymes may be elevated
Haematology	ESR	May be raised; serial measurements may be useful for monitoring
	FBC	Characteristically a neutropaenia and a lymphocytosis are seen; anaemia of chronic disease may also be apparent (usually normochromic, normocytic, with reduced serum iron and TIBC; Hb is usually $\geq 90\,g/l$). On occasion a monocytosis may be seen
Histology	Biopsy (bone marrow, lymph node, or liver) may rarely be required	Microscopy may show granulomas without caseation, thus ruling out the differential diagnoses of tuberculosis and sarcoidosis
Immunology (serology)	IgM agglutinating antibodies	May be demonstrated in acute brucellosis although significance in chronic brucellosis is unclear
	IgG and IgM	Enzyme linked immunosorbent assay (ELISA) or radio immunoassay (RIA) have now replaced the agglutination test
Microbiology	Blood cultures	Positive in up to 20% of acute presentations; usually require 3–5 days' incubation in CO_2-enriched environment but may take up to 4 weeks; pus or urine culture is also sometimes successful, and bone marrow cultures provide the highest diagnostic yield

Miscellaneous

Creutzfeldt–Jakob disease

Definition A rare, rapidly progressive neurological condition thought to be caused by a prion. Four forms of the condition have been described:

- genetic CJD – extremely rare, due to an inherited gene mutation in the prion protein gene
- iatrogenic CJD – a rare form due to transmission of the infectious agent during medical or surgical procedures
- sporadic CJD (sCJD) – the most commonly seen form of CJD, although it is still extremely rare (<80 cases/year in the UK). It primarily affects middle-aged individuals and two forms have been described; the Heiden-hain form is characterized initially by increasing visual disturbances and finally blindness before the characteristic neurological and psychiatric changes become manifest. In the Brownell–Oppenheimer form the initial presentation is of progressive cerebellar ataxia disturbance over a number of weeks prior to the appearance of the other features of the disorder
- variant CJD (vCJD) – characterized by appearance in younger individuals (usually by age 30 or so) associated with slower development of neuro-logical and behavioural symptoms. There are <30 cases/year in the UK.

Transmission Appears to be via the oral route via contamined food, but iatrogenic routes have been described and include corneal grafting, use of deep brain electrodes, implants of human dura, or use of cadaver-derived homones (growth hormone and pituitary gonadotropin).

Incubation period Unclear; may range from years to decades, but for sCJD the median illness duration is 4–6 months while for vCJD it is approximately 14 months.

Psychiatric symptoms Apathy, behavioural, cognitive, and personality changes.

Clinical signs and symptoms Prodrome – non-specific symptoms including apathy, depression, non-specific neurological symptoms, and tiredness; second stage – dementia, neurological symptoms including akinetic mutism, ataxia, cortical blindness, dysarthria, involuntary movements, limb spasticity, myoclonus, and seizures; symptoms progress rapidly and usually cause death within 6 months to 1 year.

Complications Blindness, eventual coma, movement disorders such as ataxia.

Differential diagnosis Any cause of dementia including Alzheimer's, cor-ticobasilar degeneration, effects of environmental toxins, frontotemporal dementia, HIV, hydrocephalus, hypothyroidism, leukodystrophies, Lewy body dementia, mitochondrial diseases, other prion diseases (such as fatal familial insomnia or Gerstmann–Sträussler–Scheinker disease), Parkinson's disease, Pick's dementia, psychiatric disorders, spinocerebellar degeneration, syphilis, vitamin B12 deficiency.

Laboratory investigation Magnetic resonance imaging (MRI) is a first-line investigation and the characteristic `pulvinar sign' in the posterior thalamic

Miscellaneous

region may be seen. EEG may be helpful, showing generalized bi- or triphasic periodic sharp wave complexes with a frequency of 1–2 per second. CSF analysis may also be instructive, but currently the only specific laboratory investigation is brain biopsy. Specialist advice should always be sought in cases of suspected CJD.

Table Laboratory investigations and Creutzfeldt–Jakob disease	
Investigation	*Notes*
Routine blood investigations	Routine tests such as B12, FBC, fluorescent treponemal antibody test (for syphilis), folate, LFT, TFT, U&E to rule out any obvious, treatable causes of dementia
Brain biopsy	Currently appears to be the gold standard investigation. Characteristic spongiform changes may be seen
Tonsillar biopsy	Recommended by some authorities as vCJD may be found in the lymphoid system. A specific protein, cellular prion protein (PrPSc), is measured by Western blot and/or immunohistochemistry
CSF analysis for 14-3-3	14-3-3 neuron-specific enolase is a specific brain protein which may support a diagnosis of vCJD, but *note*: a negative finding does not exclude the diagnosis

Herpes simplex
Definition Herpes simplex (HSV) is a double-stranded DNA alpha herpes virus which is generally associated with vesicular skin lesions but can also rarely cause encephalitis. The virus exists in two forms, type one (associated with orofacial lesions) and type two (associated with genital herpes).

Transmission By close interpersonal contact such as kissing for herpes simplex type one and sexual intercourse for type two.

Incubation period 3–7 days (can range up to 3 weeks).

Psychiatric symptoms Behavioural and cognitive changes (especially confusion); occasionally patients may present with psychotic symptoms. The virus is particularly associated with haemorrhagic necrotizing encephalitis affecting the temporal lobe, and hence patients may present with a temporal lobe syndrome, possibly including:

- aggressive behaviour
- auditory agnosia
- emotional lability
- memory impairments (bilateral lesions=global amnesia, immediate recall unimpaired; unilateral lesions=impaired verbal memory with dominant lesions and impaired spatial memory with non-dominant lesions)

- reduced sexual activity
- sensory dysphasia
- temporal lobe epilepsy.

Clinical symptoms Headache (severe and progressive), photophobia.

Clinical signs Papilloedema, pyrexia, reduced level of consciousness, vesicular skin lesions, vomiting.

Complications Paresis, neuropsychiatric morbidity (amnesia, mood disorders, personality change, social disinhibition).

Differential diagnosis Cerebral malaria, demyelinating disorders, space-occupying lesion, tuberculous meningitis.

Laboratory investigation

Table Laboratory investigation of herpes simplex	
Investigation	*Notes*
Antibody testing	Can demonstrate primary seroconversion with HSV but cannot distinguish between HSV types one and two
Histology	After isolation of virus in tissue culture, characteristic appearances of cells (multinucleated giant cells with eosinophilic intranuclear inclusion bodies)
PCR	Polymerase chain reaction of herpes simplex in CSF

Possible alterations in laboratory parameters in herpes simplex

Table Possible alterations in laboratory parameters (in blood) in herpes simplex		
Domain	*Parameter*	*Notes*
Clinical biochemistry	Bilirubin	May be increased
Haematology	ESR	May be increased
	Fibrinogen	May be decreased
	Platelet count	May be decreased
	Prothrombin time	May be increased

Miscellaneous

Human immunodeficiency virus

Definition   HIV is a retrovirus, which causes AIDS, defined by progressive immunodeficiency resulting in opportunistic infections and multiorgan involvement.

Transmission   Sexual transmission (main route in UK, especially anal and vaginal; oral transmission is rare); iatrogenic (e.g. from untreated blood products, such as for use in haemophilia; via infected blood (e.g. drug users sharing needles, tattoos/piercings), now rare due to heat-treatment of products); needlestick and other injuries in healthcare workers; 'vertical transmission' from mother to baby in pregnancy/breast-feeding.

Incubation period   Unclear; can be years to decades.

Psychiatric symptoms   Individuals infected with HIV may have pre-existing symptoms or develop symptoms *de novo*; adjustment, anxiety, and depressive disorders are common, with mania and psychosis rarer. Cognitive changes may initially be non-specific, and if the underlying organic cause is untreated may eventually progress to AIDS dementia. Note that some anti-retrovirals, especially efavirenz, may have psychiatric side-effects, including psychosis and *de novo* suicidal ideation (see, for example, reference 1).

Clinical symptoms

- seroconversion illness: non-specific, self-limiting flu-like symptoms may develop, such as arthralgia, diarrhoea, fatigue, fever, headache, lethargy, malaise
- primary infection: anorexia, headache, malaise, nausea, night sweats, photophobia.

Clinical signs

- seroconversion illness: may be none specific; sometimes skin rash, meningism may be seen
- primary infection: candidiasis (oral, oesophageal), lymphadenopathy, mucocutaneous ulcers, rash, vomiting, weight loss.

Complications   HIV affects every system of the body, and compliations are related to the degree of immunosuppression, especially when CD4 counts are below $100/mm^3$.

Table Possible complications of HIV

System	Condition	Notes
CNS	Cerebral toxoplasmosis	Most common CNS infection, may manifest as confusion, fever, fits, or focal neurological disturbances. MRI is probably imaging modality of choice
	Cryptococcal meningitis	May present with non-specific features such as headache, mild fever, nausea, or vomiting
	HIV encephalopathy	May resemble a depressive syndrome with non-specific cognitive changes and progressing to a dementia-type syndrome
	Peripheral myelopathy Peripheral neuropathy	May present with a range of symptoms including bladder dysfunction, diarrhoea, hypotension, impotence, and weakness
	Progressive multifocal leukoencephalopathy	Associated with ataxia, focal neurological signs, and personality change. MRI is probably imaging modality of choice
Gastrointestinal	Diarrhoea/ malabsorption	Due to effects of various infectious organisms and possible direct effects of the HIV virus on the intestinal lining. When severe, patients may experience a wasting syndrome (cachexia). Can be diagnosed when there is $\geq 10\%$ unintentional weight loss
	Hairy leukoplakia	White, raised lesions often on the tongue or in other areas of the mouth which are related to Epstein–Barr virus infection
	Oesophageal candidiasis	White, creamy lesions that can be painful and interfere with swallowing
Haematological	Thrombocytopaenia	Commonly seen and may respond to antiretroviral treatment or spontaneously remit in a minority of patients
Miscellaneous	Recurrent aphthous ulcers	Oral and genital lesions may be seen and are of two types, a herpetiform type and a painful, necrotic type
Ocular	Cytomegalovirus retinitis	May present with blurred vision or partial loss of vision in a single eye

Miscellaneous

Table Possible complications of HIV (Cont.)

System	Condition	Notes
Psychiatric	Mood disorders	May be associated with anxiety disorders and depression. Occasionally euphoria may be seen, expecially in the context of 'Lazarus syndrome' in which the patient's presentation is dramatically improved with treatment. Some antiretrovirals, especially efavirenz, are associated with a wide range of psychiatric side-effects including depression, psychosis, post-traumatic stress disorder (PTSD), and *de novo* suicidal ideation
Pulmonary	Bacterial pneumonia	May be due to a number of organisms and show atypical X-ray appearances
	Fungal infections	Mainly *Cryptococcus* spp.
	Mycobacterium avium complex	May present with non-specific symptoms and signs including abdominal discomfort, diarrhoea, fever, night sweats, and weight loss. Routine laboratory parameters may reveal abnormal liver function tests or anaemia
	Pneumocystis carinii	Symptoms may include cough, fatigue, fever, malaise, shortness of breath, and weight loss
	Tuberculosis	May not be sputum positive
Tumours	Kaposi's sarcoma	May be seen as macules or papules affecting gastrointestinal tract, lungs, mucous membranes, and skin
	Non-Hodgkin's lymphoma	Often affect CNS and present with focal neurological signs

Differential diagnosis Primary immunodeficiency disorders (e.g. Bruton's disease or X-linked agammaglobulinaemia; common variable immune deficiency, IgA deficiency, Wiscott–Aldrich syndrome); secondary immunodeficiency disorders such as with immunosuppressive drugs, lymphoproliferative disorders, malnutrition, radiotherapy, splenectomy, or systemic disease (chronic hepatic failure, chronic renal failure, diabetes mellitus, systemic malignancy).

Laboratory investigation

Table	Laboratory investigations for suspected HIV infection	
System	**Laboratory parameter**	**Notes**
Immunology	CD4	Primary means (together with viral load) of monitoring degree of immune dysfunction, disease progression, and treatment efficacy. Usually $<500\times10^6$/l ($<40\%$ of total lymphocytes) in healthy subjects, and may be $<200\times10^6$/l in AIDS (<15–20% of total lymphocytes)
	CD8	Not usually performed for diagnostic purposes. Measurement allows for monitoring degree of immune dysfunction and disease progression, especially in severely unwell individuals. Normal range approximately 275–780×10^6/l
	HIV antibody screening	May be negative in early infection; usually repeated after 3 months
Microbiology	Virus culture in peripheral blood mononuclear cells	Rarely performed
	Viral load	Test measures HIV RNA and is, together with CD4 count, the most effective means of monitoring disease progress and treatment efficacy. A low viral load is usually between 200 and 500 copies, and a high VL may be 5000–10000+

HIV and needlestick injuries   There is a relatively low risk of HIV seroconversion following needlestick injury ($<1\%$ with HIV-positive blood), although the risk for hepatitis, especially C, is much higher, possibly up to 30%.

In the event of needlestick injury, local protocols should be followed. Generally the following are advised:

* advise occupational health department as soon as possible
* encourage bleeding/wash wound thoroughly
* obtain details of patient from whom blood was taken
* store blood from both parties (serology for hepatitis B and C, HIV)
* if possible, check HIV and hepatitis status of both parties
* immediate PEP (post-exposure prophylaxis) may be appropriate as may counselling – urgent advice should be sought from occupational health department and possibly a genitourinary medicine clinic.

Miscellaneous

Infectious mononucleosis

Definition Infectious mononucleosis, also referred to as glandular fever and 'kissing' disease, is a syndrome caused by infection with the Epstein–Barr virus (EBV) and characterized by febrile illness, rash, and lymphadenopathy.

Transmission The virus is excreted in saliva and can be transmitted orally via kissing, and usually affects young adults.

Incubation period Approximately 5–6 weeks. Symptoms usually last up to 3 weeks although may be prolonged for several months in some individuals.

Psychiatric symptoms Often associated with fatigue, lethargy, and malaise; may mimic chronic fatigue syndrome.

Clinical symptoms Anorexia, difficulty swallowing (with adenoidal involvement), fever, sore throat; breathing and drinking may be compromised in severe infections involving the adenoids.

Clinical signs Dribbling (with adenoidal involvement), hepatomegaly, jaundice (occasionally), lymphadenopathy (especially axillary and cervical nodes), macular skin rash (especially in patients given penicillins), palatal petechiae, pharyngeal oedema, splenomegaly, tonsillar exudate.

Note: two patterns of clinical presentation have been described:

- anginose type, with cervical lymphadenopathy, palatal petechiae, and tonsillitis (exudative)
- juvenile type, with fever, lymphadenopathy (generalized), and sore throat.

Complications Autoimmune haemolytic anaemia, Duncan's syndrome (malignant lymphoid proliferation), hepatitis, malaise/fatigue (may persist for many months after infection), meningoencephalitis, myocarditis, pharyngeal obstruction, splenic rupture (extremely rare and usually associated with trauma), thrombocytopaenia.

Death is a rare consequence of infectious mononucleosis but may occur in Purtillo's syndrome (infectious mononucleosis with EBV-related malignant lymphoma).

Differential diagnosis Other causes of fever with generalized lymphadenopathy, e.g. cytomegalovirus infection, HIV, lymphoma, syphilis.

Note: EBV is also associated with a number of other conditions including Burkitt's lymphoma (usually presents as tumours of the jaw or occasionally of the ovaries, found in areas of Africa affected by malaria), hairy leukoplakia (in HIV-positive individuals), and nasopharyngeal carcinoma (more common in southern China).

Laboratory investigation

Table	Laboratory investigations and infectious mononucleosis	
Domain	**Laboratory tests**	**Notes**
Clinical biochemistry	CRP	May be raised
	LFT	Abnormal, non-specific LFT may be seen in a proportion of patients
Haematology	Anaemia	May be seen (secondary to autoantibodies to erythrocytes)
	Blood film	Atypical lymphocytes (misshapen nuclei with excess cytoplasm) may be seen
	ESR	May be raised
	Lymphocytosis	Important diagnostic feature of this condition
	Thrombocytopaenia	Commonly seen (secondary to autoantibodies to erythrocytes)
Immunology/serology	Anti-i cold agglutinin	Also seen in infectious mononucleosis
	EBV-associated IgM	Can confirm diagnosis
	Heterophil antibodies	Haemagglutination ('Paul–Bunnell') test is diagnostic but may not be positive until later on in the illness, often several weeks later
	Rheumatoid factor	May also be seen in infectious mononucleosis

Miscellaneous

405

Possible alterations in laboratory parameters in infectious mono-nucleosis

Table Summary of possible alterations in laboratory parameters in infectious mononucleosis		
Parameter	**Decreased**	**Increased**
Aldolase		X
ALP		X
ALT		X
Amylase		X
Antinuclear antibodies		X
Anti-smooth muscle antibodies		X
AST		X
Bilirubin		X
Cholesterol	X	
ESR	X	
GGT		X
Globulin		X
Haematocrit	X	
Haemoglobin	X	
LDH		X
Lymphocytes		X
Monocytes		X
Neutrophils		X
Rheumatoid factor		X

Lyme disease

Definition This is a tick-borne condition caused by *Borrelia burgdorferi*, a spirochaete; the disease is characterized by cardiac, joint, neurological, and skin involvement.

Transmission Transmitted by tick bites (*Ixodid* spp., especially *I. ricinus* in Europe).

Incubation period Usually 3–32 days.

Miscellaneous

Psychiatric symptoms

- early stages: non-specific (generalized malaise and fatigue)
- later stages: a wide range of presentations have been reported, including anxiety disorders, behavioural changes, cognitive changes, depression, emotional lability, hallucinations (rare), irritability, panic attacks, psychosis (rare).

Clinical symptoms Fever, headache, malaise, neck stiffness, non-specific aches and pains.

Clinical signs Erythema chronicum migrans (the main clinical marker for the disease; this is a red skin lesion at the site of inoculation which expands greatly and can affect diverse sites including the axilla, groin, and thigh), lymphadenopathy, meningeal irritation.

Complications Cardiac, including heart block (first degree or Wenckebach) of left ventricular dysfunction (cardiac involvement is usually limited but may recur); joint involvement, mainly rheumatoid factor/antinuclear antibody-negative arthritis of the knees which can recur over years; neurological, including Bell's palsy, chorea, encephalitis, meningitis; late complications may include rarely demyelinating CNS disorders or transverse myelitis.

Differential diagnosis

- infectious: babesiosis, ehrlichiosis, *Mycoplasma*, syphilis, viral infections
- non-infectious: arthritis (degenerative), B12 deficiency, diabetes mellitus, toxicity, vasculitis
- psychiatric: chronic fatigue syndrome.

Laboratory investigation

Table	Laboratory investigations and Lyme disease	
Domain	**Laboratory test**	**Notes**
Clinical biochemistry	LFT	Elevated levels of AST and GGT may be noted
	U&E	Usually normal despite possible mild microscopic haematuria/proteinuria
Haematology	ESR	May be increased, especially in the early stages of infection
	FBC	Mild anaemia and/or lymphopaenia may be seen
Immunology	Antinuclear antibody Rheumatoid factor	Only measured to rule out differentials as these are usually absent in Lyme disease
Microbiology	Antibodies	IgG usually elevated, especially when arthritis is present; can be used to rule out other rheumatological syndromes IgM can be measured by ELISA 3–6 weeks post-infection
	Cultures	Usually from skin biopsy and rarely from blood
	PCR	For spirochaete DNA

Malaria (cerebral)

Definition   Malaria is a disease due to infection with *Plasmodium* parasites (*P. falciparum, P. malariae, P. ovale, or P. vivax*) and characterized by recurrent chills and fever.

Transmission   Via bites from the *Anopheles* mosquito. When a host is infected, the parasites travel in the blood to the liver and mature in the hepatocytes where they are released and subsequently invade red blood cells. Malaria is endemic to parts of Africa, South America, and Southeast Asia.

Incubation period   Variable, but usually 8–42 days depending on *Plasmodium* species.

Psychiatric symptoms   Several neuropsychiatric syndromes associated with cerebral malaria have been identified:

1. Fluctuation of levels of consciousness leading to coma (most common presentation);
2. Personality changes with possible psychosis;
3. Depression/apathy without fever.

408

Note: use of the antimalarial medication mefloquine, especially in initial stages of treatment, can be associated with a number of psychiatric side-effects. These include anxiety, depression, disturbing dreams/nightmares, hallucinations, psychosis (rare), and sleep disturbances. Hence this medication is not recommended for use in individuals with any previous psychiatric history.

Clinical signs and symptoms Anorexia, chills, and fever (which may be cyclical, every 48 hours for *P. ovale* and *P. vivax*, 72 hours in the case of *P. malariae*, irregular with *P. falciparum*), dark urine (due to haemolysis), hypoglycaemia, nausea, pulmonary oedema (seen in patients with severe *P. falciparum* parasitaemia), retinal haemorrhage.

Complications Anaemia, coma, haemorrhage, hypotension, jaundice, malignant tertian malaria (**life-threatening** – fever, progressive, hepato-splenomegaly, extremely low RBC, haemoglobin, and serum iron), renal dysfunction (glomerulonephritis, nephritic syndrome, renal failure, shock, splenic rupture (rare, associated with *P. vivax*), splenomegaly (especially *P. malariae*)).

Differential diagnosis Other infections, especially those associated with PUI (Pyrexia of Unknown Origin), including influenza, haemorrhagic fevers, hepatitis, meningitis, and typhoid.

Miscellaneous

Laboratory investigation

Table	Laboratory investigations and acute malaria	
Domain	**Laboratory test**	**Notes**
Clinical biochemistry	Arterial blood gases	May show a metabolic acidosis – pH <7.35, HCO_3 <22 mmol/l (patient may exhibit slow, deep breathing)
	Blood glucose (fasting)	May be <2.2 mmol/l and be a treatable cause of coma
	U&E	Anuria/oliguria may be present and many patients exhibit a degree of renal impairment which may progress to renal failure
	LFT	To look for associated abnormalities of liver function such as cholestasis or hepatocellular damage
	Urinalysis	To look for hypoglycaemia and proteinuria
Haematology	ESR	May be a useful marker of disease progression
	FBC	Anaemia may be present, especially in later stages of disease
Microbiology	Dipstick antigen capture tests	Qualitative tests (e.g. OptiMAL® or ParaSight F®) that detect presence of the parasite are expensive and may not be widely available
	Fluorescent microscopy	May allow for detection of the malaria parasite in peripheral blood
	PCR	For species determination
	Serology	Not useful for diagnosis of acute malaria; may be used to detect previous infection or as an aid in the differential diagnosis of PUI
	Thick and thin blood smears	First-line investigation. Smears (EDTA blood) stained with Giemsa may allow for visualization under a light microscope. Multiple films are recommended in order to confirm the diagnosis

Summary of possible changes in laboratory parameters in malaria

Table Summary of possible alterations in laboratory parameters in malaria		
Parameter	*Decreased*	*Increased*
Albumin		X
ALP		X
ALT		X
Antinuclear antibodies		X
AST		X
Bilirubin		X
Creatinine		X
Eosinophils		X
ESR		X
Globulin		X
Haematocrit	X	
Haemoglobin	X	
Iron	X	
Leukocytes	X	
Lymphocytes		X
Monocytes		X
Neutrophils	X	
Platelets	X	
Prolactin		X
Prothrombin time		X
Reticulocytes		X
Sodium		X
TSH		X
T4		X

Meningitis
Definition A syndrome in which there is inflammation of the meninges and the intervening CSF. It is due to a number of aetiologies, but in the acute presentation is mainly due to bacterial causes.

Transmission   Usually respiratory spread, but the oral route has also been implicated.

Incubation period   1–7 days, although in acute meningitis symptom onset can be extremely rapid (<24 hours).

Psychiatric symptoms   In acute meningitis there may be personality changes (fatigue, irritability), delirium, and coma; confusional states are more likely in the elderly.

Clinical symptoms   Chills, confusion (especially in the elderly), fever, focal seizures, headache, neck rigidity, photophobia, vomiting; in some individuals there may be a prodromal upper respiratory tract infection.

Clinical signs   Brudzinski's sign (neck or hip flexion is accompanied by involuntary flexion of both hips), cranial nerve abnormalities (especially I, IV, VI, VII), Kernig's sign (knee extension in supine patient elicits neck pain), non-blanching petechial rash (non-specific), pain on neck flexion, papilloedema may be present as disease progresses.

Complications   Depression, epilepsy, hearing impairment, hydrocephalus, lethargy, mood swings, recurring headaches, shock, visual disturbances.

Differential diagnosis

- infectious: brain abscess, encephalitis, fungal infections, leptospirosis, Lyme disease, neurobrucellosis, parasitic infections, syphilis, viral infections
- non-infectious: delirium tremens, drugs (e.g. azathoprine, ibuprofen, isoniazid, trimethoprim), leukaemia, lymphoma, multiple sclerosis, sarcoidosis, SLE, subarachnoid haemorrhage.

Miscellaneous

Laboratory investigation *Note*: meningitis may be due to a number of organisms and hence speciailist advice should always be sought. The following are only suggested investigations.

Table	Suggested laboratory investigations and acute meningitis	
Domain	*Laboratory test*	*Notes*
Clinical biochemistry	CSF	Lumbar puncture is the definitive diagnostic procedure
	Glucose	To rule out reversible cause of fluctuating consciousness as well as to provide comparative marker for CSF glucose
	LFT	To rule out possible liver dysfunction
	U&E, creatinine	To determine possible dehydration and presence of SIADH
Haematology	Coagulation screen	Especially for patients with a history of chronic alcoholism or liver disease. Required if there is suspicion of disseminated intravascular coagulation
	FBC	High white cell count suggestive of bacterial infection
Microbiology	Blood, CSF cultures	To guide appropriate antibiotic therapy
	ESR	May be a useful means of assessing disease progression

Miscellaneous

Analysis of CSF in meningitis   Lumbar puncture and CSF analysis is the definitive diagnostic intervention in the investigation of meningitis.

Table Analysis of CSF in meningitis			
Parameter	**Bacterial meningitis**	**Viral meningitis**	**Fungal meningitis**
Cells	Usually raised number of polymorphs but may be normal in early stages	Monocytosis may sometimes be seen	Raised numbers of mononuclear cells may be seen
Glucose	Decreased	Normal	Usually normal but may sometimes be decreased
Organisms	Gram stain usually provides a good guide; acid-fast staining for TB may be informative	No organisms seen on staining	India ink staining may be useful for fungi
Pressure	Increased	Normal or increased	Normal or increased
Protein	Usually high	May be only moderately raised	Usually high

Neurosyphilis

Definition   Syphilis is caused by *Treponema pallidum*, a coiled gram-positive rod that is difficult to culture and is best visualized on dark-ground microscopy. Neurosyphilis may be divided into three types, asymptomatic, meningovascular, and parenchymous (see below).

Transmission   Via sexual intercourse (main route of transmission), blood transfusion, kissing, or through the placenta.

Incubation period   Appearance of chancre around 3 weeks post-exposure (ranging from 9 to 90 days), with secondary syphilis typically developing some 2–8 weeks later. Neurosyphilis is often asymptomatic but features may present many years (roughly 5–30) after initial infection.

Psychiatric symptoms   Cognitive changes, delusions, depression, euphoria, memory loss, mood swings, personality changes, poor insight and judgement, psychosis.

Clinical symptoms

- primary syphilis: often asymptomatic
- secondary syphilis: arthralgia, fever, headache, meningism, pharyngitis, weight loss

414

- neurosyphilis

  - asymptomatic: no gross symptoms
  - meningovascular: confusion, epilepsy, headache; hemi-, mono- or para-plegia
  - parenchymous: may present as 'general paralysis (paresis) of the insane' (GPI) or tabes dorsalis; GPI – epilepsy, incoordination, psychiatric symptoms as above, slurred speech, tremor, weakness; tabes dorsalis – ataxia, impotence, incontinence (bladder, rectal), sensual disturbances (deafness, 'lightning pains' (acute, stabbing pains, commonly in the legs), loss of visual acuity, paraesthesiae).

Clinical signs

- primary syphilis: may be asymptomatic or manifest as a genital or extra-genital solitary, painless, red macular lesion (chancre) which eventually ulcerates but heals within about 10 weeks; extragenital sites include eyelids, fingers, mouth and adnexae, mucous membranes, nipples. There may also be non-tender inguinal lymphadenopathy
- secondary syphilis: usually generalized maculopapular skin lesions, possibly including condylomata lata (large, coalesced papular lesions); erosions of the mucous membranes may also be present, in addition to generalized lymphadenopathy. There may rarely be associated alopecia, arthritis, cra-nial nerve palsies, eye disease (choroidoretinitis, iridocyclitis), hepatitis, meningitis, and renal damage
- neurosyphilis

  - asymptomatic: no gross neurological changes; the diagnosis is based on changes in laboratory parameters (see below)
  - meningovascular: Argyll Robertson pupil (pupils small, unequal in size, unreactive to light but reactive to accommodation), cranial nerve palsies (III, VI, and VIII), hemiplegias (rare), meningism, papilloedema
  - parenchymous: GPI – altered facial expression (may be mask-like, smiling, or vacant), convulsions, dysarthria, dyspraxia (may affect handwriting), extensor plantar responses, incoordination, loss of sphinc-ter control, optic atrophy, tremor, weakness; tabes dorsalis – absent reflexes (ankle, biceps, knee, triceps); Argyll Robertson pupil, Charcot's joints (usually painless, deformed, unstable joints with bone overgrowth at joint margins), optical changes (atrophy, palsy), perforating foot ulcers, Romberg's sign (inability to maintain balance when the eyes are shut and the feet are close together), sensory impairments (impaired pain, position, touch, and vibration sense), tabetic crises (often gastric, presenting as pain and vomiting).

Complications Cardiac involvement (aortic incompetence, aortitis, aneu-rysms, arteritis), death, dementia, gummas (granulomatous lesions usually on the face, leg, or scalp whch may ulcerate and scar); Jarisch–Herxheimer reaction (an acute febrile state with chills, headache, myalgia, and rigors which usually resolves within 24 hours; it is due to release of endotoxins following antibiotic treatment and is seen in about half of all patients with primary syphilis and up to 90% with secondary syphilis); placental transmis-sion may lead to congential syphilis.

415

Differential diagnosis   Other treponemal infections with similar presentations such as bejel (*T. endemicum*), pinta (*T. carateum*), or yaws (*T. pertenue*).

Laboratory investigation

Table	Laboratory investigations and syphilis	
Domain	*Investigation*	*Notes*
Clinical biochemistry	Glucose	Usually increased
	LFT	Hepatitis is a recognized manifestation of secondary syphilis, usually with no jaundice, but raised alkaline phosphatase is common
	U&E	Nephropathy is rare although transient nephrotic syndrome has been reported
Haematology	FBC	Anaemia may be present, and there may be leukocytosis, lymphocytosis, and monocytosis
Immunology and microbiology	ESR	Usually increased
	FTA	Fluorescent treponemal antibody test – once positive remains so for life
	IgG	Response remains high throughout course of illness
	IgM	Decreases in later stages of the disease and after treatment
	Rheumatoid factor	Usually increased
	RPR	Rapid plasma reagin test. A newer test that is similar to the older Veneral Disease Research Laboratory (VDRL) test and becomes negative post-treatment
	TPPA	*Treponema pallidum* particle agglutination test – this tests antibodies to treponemal antigens; once positive remains so for life
	Cultures	Not generally performed as the organism is difficult to grow and serological techniques are the first-line investigations of choice. Swabs (high vaginal or urethral) may be taken in order to culture other organisms associated with sexually transmitted diseases (STDs)
	Microscopy	Dark-field microscopy of fluid obtained from suspected lesions may demonstrate the organism

Miscellaneous

Analysis of CSF in syphilis CSF investigation is warranted for suspected neurosyphilis, i.e. in those individuals with positive syphilis serology and who manifest neuropsychiatric signs and symptoms.

Table CSF changes in syphilis

Parameter	Notes
Cells	Usually increased
Chloride	Usually decreased
Glucose	May be decreased
Immunoglobulins	Usually increased
Lymphocytes	Usually increased
Polymorphs	May be increased
Protein	Usually increased
RPR (rapid plasma reagin)	Usually positive

Tuberculosis

Definition Tuberculosis is a disease caused by the acid-fast bacillum *Mycobacterium tuberculosis*, although some cases may be caused by *M. kansasii* and *M. xenopi*. The disease is so-named due to the formation of tubercules or granulomata.

Transmission *M. tuberculosis* is transmitted by droplet infection from an infected individual. Overcrowding is an especially important factor in transmission. Rarely, a form of tuberculosis due to *M. bovis* can be transmitted through drinking unpasteurized milk.

Incubation period Initial exposure may be asymptomatic, but after 4–6 weeks the tuberculin skin test will be positive. Although primary infection usually resolves spontaneously, it may progress (especially in immunocompromised individuals) and/or reactivate years later.

Psychiatric symptoms Anxiety, depression, and fatigue may be associated with respiratory distress; tuberculous meningitis may present with focal neurological signs and sometimes a delirium.

Clinical symptoms

- primary: may be none
- secondary: fatigue, night sweats, tuberculous arthritis, weakness.

Clinical signs

- primary: may be none
- secondary: chronic cough possibly with haemoptysis (lung involvement), fever, lymphadenopathy (including 'scrofula', tuberculous adenitis of the cervical lymph nodes), weight loss.

Miscellaneous

Complications

- adrenal involvement (may cause Addison's disease due to destruction of adrenal cortex)
- eye involvement (choroid tubercles are pathognomonic)
- gastrointestinal TB (especially of terminal ileum)
- genitourinary TB (especially with sterile pyuria)
- miliary TB (disseminated disease with spread throughout the body; characteristic mottling pattern seen on X-ray)
- pericarditis (constrictive type, with Kussmaul's sign (an increase in jugular venous distension upon inspiration), pulsus paradoxus, and ascites/peripheral oedema)
- skin involvement (erythema nodosum, lupus vulgaris)
- tuberculous arthritis (usually involving the hip, knee, sacroiliac joints, or spine)
- tuberculous meningitis
- tuberculous osteomyelitis ('Pott's disease' is inflammation of the vertebral bodies in younger adults giving rise to kyphosis and nerve compression symptoms).

Differential diagnosis Carcinoma, diabetes mellitus, fibrotic lung disease (extrinsic allergic alveolitis, pneumoconiosis, sarcoid), lymphoma, pneumonia, pyrexia of unknown origin, Wegener's; rarely severe anorexia nervosa.

Laboratory investigation The UK NICE has published guidelines for tuberculosis (http: //guidance.nice.org.uk/CG33/niceguidance/word/English), and suggests the following laboratory investigations for diagnosis:

- active TB: at least three sputum samples for TB culture and microscopy
- active, non-respiratory TB: biopsy and TB culture of biopsy material
- latent TB: Mantoux test to be followed with interferon-γ testing in those with positive results.

Table Possible laboratory investigations and tuberculosis

Domain	Laboratory test	Notes
Clinical biochemistry	CSF analysis	For suspected tuberculous meningitis (see Table below)
	Glucose	Levels may be raised or lowered
	U&E	Hyponatraemia is common and may be indicative of SIADH; hypercalcaemia may be present
Haematology	ESR	May be raised in acute infection; serial monitoring may reflect disease progression
	FBC	Anaemia of chronic disease may be present
Microbiology	Culture	Throat/CSF culture may be helpful

Possible CSF changes in tuberculous meningitis

Table CSF changes in tuberculous meningitis

Parameter	Notes
Culture	May not be positive
Glucose	Usually decreased
Lymphocytes	Usually normal
Polymorphs	Usually raised
Pressure	Usually raised
Protein	May be raised

Possible changes in laboratory parameters in tuberculous meningitis

Table Summary of possible changes in laboratory parameters in tuberculous meningitis

Parameter	Decreased	Increased
Antidiuretic hormone		X
Chloride	X	
ESR		X
Globulin		X
Monocytes		X
Protein	X	
Rheumatoid factor		X
Sodium	X	
Urate		X

Reference

1. Foster R, Olajide D, Everall IP. Antiretroviral-therapy induced psychosis: case report and brief review of the literature. HIV Med 2003; 4: 139–44.

Miscellaneous

419

Further reading

General

Fatemi A. Neuropsychiatric Disorders and Infection. London: Taylor & Francis, 2005.
Haaheim LR, Pattison JR, Whitley RJ, eds. A Practical Guide to Clinical Virology, 2nd edn. Chichester: John Wiley & Sons, 2002.
Moore DP, Jefferson JW. Handbook of Medical Psychiatry, 2nd edn. Philadelphia: Elsevier Mosby, 2004.
Pattison JR, Gruneberg RN, Holton J et al. A Practical Guide to Clinical Bacteriology. Chichester: John Wiley & Sons, 1995.

Brucellosis

Mantur BG, Anarnath SK, Shinde RS. Review of clinical and laboratory features of human brucellosis. Indian J Med Microbiol 2007; 25: 188–202.
Yetkin MA, Bulut C, Erdinc FS, Oral B, Tulek N. Evaluation of the clinical presentations in neurobrucellosis. Int J Infect Dis 2006; 10: 446–52.

Creutzfeldt–Jakob disease

Krasnianski A, Meissner B, Heinemann U, Zerr I. Clinical findings and diagnostic tests in Creutzfeldt-Jakob disease and variant Creutzfeldt-Jakob disease. Folia Neuropathol 2004; 42 (Suppl B): 24–38.
Wall CA, Rummans TA, Aksamit AJ, Krahn LE, Pankratz VS. Psychiatric manifestations of Creutzfeldt-Jakob disease: a 25-year analysis. J Neuropsychiatry Clin Neurosci 2005; 17: 489–95.
Will RG, Ward HJ. Clinical features of variant Creutzfeldt-Jakob disease. Curr Top Microbiol Immunol 2004; 284: 121–32.

Herpes simplex

Arciniegas DB, Anderson CA. Viral encephalitis: neuropsychiatric and neurobehavioral aspects. Curr Psychiatry Rep 2004; 6: 372–9.
Steiner I, Kennedy PG, Pachner AR. The neurotropic herpes viruses: herpes simplex and varicella-zoster. Lancet Neurol 2007; 6: 1015–28.

Human immunodeficiency virus

Dube B, Benton T, Cruess DG, Evans DL. Neuropsychiatric manifestations of HIV infection and AIDS. J Psychiatry Neurosci 2005; 30: 237–46.
Hamlyn E, Easterbrook P. Occupational exposure to HIV and the use of post-exposure prophylaxis. Occup Med (Lond) 2007; 57: 329–36.
Zetola NM, Pilcher CD. Diagnosis and management of acute HIV infection. Infect Dis Clin North Am 2007; 21: 19–48.

Infectious mononucleosis

Candy B, Chalder T, Cleare AJ et al. Predictors of fatigue following the onset of infectious mononucleosis. Psychol Med 2003; 33: 847–55.
Hurt C, Tammaro D. Diagnostic evaluation of mononucleosis-like illnesses. Am J Med 2007; 120: 911.e1–8.

Lyme disease

Fallon BA, Kochevar JM, Gaito A, Nields JA. The underdiagnosis of neuropsychiatric Lyme disease in children and adults. Psychiatr Clin North Am 1998; 21: 693–703, viii.
Pachner AR, Steiner I. Lyme neuroborreliosis: infection, immunity, and inflammation. Lancet Neurol 2007; 6: 544–52.

Miscellaneous

Malaria (cerebral)

Alao AO, Dewan MJ. Psychiatric complications of malaria: a case report. Int J Psychiatry Med 2001; 31: 217–23.

Gjorup IE, Vestergaard LS, Moller K, Ronn AM, Bygbjerg IC. Laboratory indicators of the diagnosis and course of imported malaria. Scand J Infect Dis 2007; 39: 707–13.

Meningitis

Fitch MT, van de Beek D. Emergency diagnosis and treatment of adult meningitis. Lancet Infect Dis 2007; 7: 191–200.

Kaplan SL. Clinical presentations, diagnosis, and prognostic factors of bacterial meningitis. Infect Dis Clin North Am 1999; 13: 579–94.

Thomson RB Jr, Bertram H. Laboratory diagnosis of central nervous system infections. Infect Dis Clin North Am 2001; 15: 1047–71.

Neurosyphilis

Hutto B. Syphilis in clinical psychiatry: a review. Psychosomatics 2001; 42: 453–60.

Tuberculosis

Drobniewski FA, Caws M, Gibson A, Young D. Modern laboratory diagnosis of tuberculosis. Lancet Infect Dis 2003; 3: 141–7.

Yadav BS, Jain SC, Sharma G, Mehrotra ML, Kumar A. Psychiatric morbidity in pulmonary tuberculosis. Indian J Tuberc 1980; 27: 167–71.

Miscellaneous

The immunology laboratory and psychiatry

At present there are no immunological markers which are pathognomonic for any adult psychiatric disorder, and hence the immunology laboratory is used in order to monitor or diagnose disorders associated with specific autoantibodies.

Usually an autoantibody screen will be requested; this will consist of a serum sample in which antibodies to the following will be measured:

- gastric parietal cells
- liver/kidney microsomes
- mitochondria
- nuclei (antinuclear antibody)
- reticulin
- smooth muscle.

Specific psychiatric associations and immunological parameters

Althogh there are as yet no conclusive associations between psychiatric disorders and immunological parameters, various findings have been reported as summarized below, but most remain controversial. *Note*: some haematological and metabolic effects of psychotropic agents may have an immunological basis; however, the clinical implications of this remain unclear.

Table Possible psychiatric associations with immunological parameters

Psychiatric association	Reported immunological effect/parameter	Notes
Alcohol	Diverse effects on B and T cells (impaired proliferation, altered cytokine production)	Effects may be related to endocrine effects of alcohol, such as inducing higher levels of circulating glucocorticoid
	Suppression of macrophage function	Effects on macrophages may be associated with increased risk of tuberculosis
Amitriptyline	Hypersensitivity reactions reported (cutaneous lymphoid hyperplasia)	Very rare events, may be related to underlying immunodeficiency or use of immunomodulatory drugs
Cannabis	May cause or worsen immunosuppression	Effects possibly mediated via cannabinoid receptors
Carbamazepine	Humoral immune deficiency and hypersensitivity reactions reported	Rare events, may be associated with eosinophilia

Table Possible psychiatric associations with immunological parameters

Psychiatric association	Reported immunological effect/parameter	Notes
Chronic fatigue syndrome	May be associated with antigliadin/antiendomysium antibodies as part of coeliac disease	Coeliac disease is one of the differential diagnoses for CFS, and UK NICE guidelines for CFS include screening for gluten sensitivity
Clomethiazole	Anaphylaxis/hypersensitivity reactions possible	Extremely rare events
Depression	Decreased lymphocyte proliferation in response to mitogens (concavalin A, phytohaemagglutinin, pokeweed) Reduction of natural killer cell activity in some patients with depression	Unclear whether these effects are related primarily to depression or are secondary to other variables such as age, comorbidity, gender, stress, etc.
	Increased white cell counts have been reported in some patients with depression	May be associated with neutrophilia and/or lymphopaenia
Diazepam	Anaphylaxis/hypersensitivity reactions possible	Extremely rare events
Lamotrigine	Hypersensitivity reactions reported	Rare events, may be associated wih leukopaenia or thrombocytopaenia
Nitrites	Controversial association with weakened non-specific defences	Suggestion that alkyl nitrites may increase risk of transmission of HIV especially in gay men
Schizophrenia	Effect of maternal infection with neurotropic viruses	Some epidemiological evidence, no definitive association
Smoking	Suppresses some mucosal immune responses	Association of tobacco with cancer is well recognized
SSRIs	Anaphylaxis/hypersensitivity reactions possible	Very rare events, may be related to underlying immunodeficiency or use of immunomodulatory drugs; fluoxetine especially implicated
'Stress'	Wide range of effects on B and T cells	Findings difficult to interpret due to methodological limitations
Venlafaxine	Hypersensitivity reactions reported	Rare events, may include angioedema and urticaria
Zopiclone	Hypersensitivity reactions reported	Rare events, may include rashes, urticaria

Specific autoantibodies

An increasing number of medical conditions are now associated with specific autoantibodies, and the following table summarizes the most important of these. It should be noted that very few autoantibodes are fully diagnostic of any condition, that no autoantibody is currently known to be associated with any specific psychiatric disorder, and that any investigation should always be based on clinical presentation and after consultation with the appropriate expert authority.

Table Examples of antibody–disease associations		
Antibody	**Disease association**	**Notes**
Acetylcholine receptor	Myasthenia gravis	Condition associated with thymomas and other autoimmune disorders
Adrenal	Addison's disease in association with other autoimmune diseases	May be seen in approximately 50% of these patients; Addison's is associated with gastric, thyroid, and parathyroid autouimmune disease
Antinuclear (ANA)	Chronic active hepatitis	May be secondary to number of aetiologies including autoimmune, infections (hepatitis B and C), metabolic (such as Wilson's disease), toxins (alcohol, drugs), and others
	Juvenile rheumatoid arthritis	May be polyarticular or systemic (latter is known as Still's disease)
	Progressive systemic sclerosis Rheumatoid arthritis	Most commonly affect women aged between 30 and 50
	Sjögren's syndrome	Syndrome associated with conjunctival and mucosal dryness and polyarthritis in women aged between 30 and 50
	Systemic lupus erythematosus	See Chapter 6
Cardiac muscle	Myocardial infarction	Seen in Dressler's syndrome and other cardiac disorders; not usually diagnostically
Cardiolipin	Antiphospholipid syndrome	Characterized by thrombosis and thrombocytopaenia; may manifest with spontaneous miscarriage
	Systemic lupus erythematosus	See Chapter 6

Table Examples of antibody–disease associations (Cont.)

Antibody	Disease association	Notes
Centromere	CREST (a form of systemic sclerosis which is characterized by calcinosis, Raynaud's phenomenon, oesophageal involvement, sclerodactyly, and telangiectasia)	May involve intestines, kidneys, lungs, and rarely nervous system May be associated with thyroid disorders and primary biliary cirrhosis
Double-stranded DNA	Systemic lupus erythematosus	See Chapter 6
Extractable nuclear antigen (ENA)	Mixed connective tissue disease	Associated with arthralgia, hand swelling, Raynaud's, abnormalities in oesophageal motility, leukopaenia, and thrombocytopaenia
	Systemic lupus erythematosus	See Chapter 6
Endomysium	Coeliac disease	Main symptoms in adults include steatorrhoea, anaemia, and dermatitis herpetiformis. May be measured together with antigliadin to confirm a diagnosis of coeliac disease
Gastric parietal cell	Atrophic gastritis	Associated with pernicious anaemia and other autoimmune disorders including Addison's and thyroiditis
	Autoimmune thyroid disease	May manifest as hyper- or hypothyroidism (see Chapter 6)
	Pernicious anaemia	May present with hyperbilirubinaemia, macrocytic anaemia, raised LDH, and decreased B12/folate levels
Gliadin	Coeliac disease	A positive antigliadin and IgA antiendomysial antibody suggest coeliac disease
Glomerular basement membrane	Goodpasture's syndrome	Condition characterized by pulmonary haemorrhage and nephritis
Jo-1	Polymyositis	Inflammatory condition of striated muscle which presents primarily with proximal muscle weakness

Miscellaneous

Table	Examples of antibody–disease associations (Cont.)	
Antibody	**Disease association**	**Notes**
La	Sjögren's syndrome	Syndrome associated with conjunctival and mucosal dryness and polyarthritis in women aged between 30 and 50
Mitochondria	Chronic active hepatitis	May be secondary to number of aetiologies including autoimmune, viral infections (hepatitis B and C), metabolic (such as Wilson's disease), toxins (alcohol, drugs), and others
	Idiopathic cirrhosis	Cirrhosis of unknown aetiology which may present with non-specific findings
	Primary biliary cirrhosis	Usually seen in middle-aged women and may be asymptomatic or present with pruritus, jaundice, and other complications of liver disease
Neutrophil cytoplasm (ANCA)	Wegener's disease	A vasculitic disorder characterized by necrotizing granulomata in the lungs and a necrotizing glomerulonephritis. May also involve the joints, skin, heart, and nervous system
Nucleolus	Systemic sclerosis	A multisystem disorder characterized by fibrosis and vascular involvement of skin, arthralgia with effects on the gastrointestinal tract, kidney, and lungs
Reticulin	Coeliac disease	Main symptoms in adults include steatorrhoea, anaemia, and dermatitis herpetiformis
	Crohn's disease	An ulcerative condition of the whole gastrointestinal tract with multiorgan involvement
	Dermatitis herpetiformis	A pruritic, urticarial condition stongly associated with coeliac disease
Rheumatoid factor (RhF)	Felty's syndrome	Classically seen as triad of rheumatoid arthritis, splenomegaly, and neutropaenia
	Infective endocarditis	Usually bacterial, may be associated with intravenous drug use

Miscellaneous

Table Examples of antibody–disease associations (Cont.)

Antibody	Disease association	Notes
	Progressive systemic sclerosis Rheumatoid arthritis	Most commonly affect women aged between 30 and 50
	Sjögren's syndrome	Syndrome associated with conjunctival and mucosal dryness and polyarthritis in women aged between 30 and 50
	Still's disease	The systemic form of juvenile rheumatoid arthritis
	Systemic lupus erythematosus	See Chapter 6
Ro (SSA) La (SSB) (U1RNP, U1 ribonuclear protein)	Sjögren's syndrome	Syndrome associated with conjunctival and mucosal dryness and polyarthritis in women aged between 30 and 50
	Systemic lupus erythematosus	See Chapter 6
SCL-70	Systemic sclerosis	A multisystem disorder characterized by fibrosis and vascular involvement of skin, arthralgia with effects on the gastrointestinal tract, kidney, and lungs
Smooth muscle	Chronic active hepatitis Idiopathic cirrhosis Primary biliary cirrhosis	Immunological analysis may help in differential diagnosis
Striated muscle	Myasthenia gravis	Strong association with thymoma in patients with myasthenia gravis
Thyroid: microsomal	Hashimoto's thyroiditis, myxoedema	Immunological analysis may help in differential diagnosis
Thyroid: thyroid-binding	Graves' disease	

Disease associations with specific autoantibodies

Table Examples of disease–antibody associations

Condition	Main associated antibody/antibodies	Notes
Addison's syndrome	Adrenal, gastric parietal cells, thyroid	Addison's may be due to a variety of aetiologies including infection, malignancy, and sarcoid, although is usually autoimmune in Western populations. See also Chapter 6
Diabetes mellitus	Islet-cell antibodies, IgA antibodies	Antibody testing useful for diagnosis but not monitoring. See also Chapter 6
Limbic encephalitis	Antineuronal, Anti-hu (ANNA-1), anti-Ri (ANNA-2), anti-Yo	Limbic encephalitis is a rare paraneoplastic disorder associated with lung cancer, which can present with a dementia, and sometimes delirium and psychosis In rare cases, limbic encephalitis may present in patients not suffering from neoplastic disorders. In some of these, antibodies to voltage-gated potassium channels (VGKC) may be found. Patients may present with atypical seizures, delusions, and hallucinations
Pernicious anaemia	Gastric parietal cell, intrinsic factor	Strongly associated with thyroid disease; interestingly, patients may have prematurely grey hair and blue eyes. See also Chapter 8 (vitamin B12)
Rheumatoid arthritis	ANA, ENA, RhF	Antibody testing useful for diagnosis but not monitoring
Systemic lupus erythematosus	ANA, dsDNA, ENA, histone antibodies (for drug-induced SLE), ribosomal (for CNS involvement)	Other autoantibodies may be associated, including Hep-2, anticardiolipin, and organ-specific antibodies (e.g. thyroid, gastric parietal cell). See also Chapter 6
Thyroid disorders	Thyroid microsomes, thyroid-binding, thyroid-stimulating	Also consider gastric parietal cell antibodies due to association of thyroid disease with pernicious anaemia. See also Chapter 6

Further reading

Henneberg AE, Kaschka WB. Immunological Alterations in Psychiatric Diseases. Basel: Karger, 1997.

Margutti P, Delunardo F, Ortona E. Autoantibodies associated with psychiatric disorders. Curr Neurovas Res 2006; 3: 149–57.

Sperner-Unterweger B. Immunological aetiology of major psychiatric disorders: evidence and therapeutic implications. Drugs 2005; 65: 1493–520.

Spickett G. Oxford Handbook of Clinical Immunology, 2nd edn. Oxford: Oxford University Press, 2006.

Miscellaneous

System 'screens' and basic laboratory 'patterns' in selected medical presentations

System 'screens'

Below are the tests comprising standard screening of specific organs or conditions. *Note*: further investigations may be required depending on clinical findings, and should always be considered after consulting with the appropriate expert authority.

System/presentation	Laboratory tests
Amenorrhoea (secondary)	FSH, LH, prolactin
Bone	Albumin, alkaline phosphatase, calcium, phosphate
Cardiac	Creatine kinase
Clotting	APTT, prothrombin time (PT)
Dementia	Autoantibody screen, ESR, FBC, glucose, LFT, syphilis serology, TFT, U&E, urinalysis
Gastrointestinal	Albumin, alkaline phosphatase, aspartate transaminase, bilirubin, calcium, creatinine, gamma glutamyl transferase, phosphate, potassium
Haematinics	B12, folate, FBC, serum ferritin, total iron binding capacity, transferrin saturation
Hirsutism (female)	FSH, 17-hydroxyprogesterone, LH, sex hormone binding globulin (SHBG), testosterone
Hirsutism (male)	17-hydroxyprogesterone, LH, SHBG, testosterone
Infertility (female)	FSH, LH, prolactin
Infertility (male)	FSH, LH, prolactin, SHBG, testosterone
Lipids	Cholesterol, triglycerides (including HDL if appropriate)
Liver	Albumin, alkaline phosphatase, aspartate transaminase, bilirubin, gamma glutamyl transferase, total protein
'Old age'	Albumin, alkaline phosphatase, calcium, creatinine, free T4, phosphate, potassium, sodium, TSH
Porphyria	Urinary aminolevulinic acid, urinary porphobilinogen
Renal	Creatinine, glucose, sodium, potassium
Thyroid	Free T3, TSH

Laboratory 'patterns'

Below are examples of the most commonly reported alterations in routine biochemical and haematological parameters in selected presentations; for information regarding conditions or parameters not included here, see specific chapters of this book and other specialized medical and laboratory medicine texts.

Miscellaneous

Condition	Raised level of	Lowered level of	Notes*
Addison's syndrome	Potassium	Sodium	See Chapter 6
Anaemia: iron-deficiency	TIBC	MCH, MCHC, MCV, serum ferritin, serum iron	MCHC may be normal or lowered
Anaemia: sideroblastic	Serum ferritin, serum iron	MCH, MCHC, MCV	MCV may be raised in acquired sideroblastic anaemia; TIBC usually normal
Anaemia: thalassaemia	—	MCH, MCHC, MCV	Serum ferritin, serum iron, and TIBC usually normal
B12 deficiency	Serum folate (normal or raised)	Red cell folate (normal or raised), serum B12	See also folate deficiency, below
Cholestasis	ALP Bilirubin Prothrombin time Transaminases	—	Albumin, γ-globulins may be ↔ ALP ↑↑↑ Bilirubin ↑ to ↑↑↑ Prothrombin time may be ↔ to ↑ Transaminases may be ↔ to ↑
Cirrhosis	ALP ↑↑ Bilirubin γ-Globulins Prothrombin time	Albumin ↔ to ↓	Bilirubin, prothrombin time, transaminases may be ↔ ↓ α1-antitrypsin in cirrhosis due to α1-antitrypsin deficiency
Conn's syndrome	Bicarbonate Sodium	Potassium	Sodium may be ↔ Clinical features also include alkalosis and hypertension
Diabetes insipidus	Calcium Sodium	Potassium	Nephrogenic diabetes insipidus may be secondary to ↑ calcium and ↓ potassium
Diabetes mellitus	Glucose	Bicarbonate	See Chapter 6
Disseminated intravascular coagulation	Fibrinogen degradation products (FDPs)	APTT, platelet count, PT, thrombin time (TT)	May be due to anaphylaxis, infection (especially gram-negative sepsis), liver disease, malignancy, and obstetric problems

Excess alcohol intake	ALP AST Bilirubin GGT MCV Blood ethanol Carbohydrate-deficient transferrin	—	See Chapter 7
Folate deficiency	—	Serum folate, red cell folate	Serum B12 normal or borderline; see also B12 deficiency, above
Hepatitis: acute	ALP ↔ to ↑↑ Bilirubin ↔ to ↑↑ Prothrombin time ↔ to ↑ Transaminases ↑↑↑	—	Pre-icteric: transaminases ↑↑, ALK ↔, bilirubin slight ↑; Icteric: transaminases ↑, ALP slight ↑, bilirubin ↑↑
Hepatitis: chronic active	ALP Bilirubin ↔ to ↑ γ-Globulins Prothrombin time ↔ to ↑ Transaminases ↑↑	Albumin ↔ to ↓	ALP may be ↔
Hepatitis: chronic persistent	γ-Globulins Transaminases	Albumin	Albumin, ALP, bilirubin, prothrombin time may be ↔, transaminases ↑
Hyperparathyroidism	ALP Calcium	Phosphate	ALP and phosphate may be ↔
Hyperthyroidism	T4, free T4, T3	TSH	T3 helps confirm a diagnosis of hyperthyroidism
Hypoparathyroidism	Phosphate	Calcium	See Chapter 6
Hypothyroidism	TSH	T4, fT4	T3 is not considered to be a useful test in hypothyroidism
Jaundice (haemolytic)	AST Bilirubin	Haemoglobin Plasma haptoglobins	↑ Urine urobilinogen and ↑ plasma reticulocytes may also be seen

Condition	Raised level of	Lowered level of	Notes*
Liver malignancy	α-Fetoprotein ↑↑↑ ALP ↑↑ Transaminases ↔ to ↑	Albumin ↔ to ↓	Bilirubin, γ-globulins Prothrombin time may be ↔
Myocardial infarction	AST Creative kinase (CK) LDH	—	Diagnosis initially clinical with electrocardiogram (ECG), blood tests performed to confirm diagnosis and assess treatment
Osteomalacia	ALP	Calcium Phosphate	Diagnosis mainly clinical and radiological
SIADH	—	Creatinine Sodium Urea	Creatinine and urea may be ↔; see Chapter 3

↔=normal; ↑=slightly increased; ↑↑↑=markedly increased; ↓=lowered.

Further reading

General

Axford J, ed. Medicine. Oxford: Blackwell Science, 1996.
Longmore M, Wilkinson I, Turmezei T, Cheung CK, Smith E. Oxford Handbook of Clinical Medicine. Oxford: Oxford University Press, 2007.
Marshall WJ, Bangert SK. Clinical Chemistry, 5th edn. Edinburgh: Mosby, 2005.

Miscellaneous

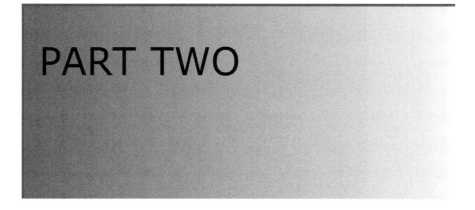

PART TWO

chapter 9

Specific laboratory parameters and psychiatry

The parameters described below are the most common that the general psychiatrist will encounter in everyday practice. Although there are many other possible laboratory tests that could be included herein, the reader is encouraged to consult appropriate specialized texts and seek expert advice for those not included in this section.

It should be noted that many of the changes associated with psychiatric illnesses and treatment described for individual laboratory parameters may be rare, idiosyncratic, or due to causes not listed herein. Where there is any doubt as to interpretation of blood tests or clinical presentation, the appropriate expert sources of help should be consulted.

For further details regarding specific biochemical and haematological effects of psychotropics see individual agents and summaries of effects in Chapters 3, 4, and 5.

For each parameter described in this section, the following information is provided:

- a brief description of function
- a commonly accepted reference range
- suggested panic/critical ranges (low and high)
- information regarding blood sampling
- details of associations with raised levels of the parameter, both psychiatric and non-psychiatric
- details of associations with lowered levels of the parameter, both psychiatric and non-psychiatric.

The following biochemical and haematological parameters as measured in blood (serum or plasma) are described:

- activated partial thromboplastin time (APTT)
- alanine transferase
- albumin
- alkaline phosphatase
- amylase
- aspartate aminotransferase
- basophils
- bicarbonate
- bilirubin
- C-reactive protein
- calcium
- carbohydrate-deficient transferrin
- chloride
- cholesterol
- creatine kinase
- creatinine
- eosinophils
- erythrocytes
- erythrocyte sedimentation rate
- ferritin
- gamma glutamyl transferase
- glomerular filtration rate
- glucose: fasting
- glucose: random
- glycated haemoglobin
- haemoglobin
- lactate dehydrogenase
- lipoproteins

  ○ low-density lipoprotein
  ○ high-density lipoprotein

- lymphocytes
- mean cell haemoglobin
- mean cell haemoglobin concentration
- mean cell volume
- monocytes
- neutrophils
- packed cell volume
- phosphate
- platelets
- potassium
- prolactin
- protein (total)
- prothrombin time/international normalized ratio
- red cell distribution width
- reticulocyte count
- sodium
- thyroid stimulating hormone
- thyroxine

440

- triglycerides
- triiodothyronine
- urate
- urea
- white cell count (total).

Activated partial thromboplastin time (APTT)

Function Test screens for deficiency in intrinsic factor and is also used for monitoring anticoagulation status when heparin is used. Also useful for screening for congenital deficiency of clotting factors (intrinsic factors II, V, VIII, IX, X, XI, XII), disseminated intravascular coagulation (DIC), haemophilia A, haemophilia B, liver failure, vitamin K deficiency, and others.

Reference range 23.8–32.2 seconds.

Suggested panic/critical ranges

- low: none identified
- high: an APTT over 70 seconds requires immediate medical attention.

Sampling Plasma specimen (sodium citrate, blue top tube); sample taken 1 hour before next dose of heparin. Not to be performed on patients with heparin infusion treatment or when heparinized catheters are in use.

Associations with increased APTT time

- psychiatric: buproprion (rare), phenothiazine treatment (especially chlorpromazine)
- other: heparin treatment, intravascular coagulation, intrinsic factor deficiency, liver disease, lupus anticoagulant, penicillin treatment, rheumatoid arthritis.

Associations with decreased APTT time

- psychiatric: buproprion, modafinil (both rare)
- other: haemolysis (in individuals with no bleeding disorders).

Alanine transferase

Function An enzyme which is measured as part of a battery of liver function tests. It is a sensitive marker of hepatocyte injury and is more specific for liver damage than AST.

Reference range 0–45 IU/l; *note*: higher levels may be found in males and obese subjects.

441

Suggested panic/critical ranges

- low: none identified
- high: none identified.

Sampling Serum (gold top tube); is stable at room temperature for 1 day and up to 3 days when refrigerated. Haemolysed samples will give erroneous results. Note that metronidazole may interfere with analysis and result in spuriously low levels.

Associations with raised levels

- Psychiatric:

  - clinical syndromes: eating disorders (especially anorexia nervosa); chronic alcoholism
  - medications (effects usually mild, transient, and reversible on cessation of implicated agent): antipsychotics – benperidol, chlorpromazine, clozapine, haloperidol, olanzapine, quetiapine, zotepine; antidepressants – duloxetine, mianserin, mirtazepine, moclobemide, monoamine oxidase inhibitors, SSRIs (especially paroxetine and sertraline), TCAs, trazodone, venlafaxine; anxiolytics/hypnotics – barbiturates, benzodiazepines, chloral hydrate, clomethiazole, promethazine; miscellaneous agents – caffeine, dexamphetamine, disulfiram, opioids; mood stabilizers: carbamazepine, lamotrigine, valproate.
    Note: many medications (both psychotropics and others), substances of abuse, and toxins may affect the liver and cause non-specific changes in all liver enzymes. See also Chapter 4 (psychotropics associated with hepatotoxicity).
  - medication syndromes: disulfiram–alcohol syndrome, neuroleptic malignant syndrome (NMS), serotonin syndrome

- Other: Addison's disease, α1-antitrypsin deficiency, coeliac disease, congestive cardiac failure, drugs (antibiotics, levodopa, oral contraceptives, phenytoin), haemolysis, hypothyroidism; liver disease – alcoholic liver disease, chronic hepatitis, haemochromatosis, hepatic cirrhosis, hepatitis, ischaemic hepatitis, Wilson's disease; muscle trauma (rhabdomyolysis, poly- and dermatomyositis); obesity.

Associations with lowered levels

- psychiatric: none known
- other: vigabatrin treatment.

Albumin

Function Most abundant plasma protein, maintains plasma oncotic pressure and acts as transport protein for hormones, calcium, fatty acids, and some medications.

Reference range 3.5–4.8 g/dl (*note*: normal range gradually decreases after age 40).

Suggested panic/critical ranges

- low: <1.5 g/dl
- high: none identified.

Sampling Serum (gold top tube); measured levels may be decreased in blood taken from patients in a supine position. Venous stasis during blood collection may lead to spurious results.

Associations with raised levels

- psychiatric: catatonic states, severe depression
  note: microalbuminuria may be a feature of metabolic syndrome secondary to psychotropic use (see Chapter 3)
- other: artefactual (rare), dehydration, intravenous administration, penicillin (interference with analytical methodology).

Associations with lowered levels

- psychiatric: chronic alcoholism, eating disorders (anorexia nervosa), may be seen in chronic, severe drug use (e.g. cocaine, amphetamines)
- other: decreased synthesis: malabsorption (e.g. Crohn's disease), malnutrition, liver disease, oedema; dilution – excessive hydration, hypoxaemia, septicaemia; increased excretion/destruction – bleeding, burns, catabolism (fever, malignancy, sepsis, trauma); gastrointestinal loss (e.g. protein-losing enteropathy); renal disease (e.g. nephritic syndrome); miscellaneous – chronic inflammatory diseases, heart failure, hyperalimentation/re-feeding, oral contraceptive use, pregancy, thyroid disease.

Alkaline phosphatase

Function Enzyme that forms part of the liver function test profile, although is also found in intestines and placenta. Provides a non-specific measure of liver and bone disease.

Reference range 50–120 IU/l.

Suggested panic/critical ranges

- low: none identified
- high: none identified.

Sampling Serum (gold top tube); sample should be taken in fasting patients. Sample should be analyzed as soon after collection as possible to avoid artefactual increases in levels. Levels will increase up to 10% within 4 hours even when refrigerated.

Associations with raised levels

- psychiatric: 'stress', fractures secondary to physical restraint, chronic alcohol use, chronic/excess caffine intake; medications (rare, idiosyncratic effects) – carbamazepine, clozapine, disulfiram, duloxetine, galantamine, haloperidol, memantine, modafinil, nortriptyline, olanzapine, phenytoin, sertraline; neuroleptic malignant syndrome
  note: many medications (both psychotropics and others), substances of abuse, and toxins may affect the liver and cause non-specific changes in all liver enzymes. See also Chapter 4
- other: artefactual (non-fasting patient, after a fatty meal); bone disease (rickets, osteomalacia, Paget's); endocrine (diabetes mellitus, hyperparathyroidism, hyperthyroidism), gastrointestinal (biliary obstruction such as cancer of the pancreas, choledocholithiasis; cirrhosis, erosive lesions of the gastrointestinal tract, hepatitis, liver tumour, peptic ulcer); miscellaneous (congestive cardiac failure, hypervitaminosis D, intravenous albumin administration; drugs, e.g. erythromycin, methyltestosterone, oestrogens, oral hypoglycaemics).

Associations with lowered levels

- psychiatric: none known
- other: hypothyroidism, pernicious anaemia, hypophosphatasia, drugs, e.g. azathioprine, clofibrate, nitrofurantoin, oestrogens; excess zinc.

Amylase

Function Enzyme produced by exocrine pancreas, which is a marker of pancreatic and general intra-abdominal damage.

Reference range <300 IU/l; caution is needed when interpreting results from patients with hypertriglyceridaemia as this may lead to spuriously low levels of amylase. In addition, amylase is produced in other organs (intestine, ovaries, parotid glands, and skeletal muscle).

Suggested panic/critical ranges

- low: none identified
- high: levels >3 times the upper limit may be thought of as significant.

Sampling Serum (gold top tube); amylase is stable at room temperature for about a week and up to 8 weeks when refrigerated. There are no differences in levels in males and females, and levels are not affected by meals or timing of sample collection.

Associations with raised levels

- psychiatric: alcohol misuse syndrome; eating disorders (especially anorexia nervosa); medications – clozapine, donepazil, olanzapine, pregabalin, rivastigmine, SSRIs (rarely), valproate; substances of abuse – methadone, opioids

- other:
  - <5 times upper limit of normal: pancreatic causes – abscess, acute pancreatitis, ascites, drugs (furosemide), neoplasms, pseudocyst, spasm of sphincter of Oddi (e.g. after morphine administration), stones in common bile duct, trauma; extrapancreatic causes – acute abdomen (aortic aneurysm, biliary tract disease, ectopic pregnancy, intestinal obstruction, perforated peptic ulcer, peritonitis), cerebral trauma, chronic renal failure, diabetic ketoacidosis, microamylasaemia, postoperative, salivary gland lesions; drugs – azathioprine, captopril, cimetidine, corticosteroids, oestrogens, ibuprofen, indometacin, methyldopa, oral contraceptives, sulphonamides, tetracyclines, thiazide diuretics
  - <10 times upper limit of normal: acute pancreatitis, ectopic secretion by metastatic tumours.

Associations with lowered levels

- psychiatric: none known
- other: cystic fibrosis (advanced), pancreatectomy, pancreatic insufficiency, severe liver disease.

Aspartate aminotransferase

Function Enzyme localized mainly to liver, heart, red blood cells, and skeletal muscle, with lower quantities in kidney, pancreas, and skin. This enzyme is important for the diagnosis of hepatobiliary disease.

Reference range 10–50 IU/l; values tend to be slightly higher in males. In severe liver injury levels peak within 24 hours and then tend to decline over the next 4 days; sustained high levels after this time require further investigation. Levels may be raised in obese subjects.

Suggested panic/critical ranges

- low: none identified
- high: none identified.

Sampling Serum (gold top tube); haemolysed samples will cause spurious results. The enzyme is stable at room temperature for approximately 72 hours and up to a week when refrigerated.

Associations with raised levels

- Psychiatric: alcoholism, deliberate self-harm involving drug overdose (e.g. paracetamol overdose); eating disorders (including malnutrition); medication-associated syndromes – malignant hyperthermia; neuroleptic malignant syndrome, serotonin syndrome; medications –
  - antipsychotics: benperidol, chlorpromazine, clozapine, fluphenazine, haloperidol, olanzapine, quetiapine, thioridazine, zotepine

445

- antidepressants: duloxetine, mianserin, mirtazepine, moclobemide, monoamine oxidase inhibitors (especially iproniazid), SSRIs (especially paroxetine and sertraline); TCAs, trazodone, venlafaxine
- anxiolytics/hypnotics: barbiturates, benzodiazepines, chloral hydrate, clomethiazole, promethazine
- miscellaneous agents: caffeine, dexamphetamine, disulfiram, modafinil, opioids
- *mood stabilizers*: carbamazepine, lamotrigine, valproate
   note: many medications (both psychotropics and others), substances of abuse, and toxins may affect the liver and cause non-specific changes in all liver enzymes. See also Chapter 4

- Other: cardiac disease (acute myocardial infarction; cardiac failure, inflammation, necrosis, trauma); drugs (isoniazid, erythromycin, methyldopa, indometacin, steroids); infections (viral hepatitis, Legionnaire's disease, typhoid fever); liver disease (all forms of hepatitis, hepatoma, obstructive jaundice); miscellaneous – cerebral infarction, haemolytic anaemia, hypothyroidism, intestinal obstruction, lactic acidosis, polymyalgia rheumatica, renal infarction, respiratory failure.

Associations with lowered levels

- psychiatric: trifluoperazine
- other: uraemia, vitamin B deficiency; drugs – metronidazole, vigabatrin.

Basophils

Function Least numerous group of white blood cells (less than 1% of total); basophils bind immunoglobulin E (IgE) and when exposed to antigen release histamine and other inflammatory mediators.

Reference range $0.0–0.10\times10^9$/l.

Suggested panic/critical ranges

- low: none identified
- high: none identified.

Sampling EDTA (ethylenediaminetetraacetic acid) tube (purple top); clotted or haemolysed specimens will give spurious results.

Associations with raised levels

- psychiatric: TCAs (especially desipramine)
- other: haemolytic anaemia (chronic), Hodgkin's disease, myxoedema, nephrosis, post-splenectomy, ulcerative colitis, viral infections (e.g. chicken pox); drugs – antithyroid medications, oestrogens.

Associations with lowered levels

- psychiatric: 'stress', especially chronic
- other: acute infection, Cushing's syndrome, hyperthyroidism, ovulation, pregnancy; drugs – chemotherapy, procainamide, steroids.

Bicarbonate

Function   Main plasma and extracellular fluid buffer which prevents increases in hydrogen ion concentrations and thus maintains blood pH.

Reference range   22–30 mmol/l.

Suggested panic/critical ranges

- low: <15 mmol/l
- high: >50 mmol/l.

Sampling   Serum (gold top tube) for non-urgent sampling; for arterial blood gases in heparin tube (green top); inadequate filling of serum tube may result in artefactually low concentrations as will excess heparin. For arterial blood gases patients are advised *not* to clench their fist, and samples should be placed on ice and analysed immediately.

Associations with raised levels

- psychiatric: deliberate self-harm (salicylate overdose); eating disorders (especially anorexia nervosa complicated by laxative use) and some forms of pica (associated with excess alkali ingestion); 'hysterical' states, hypoxia secondary to physical restraint
- other: metabolic alkalosis (plasma bicarbonate excess) – 'excess alkali ingestion, gastric aspiration or other loss of gastric acid; potassium depletion (diuresis, Cushing's, potassium-losing nephropathy, primary aldosteronism); respiratory alkalosis (decreased dissolved carbon dioxide) – early salicylate poisoning, fever, hypoxia, raised intracranial pressure.

Associations with lowered levels

- psychiatric: alcoholism, serotonin syndrome
- other: metabolic acidosis (decreased bicarbonate) – increased acid formation (diabetes mellitus, hyperthyroidism, post-trauma); decreased hydrogen ion excretion (Addison's disease, hypercalcaemia, renal failure, Wilson's disease); increased acid intake (salicylates); increased loss of alkaline fluids from body (biliary, intestinal, renal); hyperalimentation/refeeding; respiratory acidosis – congestive cardiac failure, lung disease (emphysema, pneumonia).

Bilirubin

Function   Bilirubin is a breakdown product of haem which is conjugated in the liver, excreted in bile, and converted in the small intestine to stercobilin prior to excretion.

Reference range   3–20 µmol/l (serum total bilirubin).

447

Suggested panic/critical ranges

- low: none identified
- high: none identified.

Sampling Plain tube (gold top); haemolysed samples or those exposed to light will lead to spurious results.

Associations with raised levels

- psychiatric: alcoholism, eating disorders (anorexia nervosa); drugs (rare) – amitriptyline, benzodiazepines, carbamazepine, chlordiazepoxide, chlorpromazine, clomethazole, disulfiram, imipramine, fluphenazine, meprobamate, phenothazines, phenytoin, promethazine, trifluoperazine, valproate
- other: anaemia (haemolytic, pernicious); congestive cardiac failure, liver disease (cholangitis, cirrhosis, Gilbert's syndrome, hepatitis, neoplasia, Wilson's); post-blood transfusion, pulmonary embolism, pulmonary infarct; drugs – azathioprine, erythromycin, penicillin, oral contraceptives, steroids, methyldopa, indometacin.

Associations with lowered levels

- psychiatric: none known
- other: excess ascorbic acid, possibly secondary to environmental toxins (polychlorinated biphenyls have been reported to lower blood bilirubin levels in rats); severe iron-deficiency anaemia.

C-reactive protein

Function Acute phase protein produced by hepatocytes, which serves as a non-specific marker of acute inflammation. Bacterial infections are associated with higher levels than viral infections. Levels respond rapidly (within 6 hours of change in disease activity) and C-reactive protein (CRP) can be measured in stored samples.

Reference range <10 μg/ml; postoperative levels have been reported to peak on day 3 and then return to preoperative levels within a week in the absence of complications such as infection.

Suggested panic/critical ranges

- low: none identified
- high: none identified.

Sampling Plain tube (gold top); sample should not be frozen and concurrent oral contraceptive use, haemolysed specimens, or those with lipaemia may lead to spurious results. CRP is stable when refrigerated for up to 72 hours.

Associations with raised levels

- psychiatric: alcoholism (especially when severe); buprenorphine use (rare), eating disorders, emotional stress, eosinophilia–myalgia syndrome, secondary to physical restraint
- other: inflammatory disorders (infections, inflammatory bowel disease, myocardial infarction, rheumatological disorders, etc.); tissue trauma (including post-surgery).

Associations with lowered levels

- psychiatric: none known
- other: none known.

Calcium

Function Multiple functions in the body, including acting as coenzyme for coagulation factors, acting as intracellular second messenger, important roles in muscle contraction and neurotransmitter release, and structural roles in bone and teeth.

Reference range 2.2–2.6 mmol/l (corrected calcium). *Note*: levels are affected by changes in protein concentration, with a change in albumin of 1 g/dl resulting in an associated change in calcium of up to 0.8 mmol/l; thus the 'corrected calcium' figure is often reported. Changes in blood pH may also affect calcium levels.

Suggested panic/critical ranges

- low: <1.75 mmol/l
- high: >3 mmol/l

Sampling Plain tube (gold top); ideally, a morning, fasting sample should be taken due to possible postural/diurnal effects. Levels are reported to be hightest at 20.00 and lowest at around 03.00, and standing up for over 15 minutes may cause small (4–7%) increases in levels. Spurious increases may also be seen in stored blood and with venous stasis during blood collection. Levels are reported to decrease in males from age 50.

Associations with raised levels

- psychiatric: acamprosate treatment, alcoholism (may raise or lower levels), electroconvulsive therapy (ECT) (rare, transient effect), lithium therapy (rare), physical restraint, some forms of pica
- other: alcoholic cirrhosis, dehydration, hypercalcaemia (familial, hypocalciuric, iatrogenic, idiopathic), hyperparathyroidism, infections (histoplasmosis, leprosy, tuberculosis (TB)), malignancy, Paget's disease, pheochromocytoma with parathyroid hyperplasia, sarcoidosis, vitamin D intoxication.

449

Specific laboratory parameters

Associations with lowered levels

- psychiatric: alcoholism (may raise or lower levels), chronic anticonvulsant treatment, chronic khat use (rare), eating disorders (especially anorexia nervosa), ECT (rare, transient effect), barbiturate use, haloperidol treatment
- other: acute pancreatitis, bacteraemia, blood transfusion (large amounts), chronic renal failure, cirrhosis, drugs (cimetidine, corticosteroids, phenytoin), hypoalbuminaemia, hypoparathyroidism, magnesium deficiency, malnutrition, osteomalacia, pituitary dysfunction (anterior pituitary), renal disease, vitamin D deficiency.

Carbohydrate-deficient transferrin

Function A form of transferrin (an iron transport protein) in which there are raised levels of various isoforms that provide a measure of heavy alcohol use (approximately 60 g of ethanol daily for at least 2 weeks). It is especially useful in monitoring abstinence from alcohol.

Reference range 1.9–3.4 g/l.

Suggested panic/critical ranges

- low: none identified
- high: none identified

Sampling plain tube (gold top).

Assocations with raised levels

- psychiatric: chronic alcoholism
- other: carbohydrate-deficient glycoprotein syndrome, chronic active hepatitis, chronic autoimmune hepatitis, end-stage hepatic disease, primary biliary cirrhosis.

Associations with lowered levels

- psychiatric: none
- other: none.

Chloride

Function An anion which plays a role in acid–base balance and is used to calculate the anion gap, used in the determination of metabolic acidosis.

Reference range 98–107 mmol/l.

Suggested panic/critical ranges

- low: <80 mmol/l
- high: >115 mmol/l.

Sampling Plain tube (gold top); haemolysis may cause spurious results, and the specimen should be fasting, as there is a small post-prandial decrease in chloride concentrations.

Associations with raised levels

- psychiatric: eating disorders (especially those involving laxative use and possible prolonged diarrhoea); ECT (transient increase), prolonged physical restraint, salicylate overdose
- other: adrenocortical dysfunction, ammonium chloride administration, dehydration, diarrhoea, excessive infusion of normal saline, head injury leading to hypothalamic damage, hyperparathyroidism, hyperalimentation/re-feeding, renal disease (acute renal failure, renal tubular acidosis), respiratory alkalosis.

Associations with lowered levels

- psychiatric: eating disorders (especially those involving prolonged vomiting); medications, associated with syndrome of inappropriate antidiuretic hormone secretion (SIADH) – all antidepressants, antipsychotics (clozapine, haloperidol, olanzapine, phenothiazines, pimozide, risperidone, quetiapine); carbamazepine
- other: acute intermittent porphyria, addisonian crisis, aldosteronism, burns, metabolic alkalosis, hyperhydrosis, nephritis (salt-losing), prolonged gastric secretion, prolonged vomiting, respiratory acidosis, SIADH, water intoxication.

Cholesterol

Function A structural component of cell membranes and a precursor to bile acids and steroid hormones. High levels of cholesterol are associated with increased risk of coronary heart disease (CHD).

Reference range (total cholesterol, serum) <5.2 mmol/l*.

*Note: this range is not absolute and there are a number of important factors which must be taken into account in order that the cholesterol concentration can be interpreted meaningfully; these include various risk factors for CHD such as hypertension, diabetes mellitus, smoking history, family history of vascular disease, excess weight, etc.

Suggested panic/critical ranges

- low: none identified
- high: none identified (controversial).

Sampling Plain tube (gold top); fasting sample preferred, postural changes have been noted and include decreased values (10–20%) after 20–30 minutes in recumbent position. Prolonged application of a tourniquet during blood collection may increase values by up to 5%. Patients should be on a stable diet for the preceding 3 weeks and are advised to abstain from alcohol for at least the preceding 3 days.

Some seasonal variation has also been noted (levels higher in autumn/winter than spring/summer), and emotional stress and menstruation may have inconsistent effects on levels.

Associations with raised levels

- psychiatric: alcoholism, chronic and excessive caffeine consumption (significance unclear); eating disorders (especially anorexia nervosa); metabolic syndrome; psychotropics – antipsychotic treatment, especially those implicated in the metabolic syndrome such as the phenothiazines, clozapine, olanzapine, and possibly quetiapine. Other agents rarely implicated may include aripiprazole, beta-blockers, disulfiram, memantine, mirtazepine, modanifil, phenytoin, rivastigmine, venlafaxine, and zotepine; there is generally an association with schizophrenia, although this may be secondary to lifestyle and treatment factors. Excess caffeine use has also been implicated, although this is controversial
- other: acute intermittent porphyria, diabetes mellitus, drugs (levodopa, oral contraceptives), gout, hypercholesterolaemia (primary), hyperlipidaemias, hypothyroidism, ischaemic heart disease, primary biliary cirrhosis, renal disease (chronic renal failure, glomerulonephritis, nephrotic syndrome).

Associations with lowered levels

- psychiatric: eating disorders (malnutrition), learning disability (in association with congenital syndromes), severe paracetamol overdose (hepatocellular necrosis); ziprasidone (controversial)
- other: acute and severe illness, chronic obstructive pulmonary disease, drugs (metronidazole, tetracyclines), haematological disorders (leukaemia, megaloblastic and sideroblastic anaemias, thalassaemias), hyperthyroidism, liver disease (malignancy, necrosis), malabsorption, myelofibrosis, rheumatoid arthritis.

Creatine kinase

Function Enzyme found in three forms and localized in brain, muscle (cardiac and skeletal, thyroid; levels rise in various pathological states as shown below).

Reference range (total creatine kinase, serum) <90 IU/l. *Note*: Afro-Carribeans have higher levels compared to Caucasians, with higher levels in females compared to males. Caution is therefore advised when interpreting results. Bedrest has been reported to lower levels by up to 20%.

Caucasian females are reported to have levels 20–25% lower than Caucasian males. Levels may be lower in the elderly or in those with reduced muscle mass.

Suggested panic/critical ranges

- low: none identified
- high: none identified.

Sampling Plain tube (gold top); haemolysis may give rise to spurious results, and samples are stable at room temperature for up to 8 hours. Samples may be refrigerated for up to 2 days and stored at –20° C for up to 1 month.

Associations with raised levels

- psychiatric: acute agitation (mania, psychosis), alcoholism (especially acute withdrawal/delirium tremens), complicated physical restraint (head injury, hypoxia); convulsions secondary to medication, e.g. clozapine-induced seizures; medications – clozapine (associated with seizures), donepezil, olanzapine; medication-associated syndromes – eosinophilia-myalgia syndrome, malignant hyperthermia (during ECT), neuroleptic malignant syndrome, serotonin syndrome; substances of abuse – cocaine intoxication, dexamphetamine intoxication
- other: arrhythmias, brain infarction, cardioversion, convulsions, exercise, head injury, hyperalimentation/re-feeding, hypothermia, hypothyroidism, muscle disorders (muscular dystrophy, myocarditis, polymyositis, rhabdomyolysis, trauma), myocardial infarction, neoplasms, pregnancy, pulmonary emboli, rheumatoid arthritis, steroids, surgery, trauma.

Associations with lowered levels

- psychiatric: none known
- other: low, stable body mass index (BMI) (sedentary lifestyle, small muscle mass).

Creatinine

Function An endogenous muscle breakdown product, which is measured in order to determine the glomerular filtration rate and hence possible renal impairment.

Reference range (serum) 60–110 µmol/l. Levels may be slightly lower in females.

Suggested panic/critical ranges

- low: none identified
- high: none identified.

Sampling Plain tube (gold top); haemolysis causes spurious results, and ideally a fasting sample should be taken, as ingestion of meat can cause significant rises (up to 30%) within several hours of ingestion. Strenuous exercise can also cause small, transient increases. Some drugs (ascorbic acid, methyldopa) can interfere with analysis and result in spuriously high levels.

Associations with raised levels

- psychiatric: acute agitation (e.g. psychosis), alcoholism, clozapine, lithium, thioridazine, valproate, zotepine; paracetamol overdose; dexamphetamine, caffeine, khat intoxication; physical restraint; also associated with renal failure secondary to anticonvulsant hypersensitivity syndrome and rhabdomyolysis;
- psychiatric associations with rhabdomyolysis:

  - medications: benzodiazepines, dexamphetamine, pregabalin, thioridazine
  - medication-associated syndromes: malignant hyperthermia, neuroleptic malignant syndrome
  - overdose: salicylates
  - substances of abuse: alcohol, amphetamine, anabolic steroids, cocaine, Ecstasy, ketamine, khat, methadone, morphine, phencyclidine

- other: acromegaly, catabolic states, hyperthyroidism, meat ingestion, pregnancy, reduced renal blood flow (congestive cardiac failure, dehydration, shock), renal disease, rhabdomyolysis, urinary tract obstruction.

Associations with lowered levels

- psychiatric: eating disorders (especially anorexia nervosa)
- other: decreased muscle mass, severe liver disease, small stature.

Eosinophils

Function Group of white cells thought to be involved in IgE immune responses. Also thought to have antihelminthic activity.

Reference range (plasma) $0.0-0.4\times10^9$/l (1–6% of total white cell count (WCC)).

Suggested panic/critical ranges

- low: none identified
- high: none identified.

Sampling EDTA tube (purple top); eosinophils have been reported to show a diurnal variation, with counts lowest between 10.00 and midday and highest between midnight and 04.00.

Associations with raised levels

- psychiatric: anticonvulsant hypersensitivity syndrome, disulfiram–alcohol reaction, ECT (transient effect), eosinophilia–myalgia syndrome (following ingestion of tryptophan when used as adjunct in treatment of depression); psychotropics (eosinophilia rare and reversible on cessation of putative offending agent) – amitriptyline, beta-blockers (when used for anxiety), carbamazepine, chloral hydrate, chlorpromazine, clonazepam, clozapine, donepazil, fluphenazine, haloperidol, imipramine, meprobamate, modafinil, nortriptyline, olanzapine, promethazine, quetiapine, SSRIs, tryptophan, valproate, zotepine
- other:
  - allergy: angioneurotic oedema, asthma, hay fever, urticaria
  - dermatological: dermatitis, dermatitis herpetiformis, eczema
  - haematological: leukaemia, myelofibrosis, pernicious anaemia, polycythaemia rubra vera, post-splenectomy
  - infection: aspergillosis, coccidioidomycosis, filariasis, intestinal parasitosis, scarlet fever, trichinosis, tuberculosis
  - malignancy
  - others: irradiation, lead poisoning, Loeffler's syndrome (acute pulmonary eosinophilia), rheumatoid arthritis, sarcoidosis.

Associations with lowered levels

- psychiatric: none known
- other: eclampsia, labour, major surgery, shock.

Erythrocytes

Function Transport of oxygen to tissues and carbon dioxide to lungs. Also important in blood grouping and hence transfusion.

Reference range (plasma) Males 4.5–5.8×10^{12}/l; females 3.8–5.8×10^{12}/l.

Suggested panic/critical ranges

- low: none identified
- high: none identified.

Sampling EDTA tube (purple top); haemolysed or clotted specimens will give rise to spurious results. Sample is stable at room temperature for 24 hours and 48 hours when refrigerated. Levels are lower between 17.00 and 07.00 and after meals (up to 10% lower), and prolonged venous stasis during blood collection may result in artefactually high levels. Presence of cold agglutinins may result in decreased levels.

Associations with raised levels

- psychiatric: agitation (e.g. acute psychosis)
- other: polycythaemia, haemoconcentration, high altitude, strenuous exercise.

Associations with lowered levels

- psychiatric: medications – carbamazepine, donepazil, chlordiazepoxide, chlorpromazine, meprobamate, phenytoin, trifluoperazine; prolonged recumbency (e.g. catatonia, severe depression)
- other: anaemia, G6PD deficiency, prolonged immobility; prescribed medications which cause aplastic anaemia (see current *British National Formulary* (BNF)).

Erythrocyte sedimentation rate

Function A measure of red cell tendency to aggregate and form 'rouloux', cylinders of cells. Raised levels provide non-specific evidence of disease activity and may be useful for monitoring, but are not diagnostic. Levels are usually markedly elevated in temporal arteritis. ESR levels change less rapidly than CRP and are less sensitive to small changes in disease activity.

Reference range <20 mm/hour; levels increase with age and are slightly higher in females.

Suggested panic/critical ranges

- low: none identified
- high: none identified.

Sampling EDTA tube (purple top); clotted or haemolysed specimens will cause spurious results. Sample is stable at room temperature for 2 hours and when refrigerated may result in raised levels. Prompt delivery to the laboratory is therefore mandatory.

Associations with raised levels

- psychiatric: buprenorphine abuse, dexamphetamine abuse; eosinophilia–myalgia syndrome (following ingestion of tryptophan when used as adjunct in treatment of depression); prolonged/complicated physical restraint; medications (rare, reversible effect on cessation of putative offending agent): clozapine, levomepromazine, maprotiline, SSRIs, zotepine
- other: inflammatory conditions (infection, malignancy (especially myeloma), polymyalgia rheumatica, rheumatoid arthritis, temporal arteritis); macroglobulinaemia, pregnancy, severe anaemia.

Associations with lowered levels

- psychiatric: may be low in eating disorders (anorexia nervosa)
- other: hypofibrinogenaemia, poikilocytosis, polycythaemia, spherocytosis, sickle cell disease.

Ferritin

Function Serum ferritin is a good marker of iron stores in a number of pathological states, and is mainly used to distinguish between iron-deficiency anaemias and other anaemic states.

Reference range (serum) Males 40–340 µg/l; females 14–150 µg/l. Levels increase in males up to age 50; in females postmenopausal levels may show an increase. Levels may be increased by use of oral contraceptives and may be decreased with erythropoietin (e.g. when used in treatment of chronic renal failure).

Suggested panic/critical ranges

- low: <10 µg/l (severe iron deficiency)
- high: none identified.

Sampling Plain tube (gold top); serum should be separated immediately from clot; sample is stable for up to 1 week when refrigerated and up to 6 months when frozen.

Associations with raised levels

- psychiatric: alcoholism, eating disorders (especially anorexia nervosa); starvation (e.g. in severe depression, catatonic states, or obsessive states)
- other: anaemia (haemolytic, megaloblastic, sideroblastic), inflammatory states (e.g. burns, infections, rheumatoid arthritis, SLE); iron overload (haemochromatosis, haemosiderosis, iatrogenic); leukaemias, malignancy, thalassaemia.

Associations with lowered levels

- psychiatric: none known (controversial and unproven possible link between akathisia and low serum ferritin levels)
- other: iron-deficiency due to iron-deficiency anaemia.

Gamma glutamyl transferase

Function An enzyme present in liver, kidney, and pancreas that is excreted in bile and is especially responsive to alcohol use and biliary obstruction.

Reference range (serum) 1–5 IU/l; levels in males are up to 25% higher than in females.

Suggested panic/critical ranges

- low: none identified
- high: none identified.

Sampling Plain tube (gold top); ideally, the patient should be fasted for 8 hours pre-specimen collection; certain medications associated with enzyme induction (e.g. phenytoin, phenobarbital, rifampicin) may cause raised levels. Samples are stable for up to 1 month when refrigerated and up to 1 year when stored at -20°C.

Associations with raised levels

- psychiatric: alcoholism (raised levels are *not* diagnostic and are best used for monitoring purposes); paracetamol overdose; medications (rare, idio-syncratic, and usually clinically insignificant and reversible effects): (*note*: many medications (both psychotropics and others), substances of abuse, and toxins may affect the liver and cause non-specific changes in all liver enzymes)

  ○ antidepressants: mirtazepine, SSRIs (paroxetine and sertraline impli-cated); TCAs, trazodone, venlafaxine
  ○ anticonvulsants/mood stabilizers: carbamazepine, lamotrigine, pheny-toin, phenobarbital, valproate
  ○ antipsychotics: benperidol, chlorpromazine, clozapine, fluphenazine, haloperidol, olanzapine, quetiapine, zotepine
  ○ miscellaneous: barbiturates, clomethazole, dexamphetamine, modafinil

- other: congestive cardiac failure, diabetes mellitus, drugs (oral contracep-tives, simvastatin), hyperthyroidism, infectious mononucleosis, liver disease (alcoholic liver disease, carcinoma, cholestasis, cirrhosis (especially primary biliary cirrhosis), hepatitis), myotonic dystrophy, pancreatitis, renal trans-plant, SLE, some malignancies (e.g. hepatic metastases, seminoma).

Associations with lowered levels

- psychiatric: none known
- other: chronic/heavy caffeine consumption, hypothyroidism, treatment of hypertriglyceridaemia.

Glomerular filtration rate

(See also Chapter 8 'Chronic renal failure'.)

Function The (estimated) glomerular filtration rate (eGFR) is a rough measure of excretory function of the kidney and is a useful marker in chronic renal failure. It is calculated using the following formula:

eGFR (ml/l/1.73 m^2)$=186\times\{[$serum creatinine (μmol/l)/88.4$]^{-1.154}\}\times$age (years)$^{-0.203}\times a$

where:

$a=1$ (for males)
$a=0.742$ (for females)
$a=1.21$ (for African-Carribbeans).

Reference range (whole blood)   >90 ml/l/1.73 m^2.

Suggested panic/critical ranges

- low: 60–89 ml/l/1.73 m^2 suggests mild impairment if accompanied by signs of kidney damage (see Chapter 8); <15 ml/l/1.73 m^2 suggests established ('end-stage') renal failure.
- high: none.

Sampling   Plain tube (gold top); haemolysis causes spurious results, and ideally a fasting sample should be taken, as ingestion of meat can cause significant rises (up to 30%) within several hours of ingestion. Strenuous exercise can also cause small, transient increases. Some drugs (ascorbic acid, methyldopa) can interfere with creatinine determinations and result in a spuriously high eGFR.

Associations with raised/lowered levels   See creatinine above.

Glucose: fasting

Function   Glucose is an important metabolic substrate and source of energy for psychological processes. Its measurement is used to evaluate disorders of carbohydrate metabolism.

Reference range (whole blood)   2.8–6.0 mmol/l; plasma levels are up to 15% higher than in whole blood and arterial concentrations are higher than in venous samples. Finger-prick samples should be analysed immediately.

Suggested panic/critical ranges

- low: <2.2 mmol/l
- high: >22 mmol/l.

Sampling   Fluoride oxalate tube (grey top); *note*: for routine profiles, a plain tube (gold top) may also be used, but due to continuing red cell metabolism, glucose levels will fall over time (approximately 0.25–0.5 mmol/l per hour). Patients should fast for 8 hours prior to blood sampling. Haemolysed samples will produce spurious results. High levels of ascorbic acid may interefere with analysis and result in spuriously lower levels.

Associations with raised levels

- psychiatric: acute agitation, alcoholism (especially Wernicke's encephalopathy), eating disorders; ECT (transient effect); metabolic syndrome (variable effects on glucose levels reported), strong emotional stress; medications:

  - antidepressants: MAOIs, SSRIs, TCAs*
  - antipsychotics: aripiprazole, chlorpromazine, clozapine, olanzapine,* quetiapine, zotepine*

Specific laboratory parameters

○ substances of abuse: methadone, opioids

• other: acanthosis nigricans, acromegaly, artefactual (e.g. non-fasting sample, haemolysis), beta-blockers, buproprion, cerebrovascular accident (CVA), chronic liver disease, chronic renal disease, Cushing's disease, cystic fibrosis, diabetes mellitus, donepazil, galantamine, general anaesthesia, glucagonoma, haemochromatosis, lithium, malignancy (e.g pancreatic), myocardial infarction, pancreatitis, phaeochromocytoma, pregabalin, pregnancy, somatostatinoma, thyrotoxicosis, trauma; many medications (including cimetidine, furosemide, oral contraceptives, phenytoin, thiazide diuretics; see BNF for complete list).

*May also be associated with hypoglycaemia.

Associations with lowered levels

• psychiatric: alcohol poisoning, chronic, heavy caffeine consumption; chronic malnutrition states; drugs (dextropropoxyphene), eating disorders (surreptitious injection of insulin); metabolic syndrome (variable effects on glucose levels reported), paracetamol overdose, salicylate overdose medications – hypoglycaemia has been reported with beta-blcokers, duloxetine, haloperidol, olanzapine, pregabalin, TCAs, zotepine
• other: Addison's disease, artefact (haemolysis), congestive cardiac failure (severe), diabetes mellitus (excess insulin), (hypopituitarism, hypothyroidism, insulin excess (extrahepatic tumours, insulinoma), haemolysis, liver damage (hepatitis, necrosis), malignancy (secondary to increased production of insulin-like growth factors), post-gastrectomy, starvation states.

Glucose: random

Function   Glucose is an important metabolic substrate and source of energy for psychological processes. A random blood glucose determination is useful in the evaluation of disorders of carbohydrate metabolism and symptoms such as dehydration. In addition, monitoring may be a useful predictor of neurological recovery in myocardial infarction as increased levels may be suggestive of severe brain ischaemia and hence complicated resuscitation.

Reference range (whole blood)   >11.1 mmol/l may support a diagnosis of diabetes mellitus. *Note*: timing and content of meals will affect this result, as will stress and physical activity. Samples should be analysed immediately. Values for males are slightly higher than for females.

Suggested panic/critical ranges

• low: <2.2 mmol/l
• high: >22 mmol/l.

Sampling   Fluoride oxalate tube (grey top); *note*: for routine profiles, a plain tube (gold top) may also be used, but due to continuing red cell metabolism glucose levels will fall over time (approximately 0.25–0.5 mmol/l per hour). High levels of ascorbic acid may interfere with analysis and result in spuriously lower levels.

Associations with raised levels   See glucose: fasting above.

Associations with lowered levels   See glucose: fasting above.

Glycated haemoglobin

Function   Glycated haemoglobin (HbA1c) allows a general measure of glycaemic control in diabetic patients covering the 8–12 weeks prior to testing.

Reference range (whole blood)   3.5–5.5% (4–6% in diabetics).

Suggested panic/critical ranges

- low: none identified
- high: >8% (increased risk of microalbuminaemia).

Sampling   EDTA tube (purple top); samples are stable for up to 1 week at 4°C and up to 1 month at −70°C.

Associations with raised levels

- psychiatric: all antipsychotics associated with hyperglycaemia (excluding amisulpride, and ziprasidone); galantamine, methadone, morphine, TCA
- other: diabetes mellitus (especially insulin-dependent, IDDM); medications including indapamide, propranolol, steroids (especially high dose).

Associations with lowered levels

- psychiatric: lithium, MAOIs, SSRIs
- other: chronic blood loss, chronic renal failure, haemolysis, haemolytic anaemia, pregnancy; medications including insulin, oral hypoglycaemics.

Haemoglobin

Function   Haemoglobin is the main constituent of red blood cells and has a number of important functions, including the transport of oxygen and the buffering of carbon dioxide during metabolic processes.

Reference range   Male 13.0–16.5 g/dl; female 11.5–15.5 g/dl.

Suggested panic/critical ranges

- low: <6 g/dl
- high: >18 g/dl.

461

Specific laboratory parameters

Sampling EDTA tube (purple top); clotted or haemolysed samples will result in spurious results; stable up to 6 hours at room temperature and up to 24 hours when refrigerated. Blood tube should be mixed by gentle inversion only. Note that hyperlipidaemic samples, those with grossly raised white cell counts ($>50 \times 10^9$/l), and prolonged stasis during blood collection may produce spuriously raised haemoglobin levels. Haemoglobin is affected by circadian rhythms and levels are highest in the morning.

Associations with raised levels

- psychiatric: acute agitation, eating disorders (especially those with severe vomiting)
- other: haemoconcentration (burns, dehydration, intestinal obstruction, severe vomiting), polycythaemia, strenuous exercise.

Associations with lowered levels

- psychiatric: catatonic states (e.g. schizophrenia, severe depression); prolonged recumbency (e.g. catatonia, severe depression), theoretical effect of physical restraint; medications – aripiprazole, barbiturates, bupropion, carbamazepine, chlordiazepoxide, donepazil, duloxetine, galantamine, MAOIs, memantine meprobamate, mianserin, phenytoin, promethazine, rivastigmine, trifluoperazine, zotepine
- other: anaemia, prolonged recumbency.

Lactate dehydrogenase

Function An enzyme found in five forms (isoenzymes) that catalyses the lactate/pyruvate interconversion pathway. It is a non-specific indicator of disease activity, although specific isoenzymes are useful in the differential diagnosis of acute myocardial infarction and certain anaemias (see specialized texts for further details).

Reference range (serum) 90–200 U/l; levels rise gradually with age although are lower in childhood.

Suggested panic/critical ranges

- low: none identified
- high: none identified.

Sampling Plain tube (gold top); haemolysed samples should be avoided (causes artefactually high results). Samples are stable at room temperature for up to 3 days.

Associations with raised levels

- psychiatric: alcoholism, methadone (rare), neuroleptic malignant syndrome; medications – TCAs (especially imipramine), valproate
- other: acute pancreatitis, anaemia (haemolytic, megaloblastic), cerebrovascular accident, head trauma, hypotension, hypothyroidism, inflammatory

states, intestinal obstruction, leukaemia, liver disease (cirrhosis, obstructive jaundice, viral hepatitis), lung disease (hypoxia, pulmonary infarct), malignant hyperthermia, meningitis, muscular dystrophy, myocardial infarct, neoplastic syndromes, renal infarct, seizures, shock.

Associations with lowered levels

- psychiatric: none known
- other: rare, congenital disorders.

Lipoproteins

Function   Lipoproteins are the main transporters of lipids (excluding free fatty acids) in the circulation. There are two main subtypes, namely low-density lipoprotein (LDL) and high-density lipoprotein (HDL). Lipoproteins are usually measured as part of a lipid profile.

Reference range (serum)   LDL (serum) <3.5 mmol/l,∗ HDL (serum) >1.2 mmol/l.∗

∗*Note*: the above ranges are 'ideal', and a great number of individual factors must be taken into account in order to accurately interpret lipoprotein levels (see also cholesterol, above, for further comments regarding reference ranges).

Suggested panic/critical ranges

- low: none identified
- high: none identified (controversial – increased levels associated with coronary artery disease).

Sampling   Plain tube (gold top); samples are stable at several days at 4°C and for several weeks at −20°C. (See also cholesterol, above, for comments on sampling.)

Low-density lipoprotein
Associations with raised levels

- psychiatric: anabolic steroid use, anorexia nervosa; caffeine (controversial), medications – aripiprazole, beta-blockers, chlorpromazine, clozapine, memantine, mirtazepine, modafinil, olanzapine, quetiapine, risperidone; rivastigmine, venlafazine, zotepine.
- other: coronary heart disease/atherosclerosis (increased risk associated with raised LDL), Cushing's syndrome, diabetes mellitus, diet (high cholesterol or high saturated fat), hypothyroidism, liver disease (including hepatocellular and obstructive), medications (androgens, beta-blockers, diuretics, steroids, progestins), porphyria, pregnancy, renal disease (chronic renal failure, nephrotic syndrome).

463

Associations with lowered levels

- psychiatric: none known
- other: anaemia (chronic), burns, chronic pulmonary disease, diet (low cholesterol, low saturated fat or high polyunsaturated fat), hyperthyroidism, medications (aspirin, ketokonazole, niacin, oestrogens, statins, thyroxine), myeloma, systemic illness causing actute stress, Tangier disease (extremely rare syndrome with very low HDL, low cholesterol, and low LDL).

High-density lipoprotein

Associations with raised levels

- psychiatric: medications (carbamazepine, phenobarbital, phenytoin)
- other: balanced diet, exercise, medications (clofibrate, oestrogens, oral contraceptives, statins), moderate alcohol intake.

Associations with lowered levels

- psychiatric: anabolic steroids (may raise or lower levels); medications, e.g. olanzapine (controversial), phenothiazines, valproate (especially in women with hyperandrogenism, obesity, or polycystic ovary syndrome)
- other: diabetes mellitus, glucose intolerance, hypertension, hypoalphalipoproteinaemia, increased risk of coronary heart disease/atherosclerosis, left ventricular hypertrophy, male gender, medications (beta-blockers (non-selective), diuretics, neomycin, steroids, thiazides), obesity (especially in males), smoking, Tangier disease (extremely rare syndrome with very low HDL, low cholesterol, and low LDL), uraemia, zinc (excess).

Note: risk of coronary artery disease is *directly* correlated with LDL and *inversely* correlated with HDL.

Lymphocytes

Function   Lymphocytes play important roles in immune defence and are of two types. B cells bind soluble antigens and secrete lymphokines while T cells are involved in both cell-mediated and antibody-mediated immune responses.

Reference range (plasma) $1.3–4.0 \times 10^9$/l.

Suggested panic/critical ranges

- low: none identified
- high: none identified.

Sampling   EDTA tube (purple top); clotted or haemolysed specimens should be rejected. Samples are stable for up to 24 hours when stored at 4°C.

Associations with raised levels

- psychiatric: drug abuse (opioids), valproate (rare)
- other: autoimmune disorders, haematological disorders (acute/chronic lymphocytic leukaemia, certain lymphomas, 'heavy chain' disease), toxoplasmosis, tuberculosis, viral infections.

Associations with lowered levels

- psychiatric: chloral hydrate, lithium treatment
- other: acute infections including miliary tuberculosis, advanced cancers, acquired immunodeficiency syndrome (AIDS), aplastic anaemia, bone marrow failure, drugs (azathioprine, corticosteroids), Hodgkin's disease, renal failure, systemic lupus erythromatosus.

Mean cell haemoglobin (see also Haemoglobin)

Function This refers to the total haemoglobin content of the average red cell and can aid in the diagnosis of anaemia.

Reference range 25–34 pg. Levels are slightly higher in males and may be raised in the elderly.

Suggested panic/critical ranges

- low: none identified
- high: none identified.

Sampling EDTA tube (purple top); sample stable at room temperature for about 10 hours and roughly 18 hours at 4°C. Haemolysed or clotted specimens should be rejected.

Associations with raised levels

- psychiatric: alcoholism, eating disorders (occasionally seen), medications associated with megaloblastic anaemia, e.g. anticonvulsants
- other: anaemia (aplastic, haemolytic, pernicious); B12 deficiency, folate deficiency, hereditary spherocytosis, hypothyroidism, liver disease, malignancy (especially disseminated), smoking.

Associations with lowered levels

- psychiatric: none known
- other: anaemia of chronic disease, iron-deficiency anaemia, some haemoglobinopathies, thalassaemias.

465

Mean cell haemoglobin concentration (see also Haemoglobin)

Function   MCHC is the average haemoglobin concentration in a given volume of packed red cells and aids in the diagnosis of anaemia.

Reference range   32.0–37.0 g/l

Suggested panic/critical ranges

- low: none identified
- high: none identified.

Sampling   EDTA tube (purple top); sample stable at room temperature for about 10 hours and roughly 18 hours at 4°C. Haemolysed or clotted specimens should be rejected.

Associations with raised levels

- psychiatric: alcoholism, eating disorders (?), medications associated with megaloblastic anaemia, e.g. anticonvulsants
- other: hereditary spherocytosis, warm antibody immunohaemolytic anaemia.

Associations with lowered levels

- psychiatric: none known
- other: iron-deficiency anaemia, haemoglobinopathies (example), thalassaemias.

Mean cell volume

Function   The MCV provides a measure of the size (volume) of the average red cell and is a key investigation in the evaluation of anaemia.

Reference range   77–95 fl.

Suggested panic/critical ranges

- low: none identified
- high: none identified.

Sampling   EDTA tube (purple top); sample is stable for approximately 6 hours at room temperature and 24 hours at 4°C.

Associations with raised levels

- psychiatric: alcoholism (chronic and acute); medications including anticonvulsants

- other: acute blood loss, plastic anaemia, haemolytic anaemia, hypothyroidism, liver disease, malignancy (disseminated), megaloblastic anaemias (B12 deficiency, folate deficiency), smoking; medications (including acyclovir, azothiaprine, cycloserine, hydroxyurea, isoniazid, mefenamic acid, metformin, methotrexate, neomycin, oral contraceptives, trimethoprim).

Associations with lowered levels

- psychiatric: none known
- other: anaemia of chronic disease, hyperthyroidism (occasionally), iron-deficiency anaemia, thalassaemias.

Monocytes

Function   The largest subset of white cells, accounting for 3–9% of leukocytes. Monocytes leave the circulation via a process known as diapedesis to form macrophages which are involved in non-specific immune responses.

Reference range $0.2–1.0\times10^9/l$.

Suggested panic/critical ranges

- low: none identified
- high: none identified.

Sampling   EDTA tube (purple top); sample is stable for approximately 6 hours at room temperature and 24 hours at 4°C.

Associations with raised levels

- psychiatric: haloperidol treatment
- other: heat stroke, Hodgkin's lymphoma, infections (bacterial, fungal, protozoal, rickettsial, viral, especially endocarditis, tuberculosis, typhoid); leukaemias, lymphomas, multiple myeloma, myelodysplasia, polyarteritis nodosa, rheumatoid arthritis, sarcoidosis, systemic lupus erythematosus, ulcerative colitis; medications (griseofulvin, prednisone).

Associations with lowered levels

- psychiatric: none known
- other: aplastic anaemia, hairy cell leukaemia.

Neutrophils

Function   A granulocytic white blood cell subset involved in non-specific immune defences.

Reference range $2.2–6.3\times10^9/l$.

467

Suggested panic/critical ranges

- low: none identified
- high: none identified.

Sampling EDTA tube (purple top); sample is stable for approximately 6 hours at room temperature and 24 hours at 4°C. Note that Afro-Carribbeans may have lower neutrophil counts (benign ethnic neutropaenia).

Associations with raised levels

- psychiatric: ECT (transiently), extreme emotion (anger, euphoria, fear; transient increases possible); anticonvulsant hypersensitivity syndrome, physical restraint; medications associated with leukocytosis – bupropion, carbamazepine,* citalopram, chlorpromazine, clozapine,* duloxetine, fluphenazine, haloperidol, lithium, olanzapine, quetiapine, risperidone, rivastigmine, trazodone, venlafaxine, zotepine
- other: cold, colitis, dermatitis, diabetes mellitus, eclampsia, exercise, haemolytic anaemia, haemorrhage, heat, infections (especially bacterial), myeloproliferative disorders, nausea/vomiting, nephritis, pancreatitis, post-splenectomy, pregnancy/labour, rheumatoid arthritis, smoking, thyroiditis, trauma, uraemia.

*Usually associated with leukopaenia.

Associations with lowered levels

- psychiatric: disulfiram–alcohol syndrome; medications (see also Chapter 4):

  o agents associated with agranulocytosis: amitriptyline, amoxapine, aripiprazole, barbiturates, carbamazepine, chlordiazepoxide, chlorpromazine, clomipramine, clozapine,* diazepam, fluphenazine, haloperidol, imipramine, meprobamate, mianserin, mirtazepine, nortriptyline, olanzapine, prourethazine, tranylcypromine, valproate*
  Note: in rare cases clozapine has been associated with a 'morning pseudoneutropaenia' with lower levels of circulating neutrophil levels. As neutrophil counts may show circadian rhythms, repeating the FBC at a later time of day may be instructive
  o agents associated with leukopaenia: amitriptyline, amoxapine, bupropion, carbamazepine, chlorpromazine, citalopram, clomipramine, clonazepam, clozapine, duloxetine, fluphenazine, galantamine, haloperidol, lamotrigine, lorazepam, MAOIs, memantine, meprobamate, mianserin, mirtazepine, modafinil, nefazodone, olanzapiae, oxazepam, pregabalin, promethazine, quetiapine, risperidone, tranylcypromine, valproate, venlafaxine, zotepine
  o agents associated with neutropaenia: trazodone, valproate

- other: anaphylactic shock, aplastic anaemia, Chediak–Higashi syndrome (an autosomal recessive disorder characterized by albinism, ataxia, epilepsy, frequent infections, impaired vision, mental retardation, photophobia, and other features), cyclical neutropaenia (a rare condition with a periodicity of 2–4 weeks; neutrophilia is temporary but extreme, and there may be an associated monocytosis), hepatic cirrhosis, hypersplenism,

hypothyroidism, iron-deficiency anaemia, leukaemia, megaloblastic anaemia, overwhelming infection in debilitated individuals (elderly, immunosuppressed)
- non-psychiatric medications: a wide range of medications cause idiosyncratic reductions in neutrophil counts including analgesics, anticonvulsants, antihistamines, antimicrobials, antineoplastic agents, antithyroid drugs, antivirals, cardiovascular drugs, hypoglycaemics, and more. For further details the reader is advised to consult other sources of information such as the latest BNF or equivalent.

Packed cell volume (haematocrit)

Function   The percentage of whole blood that is made up of red cells. Measurement of the packed cell volume is useful in the evaluation of anaemia.

Reference range   Adult males 42–52%; adult females 35–47% (levels slightly lower in pregnant versus non-pregnant women).

Suggested panic/critical ranges

- low: none identified
- high: none identified.

Sampling   EDTA tube (purple top); sample is stable for approximately 6 hours at room temperature and 48 hours at 4°C. Clotted or haemolysed samples should be rejected. Levels are lower between 17.00 and 07.00 hours and are reported to be up to 10% lower after meals.

Associations with raised levels

- psychiatric (rare): acute, sustained agitation
- other: extreme physical exercise, haemoconcentration, heavy smoking, high altitude, polycythaemia; high levels are associated with increased risk of cardiovascular morbidity including stroke.

Associations with lowered levels

- psychiatric (rare): chronic catatonic states, complicated physical restraint (especially involving prolonged recumbency), severe depressive illness involving prolonged recumbency
- other: anaemia, post-prandial, prolonged recumbency.

Phosphate

Function   Phosphate is the principal urinary buffer and plays a pivotal role in the maintenance of body pH.

Reference range (serum)   0.8–1.4 mmol/l.

Suggested panic/critical ranges

- low: <0.4 mmol/l
- high: none identified.

Sampling Plain tube (gold top); patients should be fasting as phosphate levels are lower after meals. Levels are highest in the late morning and lowest in the evening, with seasonal variations noted (levels highest in May/June and lowest in winter). Haemolysed samples should be rejected and venous stasis should be avoided. Spun/separated samples are stable for several days at 4°C and for several months when frozen at –20°C.

Associations with raised levels

- psychiatric: eating disorders not associated with severe malnutrition, hyperpyrexia (possible extreme agitation/excitement, neuroleptic malignant syndrome, malignant hyperthermia), physical restraint; acamprosate, carbamazepine, dexamphetamine
- other: acidosis (lactic, respiratory), acromegaly, acute renal failure, bone tumours, diabetes mellitus, healing fractures, hypoparathyroidism, milk–alkali syndrome, portal cirrhosis, pseudohypoparathyroidism, pulmonary embolism, sarcoidosis, uraemic encephalopathy, vitamin D intoxication.

Associations with lowered levels

- psychiatric: acute alcohol intoxication, deliberate self-harm (diuretic phase of severe, self-inflicted burns; salicylate poisoning), eating disorders associated with severe malnutrition, especially anorexia nervosa, involving re-feeding; controversial association with behavioural changes such as irritability and possibly coma or delirium; khat (rare)
- other: alkalosis (respiratory), diarrhoea (severe), Fanconi's syndrome (a disturbance in renal transport characterized by aminoaciduria, glycosuria, osteomalacia, phosphaturia, renal tubular acidosis type 2); growth hormone deficiency, hyperalimentation/re-feeding, hypokalaemia, malabsorption, osteomalacia, primary hyperparathyroidism, renal tubular acidosis, respiratory infections, septicaemia (especially gram-negative), steatorrhoea, vomiting, Wilson's disease.

Platelets

Function Platelets play key roles in the formation of clots to prevent haemorrhage in addition to releasing a number of mediators involved in immune and other responses. Generally, the lower is the platelet count, the more is the risk of bleeding.

Reference range $150–400\times10^9$/l.

Suggested panic/critical ranges

- low: $<50\times10^9$/l.
- high: $>1000\times10^9$/l.

Sampling EDTA tube (purple top); clotted specimens should be discarded. Samples are stable for several hours at room temperature or for up to 24 hours at 4°C.

Associations with raised levels

- psychiatric: acute agitation (transient), lithium treatment
- other: anaemia (haemolytic, haemorrhagic, iron-deficiency), chronic myelogenous leukaemia, lymphoma, myeloproliferative disorders, polycythaemia vera, post-splenectomy, rheumatoid arthritis, tuberculosis, ulcerative colitis.

Associations with lowered levels

- psychiatric: disulfiram–alcohol syndrome

  ○ medications: acetylcysteine, amitriptyline, barbiturates, bupropion, carbamazepine, clomipramine, chlordiazepoxide, chlorpromazine, clonazepam, clozapine, diazepam, donepazil, duloxetine, fluphenazine, imipramine, lamotrigine, MAOIs, memantime, meprobamate, mirtazepine, olanzapine, promethazine, risperidone, rivistigmine, sertraline, tranylcypromine, trazodone, trifluoperazine, valproate, zotepine
  ○ agents which are associated with impaired platelet aggregation: chlordiazepoxide, citalopram, diazepam, fluoxetine, fluvoxamine, paroxetine, sertraline
  ○ substances of abuse: cocaine, methadone

- other:

  ○ acquired disorders: aplastic anaemia, congestive cardiac failure, hyperthyroidism, hypothyroidism, idiopathic thrombocytopaenic purpura, infections, liver disease, systemic lupus erythematosus, severe iron-deficiency anaemia, splenomegaly, uraemia
  ○ congenital, e.g. Chediak–Higashi syndrome (oculocutaneous albinism with mental retardation, paraesthesia photophobia, mental retardation, recurrent infections, and seizures), Fanconi's syndrome (a disturbance in renal transport characterized by aminoaciduria, glycosuria, osteomalacia, phosphaturia, renal tubular acidosis type 2).

Potassium

Function Potassium is a major intracellular cation and plays important roles in nerve impulse propagation and muscle contraction. Hyperkalaemia (K+ >6.5 mmol/l) is especially associated with cardiac arrhythmias, while hypokalaemia is associated with hypotonia, muscle weakness, and tetany.

Reference range plasma 3.5–5.0 mmol/l.

Suggested panic/critical ranges

- low: <2.5 mmol/l
- high: >6.5 mmol/l.

471

Sampling Plain tube (gold top); small needles should be avoided (increased risk of haemolysis with spuriously increased potassium concentrations) as should stasis, use of a tourniquet, and hand-clenching.

Associations with raised levels

- psychiatric: anorexia nervosa (with severe, acute starvation), extreme agitation/activity, malignant hyperpyrexia (e.g. following anaesthesia for ECT); medications – pregabalin
- an organic brain syndrome has been described with the following features: weakness, dysarthria, neurological symptoms, muscle weakness which may mimic neurosis; in severe hyperkalaemia, delirium and paralysis (flaccid, ascending) may occur
- in addition, a condition known as hyperkalaemic periodic paralysis has been described. This is an autosomal dominant disorder in which the affected individual can suffer episodes of hyperkalaemia and paralysis, usually of the muscles of the lower extremities, lower trunk, and arms. These episodes typically last up to an hour and can occur after exercise. They can also occur following excess dietary intake and in some cases may mimic neurosis
- other:
  - decreased potassium loss (Addison's disease, adrenalectomy, drugs (such as potassium-sparing diuretics), renal failure, tissue ischaemia)
  - excessive potassium intake (iatrogenic, oral, transfusion)
  - transcellular potassium movement (acidosis, dehydration, status epilepticus, systemic acidosis, tissue damage)
  - miscellanous (contamination, haemolysis, laboratory error)
  - medications associated with hyperkalaemia include amiloride, angiotensin converting enzyme (ACE) inhibitors, digoxin, heparin, mannitol, methicillin, non-steroidal anti-inflammatory drugs (NSAIDs), penicillin, spironolactone, tetracycline.

Associations with lowered levels

- psychiatric: disorders associated with chronic starvation (eating disorders, major depressive episode, possibly some dementias); bulimia nervosa; medication – haloperidol, lithium, mianserin, reboxetine, rivastigmine; substances of abuse – alcohol, caffeine, cocaine
- a hypokalaemic organic brain syndrome has been described, which presents with neurological symptoms including paralysis, muscle weakness, and lassitude; in severe deficiency, delirium may occur
- in addition, a condition known as periodic hypokalaemic paralysis has been described. This manifests with weakness and paralysis that is episodic and may not have a clear precipitant, although it may occur following excess carbohydrate intake. In some cases it may resemble a hysterical conversion disorder
- other: aldosteronism (primary and secondary), alkalosis, Cushing's syndrome, cystic fibrosis, diabetic ketosis, Fanconi's syndrome, hyperalimentation/re-feeding, hyperglycaemia, hypothermia, muscle weakness, postoperative states, prolonged diarrhoea and vomiting; renal tubular

acidosis; medications associated with hypokalaemia include carbenoxolone, cholestyramine, diuretics, insulin, licorice, salbutamol, theophylline.

Prolactin

Function   A hormone secreted by the anterior pituitary which is involved in the initiation and maintenance of lactation. Prolactin is inhibited by dopamine, and levels may rise secondary to dopamine antagonism, as occurs with certain antipsychotics.

Reference range   Normal <350 mU/l; abnormal >600 mU/l.

Suggested panic/critical ranges

- low: none identified
- high: none identified.

Sampling   Plain tube (gold top); patients should be fasted overnight prior to sampling and levels should be collected between 08.00 and 10.00, ideally in a chilled tube. Venepuncture may actually cause rises in prolactin levels. The sample is stable for up to 3 months at –20°C.

Associations with raised levels

- psychiatric: antidepressants (especially MAOIs and TCAs, venlafaxine also implicated); antipsychotics, e.g. amisulpride, haloperidol, paliperidone, pimozide, risperidone, sulpiride, zotepine (*note*: aripiprazole, clozapine, olanzapine, quetiapine, and ziprasidone have been reported to have minimal effects on prolactin levels); eating disorders (especially anorexia nervosa); carbamazepine, opioids
- other: adrenal insufficiency, Argonz–Del Castillo syndrome (galactorrhoea–amenorrhoea in absence of pregnancy – oestrogen deficiency and decreased urinary gonadotropin levels seen), amyloidosis, Chiari–Frommel syndrome (persistent galactorrhoea and amenorrhea postpartum), chronic renal failure, drugs (e.g. methyldopa, metoclopramide, oestrogens, reserpine), ectopic secretion, empty sella syndrome, histiocytosis X, hypothyroidism, insulin-induced hypoglycaemia, irradiation, liver disease, pituitary tumours (craniopharyngioma, dysgerminoma, metastases, meningioma, non-secreting macroadenomas with suprasellar extension), polycystic ovary syndrome, post-coitus, pregnancy, renal failure, sarcoidosis, sleep (levels peak early in the morning), stress, suckling, surgery, Rathke's cyst.

Note: antipsychotics and prolactin-secreting tumours may raise levels into the thousands.

Associations with lowered levels

- psychiatric: none known
- other: Sheehan's syndrome (pituitary infarction).

Protein (total)

Function Total serum protein measures a number of important proteins which collectively act as surrogate markers of nutritional status and conditions that alter protein metabolism.

Reference range (serum) 60–80 g/l; *note*: a number of variables will result in increased total protein concentrations, including prolonged application of a tourniquet, upright posture/ambulation for at least 1 hour. Associations with lowered total protein values include intravenous infusions (due to haemodilution), pregnancy (third trimester), and recumbency (especially when prolonged).

Suggested panic/critical ranges

- low: none identified
- high: none identified.

Sampling Plain tube (gold top); sample is stable for up to 3 days when stored at 4°C and up to 6 months at –20°C. Haemolysed samples should be rejected.

Associations with raised levels

- psychiatric: none reported
- other: chronic infection/inflammation, dehydration, haemoconcentration, liver disease (autoimmune hepatitis, occasionally cirrhosis), myeloma, sarcoidosis, SLE.

Associations with lowered levels

- psychiatric: chronic alcoholism, eating disorders (especially anorexia nervosa), prolonged recumbency (e.g. catatonic states, severe depression, possibly in prolonged physical restraint)
- other: burns, catabolic states, haemodilution, hyperthyroidism, inflammatory bowel disease (Crohn's disease, ulcerative colitis), intravenous infusions, liver disease (such as cirrhosis), malabsorption/malnutrition, neuropathy, pregnancy, renal disease (glomerulonephritis, nephritic syndrome).

Prothrombin time/international normalized ratio

Function The prothrombin time (also known as INR – international normalized ratio) is a measure of evaluation of the extrinsic clotting system and is used mainly to monitor the effects of the anticoagulant warfarin, which is used in the treatment of conditions such as atrial fibrillation, pulmonary embolus, and others.

Reference range (plasma) 10.3–13.3 seconds.

Reference ranges for INR 2–2.5 prophylaxis for deep venous thrombosis (DVT); 2–3 treatment of atrial fibrillation, DVT, myocardial infarction; 3–4.5 treatment of recurrent DVT, pulmonary embolus.

Suggested panic/critical ranges

• low: none identified
• high: >20 seconds (non-anticoagulated); >3×control (anticoagulated).

Sampling Sodium citrate (blue top) tube; sample should be analysed immediately as it is only stable for about 2 hours at room temperature and up to 4 hours at 4°C. Haemolysed, clotted, icteric, or lipaemic samples should be rejected. Inadequately filled tubes should also be rejected.

Associations with raised levels

• psychiatric: psychotropics including fluoxetine, fluvoxamine; disulfiram; bupropion
• other: fibrinogen disorders (afibrinogenaemia, dysfibrinogenaemia, hypo-fibrinogenaemia), clotting factor deficiencies (II, VII, X), intravascular coagulation, liver disease, vitamin K deficiency, warfarin treatment.

Associations with lowered levels

• psychiatric: medications including barbiturates, carbamazepine, phenytoin
• other: medications (e.g. cholestyramine, griseofulvin, oral contraceptives, primidone, rifampicin, sucralfate).

Red cell distribution width

Function This refers to the variation in red cell size, with higher figures suggesting greater size variation. The red cell distribution width is used in the evaluation of anaemia.

Reference range (whole blood) 11.0–15.0%.

Suggested panic/critical ranges

• low: none identified
• high: none identified.

Sampling EDTA tube (purple top); clotted samples should be rejected.

Associations with raised levels

• psychiatric: psychotropics associated with anaemia, such as carbama-zepine, chlordiazepoxide, citalopram, clonazepam, diazepam, lamotrigine,

475

mirtazepine, nefazodone, sertraline, tranylcypromine, trazodone, valproate, venlafaxine
- other: anaemias (especially iron-deficiency, pernicious, vitamin B12/folate deficiency), reticulocytosis.

Associations with lowered levels

- psychiatric: none reported
- other: none reported.

Reticulocyte count

Function   Reticulocytes are immature red blood cells which usually remain in the bone marrow with only small numbers found in circulating blood. Reticulocytosis occurs with increased erythropoiesis, such as after severe bleeding.

Reference range (whole blood) 0.2–2.2%.

Suggested panic/critical ranges

- low: none identified
- high: none identified.

Sampling   EDTA tube (purple top); samples may be stored at room temperature for up to 2 days or up to 3 days at 4°C.

Associations with raised levels

- psychiatric: severe self-harm involving massive blood loss
- other: anaemia (haemolytic, secondary to blood loss); anaemia under treatment (iron-deficiency, megaloblastic).

Associations with lowered levels

- psychiatric: psychotropics including carbamazepine, chlordiazepoxide, chlorpromazine, meprobamate, phenytoin, trifluoperazine
- other: aplastic anaemia, endocrine disease, red cell aplasia, renal disease.

Sodium

Function   Sodium is the major cation found in extracellular fluid and plays an important role in maintenance of water and osmotic pressure in the cell.

Reference range (serum)   135–145 mmol/l.

Suggested panic/critical ranges

- low: <120 mmol/l
- high: >160 mmol/l.

Sampling Plain tube (gold top); sample should be kept at room temperature. Haemolysed samples should be rejected.

Associations with raised levels

- psychiatric: excess ingestion of sodium chloride (as rare form of pica); Munchausen's syndrome (rare)
- other: azotaemia, Cushing's syndrome, dehydration, diuretic use, hyperalimentation, lactic acidosis, nephrogenic diabetes insipidus, primary aldosteronism.

Associations with lowered levels

- psychiatric: cachexia (alcoholism, anorexia nervosa, depression; may be rarely associated with severe obsessive–compulsive disorder (OCD)); psychogenic polydipsia; Ecstasy use; medications – benzodiazepines, carbamazepine, chlorpromazine, donepezil, duloxetine, haloperidol, lithium, memantine, mianserin, phenothiazines, reboxetine, rivastigmine, SSRIs, tricyclic antidepressants (amitriptyline)
  note: the UK Committee on Safety of Medicines (CSM) advises that hyponatraemia should be considered in any patient on an antidepressant who develops confusion, convulsions, or drowsiness
- other: acute intermittent porphyria, Addison's disease, cachexia, cirrhosis, congestive cardiac failure, cystic fibrosis, diabetes mellitus, drugs (clofibrate, diuretics, steroids), hyperalimentation/re-feeding, hypopituitarism, hypothyroidism, liver disease, malnutrition, nephrotic syndrome, SIADH.

Note: 'pseudohyponatraemia' may occur in severe hypertriglyceridaemia, severe hyperglycaemia, and severe hyperproteinaemia such as in Waldenström's macroglobulinaemia (a B cell malignancy found especially in older men, in which IgM paraprotein is secreted).

Note: low blood levels (<110 mmol/l) may result in neurological and neuropsychiatric symptoms (bulbar/pseudobulbar palsy, water intoxication), and over-rapid correction of hyponatraemia may lead to central pontine myelinolysis (variable clinical manifestations which may include coma, delirium, eye involvement (horizontal gaze paralysis, vertical ophthalmoparesis), 'locked-in' syndrome, pseudobulbar palsy, or spastic quadriplegia).

Thyroid stimulating hormone

Function Thyroid stimulating hormone (TSH) (thyrotropin) is produced by the anterior pituitary gland and stimulates secretion of T3 (triiodothyronine) and T4 (thyroxine) from the thyroid gland.

Reference range 0.3–4.0 mU/l; TSH exhibits diurnal rhythm, with the highest level at around 23.00.

Suggested panic/critical ranges

- low: none identified
- high: none identified.

Sampling Plain tube (gold top); samples are stable for up to 4 days when refrigerated.

Associations with raised levels

- psychiatric: aripiprazole, carbamazepine, lithium, rivastigmine
- other: hypothyroidism (primary).

Associations with lowered levels

- psychiatric: moclobemide
- other: hypothyroidism; drugs, e.g. dopamine, glucocorticoids, octreotide.

Thyroxine

Function The main hormone produced by the thyroid gland. It is converted to triiodothyronine (T3).

Reference range (serum) Free 9–26 pmol/l; total: 60–150 nmol/l; total thyroxine depends on thyroid activity as well as plasma binding and has now been superseded by free thyroxine measurements.

Suggested panic/critical ranges (total)

- low: <26 nmol/l (risk of myxoedema coma)
- high: >257 nmol/l (risk of thyroid storm).

Sampling Plain tube (gold top); samples are stable for up to 1 week at room temperature.

Associations with raised levels (free T4)

- psychiatric: anxiety, apathy (especially in older patients), delirium, depression, emotional lability, overactivity syndrome (increased appetite, irritability, nervousness, overactivity, sleep disturbance), psychosis (rare); dexamphetamine and moclobemide may rarely be associated
- other: acute intermittent porphyria, drugs (beta-blockers, oral contraceptives), primary biliary cirrhosis, Graves' disease, pregnancy, thyroiditis (first stage).

Associations with lowered levels (free T4)

- psychiatric: cognitive changes (impaired concentration, poor memory), delirium/dementia, depression, eating disorders (especially anorexia

nervosa), fatigue, psychosis (possible paranoid delusions and hallucinations); drugs – lithium treatment (causes decreased T4 secretion); heroin, methadone (increased serum thyroxine-binding globulin); carbamazepine, phenytoin treatment. Aripiprazole, quetiapine, and rivastigmine may rarely be associated
- other: drugs (methimazole, propylthiouracil, salicylates), hypothyroidism, treated hyperthyroidism (iodine, radiation); secondary causes such as pituitary tumours, Sheehan's syndrome.

Triglycerides

Function Triglycerides are the major fatty substances in blood and are derived both from dietary sources and from carbohydrate metabolism in the liver.

Reference range (serum) 0.4–1.8 mmol/l. Patients should be fasting and have been on a stable diet for the previous 3 weeks. Alcohol should be avoided for at least 3 days prior to sampling.

Suggested panic/critical ranges

- low: none identified
- high: none identified (controversial).

Sampling Plain tube (gold top); non-fasted samples should be rejected. Samples are stable for up to 7 days when refrigerated and for up to 3 months at –20°C.

Associations with raised levels

- psychiatric: anorexia nervosa, chronic alcoholism, metabolic syndrome, 'stress'; medications – aripiprazole, beta-blockers, chlorpromazine, clozapine, memantine, mirtazepine, modafinil, olanzapine, quetiapine, phenothiazines, rivastigmine, valproate, venlafaxine, zotepine
- other: acute intermittent porphyria, diabetes mellitus, drugs (e.g. beta-blockers, oestrogen, oral contraceptives, thiazide diuretics), hyperlipoproteinaemias, hypertension, hypothyroidism, impaired glucose tolerance, liver disease (cirrhosis, viral hepatitis), metabolic syndrome, myocardial infarction (acute), nephritic syndrome, obesity, pancreatitis, pregnancy, renal disease (chronic renal failure, nephrotic syndrome).

Associations with lowered levels

- psychiatric: disorders associated with malnutrition (not starvation); ziprasidone (controversial)
- other: brain infarction, chronic obstructive lung disease, hypoproteinaemias, hyperparathyroidism, hyperthyroidism, malabsorption.

479

Triiodothyronine

Function   The active hormone resulting from the conversion of the prohormone thyroxine. It has greater biological activity than thyroxine.

Reference range (serum)   Free 3.0–8.8 pmol/l; total 1.2–2.9 nmol/l; like thyroxine, T3 exists in two forms, free and bound (to plasma proteins). Note that pregnancy increases T3 concentrations.

Suggested panic/critical ranges

- low: none identified
- high: none identified.

Sampling   Plain tube (gold top); sample is stable for up to 2 weeks at room temperature.

Associations with raised levels

- psychiatric: heroin, methadone; moclobemide
- other (free T3): hyperthyroidism, T3 toxicosis.

Associations with lowered levels

- psychiatric: eating disorders, chronic alcoholism; drugs (free T3: valproate; total T3: carbamazepine, lithium)
- other (free T3): hypothyroidism, pregnancy (third trimester), sick euthyroid syndrome (abnormal thyroid function in patients with non-thyroidal illness; may occur in chronic disease, infections, malignancy, myocardial infarction, post-surgery, and other conditions).

Urate (uric acid)

Function   Urate is the end product of the metabolism of a number of related compounds (adenine, guanine, hypoxanthine, xanthine) known collectively as purines.

Reference range (serum)   0.1–0.4 mmol/l. *Note*: raised levels of urate may be seen with exercise, increased dietary intake of purines (especially anchovies, kidneys, livers, sardines), increased body mass, and stress.

Suggested panic/critical ranges

- low: none identified
- high: >0.7 mmol/l.

Sampling   plain tube (gold top); patients should be fasting, and levels show diurnal variation, higher in the morning than in the evening. Samples are stable for up to 3 days at room temperature, up to 1 week at 4°C, and up to 12 months at −20°C.

Associations with raised levels

- psychiatric: anorexia nervosa, chronic alcohol consumption, zotepine (rare), rivastigmine (rare); increased levels may be seen in some congenital syndromes such as Down's and Lesch–Nyhan
- other: acidosis, anaemia (haemolytic, pernicious), drugs (e.g. low dose aspirin, diuretics, propranolol, and many more), endocrine disorders (Addison's, hyper- and hypoparathyroidism, hypothyroidism, nephrogenic diabetes insipidus), gout, lead poisoning, neoplasia (leukaemia, lymphoma), pregnancy, psoriasis, renal disease.

Associations with lowered levels

- psychiatric: none specific
- other: acute intermittent porphyria, caffeine consumption, diabetes mellitus, drugs (e.g. high dose aspirin, corticosteroids, probenecid, high doses of vitamin C), Fanconi's syndrome, Hodgkin's disease, liver disease (severe), low purine diet, SIADH, Wilson's disease (late finding).

Urea

Function   Urea is synthesized in the liver and is the end product of protein metabolism.

Reference range (serum)   5–20 mg/dl (1.8–7.1 mmol/l). *Note*: levels increase slightly after age 40.

Suggested panic/critical ranges

- low: none identified
- high: >35.7 mmol/l.

Sampling   Plain tube (gold top); samples are stable for 1 day at room temperature, 3 days at 4°C, and up to 3 months at −20°C.

Associations with raised levels

- psychiatric: anticonvulsant hypersensitivity syndrome, hyperalimentation with anorexia nervosa and occasionally severe depression; uraemic encephalopathy (see Chapter 6). May also occur in situations involving acute stress such as physical restraint or rhabdomyolyis (see creatinine above)
- other: acute myocardial infarction, burns, catabolic states, diabetes mellitus, gastrointestinal bleeding, high protein diet, hyperalimentation/re-feeding, medications (corticosteroids, nephrotoxic agents such as salicylates, tetracyclines, excess thyroxine), renal disease, severe congestive cardiac failure, severe salt/water depletion (diarrhoea, diuresis, vomiting).

Specific laboratory parameters

Associations with lowered levels

- psychiatric: eating disorders with decreased protein intake; chronic alcoholism
- other: acromegaly, celiac disease, dietary insufficiency (e.g. vegetarian/vegan diets), iatrogenic (growth hormone administration), pregnancy (third trimester), severe liver damage.

White cell count (total)

Function Measurement of all types of white cells in blood can provide important imformation regarding disease states, especially those involving infection or neoplasm.

Reference range (whole blood) $4.5–11.0 \times 10^9$/l.

Suggested panic/critical ranges

- low: $<2.5 \times 10^9$/l
- high: $>30.0 \times 10^9$/l.

Sampling EDTA tube (purple top); clotted or haemolysed samples should be rejected. Sample is stable for approximately 6 hours at room temperature and 24 hours at 4°C.

Associations with raised/lowered levels See neutrophils above.

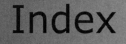

Index

484

485

486

Guillain–Barré syndrome 327
Gynaecomastia 136

Haemagglutination test 405
Haematocrit (packed cell volume/PCV) 406, 411, 469
Haemochromatosis 257
Haemoglobin 461–2
    function 461
    glycated (HbA1c) 212, 265, 461
    lowered levels 207, 216, 218, 226, 234, 235, 462
    raised levels 232, 462
    reference range 461
    sampling 462
    urine 332
    see also Mean cell haemoglobin concentration (MCHC); Mean cell haemoglobin (MCH)
Haemolysis, Wilson's disease 243
Haemolytic jaundice 433
Hair, drug testing 249
Hairy leukoplakia 401, 404
Hallucinosis, alcoholic 260, 262
Haloperidol 124–5
    indications and cautions 124
    side effects 125, 168, 361
    therapeutic monitoring/reference range 125, 201
Halothane 87
Halothane–caffeine contracture test 88
Haptoglobin 235
Hartnup's disease 344
Hashimoto's thyroiditis 224, 427
HbA1c, see Glycated haemoglobin
Heat exposure 372
Hepatic encephalopathy 300, 302
Hepatic failure 299–304
    classification 302–3
    cocaine use 276
    drugs causing 102, 104, 105, 114
    laboratory features 300–1
Hepatic fibrosis 255, 280
Hepatitis
    alcoholic 255
    anticonvulsant hypersensitivity syndrome 79
    cholestatic 291
    chronic active 424, 426, 433
    chronic persistent 433
    drugs associated 79
        opioids 286
        SSSIs 111
    secondary syphilis 416
    serological testing 393
Hepatocellular injury 165
Hepatorenal syndrome 79, 300
Hepatotoxicity
    drugs (therapeutic) associated with 164–5
    substances of abuse 268, 294
Herpes simplex (HSV) 398–9
High-density lipoprotein (HDL) 89, 213, 464

Hirsuitism, standard 'screens' 430
Homocysteine 28, 38
Homovanillic acid 61
5-HT (serotonin, 5-OH-tryptamine) 43
Human chorionic gonadotropin (hCG) 316
Human immunodeficiency virus (HIV) 393, 400–3
Human placental lactogen 316
Hunter Serotonin Toxicity Criteria 92
Huntington's chorea 211
8-Hydroxyamoxapine 117, 200
Hydroxycorticosteroids 70, 264
5-Hydroxyindoleacetic acid (5-HIAA) 43, 56, 61
21-Hydroxylase, antibodies 208
Hydroxymethoxymandelic acid 232
Hydroxyproline 216
Hyoscine 150, 167
Hyperalimentation 363–5
Hypercalcaemia 206, 209, 215, 216, 224, 232, 433, 449
Hypercholesterolaemia, see Cholesterol, raised levels
Hyperglycaemia 10, 209, 218, 238, 243
    drugs associated with 107, 161
    non-ketotic 213
Hyperkalaemia 206, 213, 238, 432, 472
Hypernatraemia 309, 411, 477
Hyperparathyroidism 215–16, 433
Hyperphosphataemia 220, 238, 470
Hyperpyrexia 279, 280, 289
Hypersensitivity reactions 422, 423
Hypertension 89
    in cocaine use 276
Hyperthermia 274
    drugs associated with 88, 280, 289
    laboratory effects 372
    malignant 87–8
Hyperthyroidism 217–18
    drugs associated with 171
    laboratory 'patterns'/results 218, 433
    laboratory tests 217
    signs and symptoms 217
Hypertriglyceridaemia 70, 89, 182, 209, 213, 238, 257, 479
Hyperuricaemia 238
Hyperventilation 372
Hypervitaminosis A 338
Hypervitaminosis K 350
Hypnotics 141–4, 170
Hypocalcaemia 213, 220, 238, 243, 433, 450
Hypochondriasis 62
Hypoglycaemia 10, 161
    Addison's syndrome 206
    alcoholism 258
    diabetes mellitus 213
Hypokalaemia 109, 206, 209, 232, 271, 277, 432, 472–3
Hyponatraemia
    dehydration 309
    dilutional 107, 222

490

491

lowered 218, 226, 234, 467
raised 218, 224, 263, 265, 466–7
Medical conditions
  causing anxiety 16
  differentiation from dementia 35
  and schizophrenia 59
  and weight gain/loss 357–8
  see also named medical conditions
Mees' lines 376
Melanocyte stimulating hormone 316
Memantine 147–8, 166
Memory loss, in dementia 34
Menaquinone 349
Meningitis 327, 411–14
  cryptococcal 401
  definition 411
  laboratory investigations 413–14
    CSF analysis 326, 327
  signs and symptoms 412
  tuberculous 419
Menorrhagia 314
Menstrual disorders 312–14
Meprobamate 139–40
  blood reference range 140, 202
  cautions 139
  indications 139
  side effects 140, 169
Mercury 65, 383–4
Metabolic syndrome 22, 61, 89
  laboratory features 89
  olanzapine therapy 22, 194, 195
Metachromatic leukodystrophy 227
Methadone 157–9
  indications and cautions 157
  side effects 158, 169
  testing for 248, 249
Methaemoglobinaemia 284
3-Methoxy-4-hydroxyphenylglycol 24, 43
Methylene chloride 294
3,4-Methylenedioxymethamphetamine
    (MDMA), see Ecstasy
Metyrapone test 210
Mianserin 103–4, 167
  blood reference range 104, 200
  indications and cautions 103
  side effects 104, 361
  therapeutic monitoring 104
Microalbuminuria 89, 214, 333
Microbiology testing 390
  brucellosis 396
  HIV 403
  Lyme disease 408
  malaria 410
  meningitis 413
  syphilis 416
  tuberculosis 418
  urine 335–6
Midazolam 136, 137, 201
Mineralocorticoids 208
Mirtazepine 104–5
  blood reference range 200

indications and cautions 104
monitoring 105
side effects 105, 167
Mitochondrial antibodies 426
Moclobemide 105–6
  blood reference range 200
  cautions 106
  indications 105
  monitoring 106
  side effects 106, 167
Modafinil 152–3, 169
Model for End-Stage Liver Disease
    (MELD) 303
Monoamine oxidase, platelet 56
Monoamine oxidase inhibitors (MAOIs) 93,
    106–8
  indications and cautions 107
  monitoring requirements 108
  side effects 107–8, 167, 361
Monocytes 467
  lowered levels 411, 467
  raised levels 164, 391, 406, 467
  reference range 467
Mood disorders
  in HIV infection 402
  see also Anxiety; Depression
Mood stabilizers 144–5
  nephrotoxicity 166
  weight gain risk 361
  see also named agents
Morning pseudoneutropaenia 182
Morphine
  blood/urine concentrations 288
  see also Opioids
Multiple endocrine neoplasia, type 1
    (MEN-1) 212
Multiple sclerosis 228–9
Munchausen's syndrome 62
Myalgic encephalomyelitis (ME), see Chronic
    fatigue syndrome
Myasthenia gravis 190, 424, 427
Mycobacterium avium 402
Mycobacterium bovis 417
Mycobacterium tuberculosis 336, 417
Myelopathy, peripheral 401
Myocardial infarction 276, 424
  laboratory 'patterns' 434
Myocarditis 181, 185, 276
Myoclonic jerks 277
Myoglobin, serum 70, 283
Myoglobinuria 283, 287
Myopathy, alcoholism 259
Myositis, caffeine consumption 271
Myxoedema 427

Naloxone 159
Naltrexone 159, 169
Nasopharyngeal carcinoma 404
Needlestick injuries 403
Nephritis 236
Nephropathy, diabetic 214

493

Papilloedema 412, 415
Paracetamol overdose 71–3, 154
ParaSight F® 410
Parathyroid hormone (PTH) 216, 220, 264, 265
Paresis, general of the insane (GPI) 415
Parkinsonism 82
  drug treatments 149–51
Parkinson's disease 321
Paroxetine
  side effects 111, 112, 361
  therapeutic monitoring 113
  see also Selective serotonin reuptake inhibitors (SSRIs)
Partial thromboplastin time (PTT) 235
Paterson–Kelly (Plummer–Vinson) syndrome 225, 380
'Patterns', laboratory 432–4
Paul Bunnell test 405
Pellagra 344
Perazine 201
Pericarditis, tuberculosis 418
Pericyazine 126, 168, 201
Peripheral neuropathy 260, 401
Pernicious anaemia 425, 428
Perphenazine 168, 201
Personality disorders 54–6
Pethidine 93
Phaeochromocytoma 106, 231–2, 332
Phencyclidine
  blood/urine testing 248, 289
  clinical features of intoxication 251, 288
  possible laboratory sequelae 289
  withdrawal 288
Phenelzine 107–8, 361
Phosphate 469–70
  functions 469
  lowered levels (hypophosphataemia) 206, 216, 232, 258, 264, 283, 433, 434, 470
  raised levels (hyperphosphataemia) 220, 238, 470
  reference range 469
pH, urine 50, 333
  see also acidosis; alkalosis
Phylloquinone 349
Physical restraint 97–8
Pica
  definition 44
  diagnostic criteria 45
  laboratory investigations 48–9
Pimozide 127, 168, 201
Pipotiazine 127, 168
Pituitary function, 'combined' test 222
Plasma factor V 302
Plasma osmolality 111, 119
Plasmodium spp. 408, 409
Platelet monoamine oxidase 56
Platelets 470–1
  dysfunction, drugs associated with 112, 163
  functions 470

lowered levels 112, 136, 164, 265, 411, 471
raised levels 164, 212, 471
reference range 470
sampling 471
Plumbism 381
Plummer–Vinson (Paterson–Kelly) syndrome 225, 380
Pneumocystis carinii 402
Pneumomediastinum 278
Pneumonia, in alcoholism 261
Pneumonitis 278
Polychlorinated biphenyls (PCBs) 448
Polycystic ovary syndrome 314, 358
Polycythaemia 209
Polydipsia 59
  psychogenic 239–40
Polymorphs, CSF 417, 419
Polymyositis 425
'Poppers', see Nitrites
Porphobilinogen deaminase 234
Porphyria 233–4
  definition 233
  drug associations 137, 177
  laboratory tests 234, 430
  signs and symptoms 233
Porphyrin, urinary 234
Potassium 471–3
  critical/panic range 471
  function in body 471
  lowered levels (hypokalaemia) 109, 209, 232, 265, 271, 277, 432, 472–3
  raised levels (hyperkalaemia) 206, 213, 238, 432, 472
  reference range 471
  urine 331
Pott's disease 418
Pregabalin 141, 145
Pregnancy 314–16, 360
  diagnosis 315
Proaccelerin (plasma factor V) 302
Prochlorperazine 127–8, 168
Procollagen type III 302
Procyclidine 150–1, 167
Progressive multifocal leukoencephalopathy 401
Proinsulin 212
Prolactin
  after electroconvulsive therapy 322
  function 473
  in lactation 317
  lowered levels 473
  raised levels 16, 70, 207, 224, 314, 317, 319, 411, 473
  drugs associated with 107, 111, 119, 286
  reference range 473
  sampling 473
Prolactinoma 314, 319
Promazine 128, 168
Prostaglandins 43, 61

497

498